CARDIOLOGY RESEARCH AND CLINICAL DEVELOPMENTS

SUDDEN DEATH

CAUSES, RISK FACTORS AND PREVENTION

CARDIOLOGY RESEARCH AND CLINICAL DEVELOPMENTS

Additional books in this series can be found on Nova's website under the Series tab.

Additional e-books in this series can be found on Nova's website under the e-book tab.

PUBLIC HEALTH IN THE 21ST CENTURY

Additional books in this series can be found on Nova's website under the Series tab.

Additional e-books in this series can be found on Nova's website under the e-book tab.

CARDIOLOGY RESEARCH AND CLINICAL DEVELOPMENTS

SUDDEN DEATH

CAUSES, RISK FACTORS AND PREVENTION

JIASHIN WU
EDITOR
AND
JESSICA WU
ASSISTANT EDITOR

NOVA BIOMEDICAL

New York

For permission to use material from this book please contact us:
Telephone 631-231-7269; Fax 631-231-8175
Web Site: http://www.novapublishers.com

Library of Congress Cataloging-in-Publication Data

ISBN: 978-1-62618-825-9

Library of Congress Control Number: 2013938101

Published by Nova Science Publishers, Inc. † New York

Contents

Preface

Sudden death is a broad topic, so as this book. Cardiac dysfunctions are major causes of sudden death. Among cardiac dysfunctions, ventricular fibrillation is typically the direct cause of death. This book dedicates the first seven chapters to cardiac electrophysiological dysfunction that can lead to ventricular fibrillation and sudden death. The next six chapters expand the topics of sudden death to other causes.

Brugada Syndrome has been under intensive investigation since the syndrome of sudden death, right bundle branch block and ST segment elevation in electrocardiogram, was first reported about 25 years ago. Because it is considered the top cause of non-traumatic sudden death in young males, especially in peoples of Southeastern Asian and southern European origins, it also becomes one of the major topics of this book. In Chapter 1, Dr. Martini et al. extensively reviewed the history and current status of this syndrome and discussed the gaps in the current knowledge. This chapter is a significant work, and prompts re-thinking of many current concepts and understandings about Brugada Syndrome. Chapter 2 concentrates on current understandings of the mechanisms of arrhythmia in Brugada Syndrome, as unveiled by experimental studies. It also summarized the currently recognized gene mutations of Brugada syndrome. Chapter 3 presents original clinical studies in China on the A1180V (with 25 years patient follow-up) and R1193Q mutations of the cardiac sodium channel gene, SCN5A. The authors identified clinical phenotypes and their pathophysiology of A1180V mutation. Their results on R1193Q mutation may change our views on the genetic bases of Brugada and long QT syndromes. The authors identified R1193Q mutation in 12.8%-16% of the general Chinese population, much higher than 0.2% in Whites and 2% in Japanese. The majority of these Chinese R1193Q mutation carriers did not manifest Brugada or Long QT Syndrome, although R1193Q is pathogenic in patients of other ethnicities. Now, the question becomes, "Are SCN5A mutations still the top genetic bases of Brugada and long QT syndromes?" If the answer is still a yes, what protects these Chinese mutation carriers from manifesting the syndromes? Chapters 4 and 5 cover the general topics of sudden cardiac death. These two chapters discussed the pathophysiology causes, risk factors, predictors, prevention, and possible therapeutical strategies of sudden cardiac death. Chapter 6 reviews the scope and causes of sudden cardiac death in athletics. Chapter 7 is dedicated to the roles of electrical cardiac systole in sudden death.

In addition to cardiac arrhythmias and ventricular fibrillation, sudden death can also be caused or triggered by other pathophysiological causes. Chapter 8 reviews the clinical and pathological characteristics of the sudden death related to cardiac and brain tumors, pulmonary tumor embolism, asphyxia, massive exsanguinations, and their pathophysiology. Chapter 9 summarizes the pathophysiology of sudden death caused by myocardial tuberculosis. Although it primarily involves the pulmonary system, around 1-2% of tuberculosis patients also have cardiovascular involvement. Chapter 10 introduces bath-related sudden death, which occurs commonly in elderly people with a medical history of diabetes or hypertension, especially during the winter season in Japan. The bath-related sudden deaths are presumed to be related to Japanese bathing practices of spending long amounts of time in a deep bathtub filled with hot water. This chapter discussed the pathological responses that lead to sudden death in response to the prolonged exposure to hot temperature and hydrostatic pressure during bathing. Chapter 11 discusses air pollution as a trigger of sudden death. Exposure to air borne particulate matter can affect cardiac ion channels and vascular epithelium directly, and increase the generation of reactive oxygen species and release of pro-oxidative and pro-inflammatory mediator. In addition, air pollution has also been associated with pulmonary inflammation, autonomic nervous system and central nervous system imbalance, pulmonary oxidative stress, and increase in the number and severity of asthma attacks. This chapter further discussed possible pharmacological strategy to manage the pathological responses and prevent sudden death triggered by air pollution. Chapter 12 presents biochemical, cytological and histopathological examination of sudden unexpected death in infancy. The last chapter of the book, Chapter 13, reviews postmortem cardiac markers in different body fluids and their application in forensic pathology diagnosis of sudden cardiac death. In combination, these chapters give broad and balanced views on the topic of sudden death.

In: Sudden Death
Editors: Jiashin Wu and Jessica Wu

ISBN: 978-1-62618-825-9

Chapter I

A Rare Lethal Syndrome in Search of Its Identity: Sudden Death, Right Bundle Branch Block and ST Segment Elevation

***Bortolo Martini,*[1,*] *Jiashin Wu*[2] *and Andrea Nava*[3]**
[1]Director of the Cardiovascular Unit, Boldrini Hospital, Thiene, Italy
[2]University of South Florida, Tampa, FL, US
[3]Associate Professor of Cardiology, University of Padua, Italy

Abstract

Twenty five years ago a group of doctors from the Padua Medical School described a new familial syndrome characterized by sudden or aborted death, and a strange ECG pattern on the precordial leads, namely an elevated J point and a coved ST segment elevation. A PR interval prolongation, left axis deviation, prolonged HV interval and late potentials at the right ventricular outflow tract (RVOT) clearly indicated a conduction delay. Ventricular fibrillation was easily inducible from the above area. Some minor structural abnormalities of the right ventricle could be evidentiated, and further confirmed by a necropsy study. The syndrome was lately called Brugada syndrome (BS), as more patients with the same ECG pattern and clinical symptoms were identified by these authors, who claimed a new entity not related to a structural abnormality, but with the same phenotypic traits. An explosion of published papers on this topic was seen in the following years, mostly devoted to confirm a functional disease rather than to investigate the underlying etiology; necropsy studies were so rarely described, and not one was consistent with a normal heart. This mistake led to a severe overestimation of the true patients, as the isolated ECG, that is not so rare, was considered itself the disease, following an unjustified J-ICD reflex (ICD implant following the casual detection of a

* Corresponding author: Dr Bortolo Martini, Via Gioberti 9, 36016 Thiene (VI), Tel: +39 0445 5719891; Fax; +39 0445 571928; E-mail: bortolo.martini@gmail.com.

precordial J-ST elevation) in healthy people. Recently, more accurate series are confirming that the true syndrome is so rare, and linked to an underlying right ventricular disease causing a conduction disease at the RVOT. The correct definition of this structural anomaly and of its genetic origin, is still needed to transform an ECG into a disease.

Keywords: Brugada syndrome, sudden death, right bundle branch block and ST elevation, ventricular fibrillation, molecular genetics, arrhythmogenic right ventricular cardiomyopathy

Introduction

The syndrome of sudden death, right bundle branch block and ST segment elevation was introduced as a new medical entity 25 years ago [1-5], but became popular after the description by the Brugada brothers [5].

The typical expression describes a middle aged man with a coved ST segment elevation in the precordial leads, and sometime with a family history of cardiac event, that suddenly collapses because of Polymorphic Ventricular Tachycardia (PVT), degenerating into Ventricular Fibrillation (VF). The event occurs usually at rest, sometime at night-time.

Asians are reported to have a high prevalence of this syndrome where it may be the cause of the nocturnal sudden unexplained death syndrome in young males (Pokkurry death, Bangucut disease).

The data are, however, controversial, because of the limited availability of clinical and necropsy studies. The syndrome is still retained a typical expression of a functional idiopathic VF in normal hearts, with an underlying repolarization abnormalities possible linked to genetic disorders of ion channels, especially the sodium and calcium channels.

These latter theories lack of a serious documentation and the evidence based data are little by little confirming that the disorder has some underlying structural and not functional abnormality.

Anecdotes

On 20 October 1984 a 42 years old healthy and previous asymptomatic cook, quietly talking with the post officer outside his restaurant (http://digilander.libero.it/martini_ syndrome/slide.htm) suddenly collapsed but was so fortunate that an ambulance arrived promptly and a successful defibrillation was performed [1, 2]. The electrocardiogram (ECG) taken showed an ST elevation in the precordial leads (Figure 1), and acute myocardial infarction was diagnosed.

Coronary heart disease was ruled out at angiography. The patient is still alive and asymptomatic on beta blockers therapy. Twenty-eight years later all the interns, fellows and doctors working in the emergency departments are so aware and frightened of this new (lately called) Brugada Syndrome (BS) that they look carefully for similar typical and atypical ECG abnormalities in patients admitted because of syncope.

The entity has become so popular that also Dr. House in his television series has discussed it as one of his brilliant diagnoses, and it also inspired Wes Craven in the film *A Nightmare on Elm Street.*

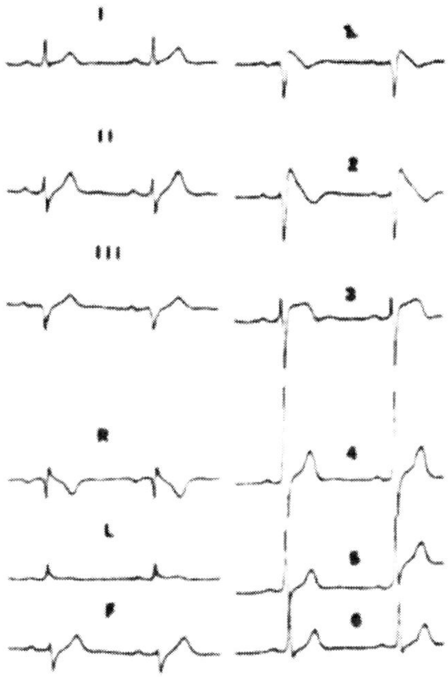

Figure 1. This ECG (now called "Brugada sign") is the first published trace of the syndrome in 1988, [1]. It shows the most typical pattern: slightly prolonged PR interval, left axis deviation, coved ST elevation starting from the J point, in the precordial leads, with inverted t waves in V1-V2 and reduced s1 wave in V6.

In 2004 in "The New York Times" journalist Sandeep Jauhar, reported a scientists note that as many as 12% of all sudden deaths and roughly 20% of deaths in patients with structurally normal hearts were attributed to the disease.

All this uncontrolled informations have created a lot of unjustified nightmares in doctors and their healthy patients with some similar ECG waves. A J-ICD reflex (Implantable Cardiac Defibrillator when a J wave in V1 is seen), is still believed to be a guideline . At the present time however, the evidence-based data have only clarified that this syndrome is an extremely rare lethal disease, characterized by a not so rare, typical or similar healthy ECG pattern. This syndrome is slowly reaching his third decade but we do not yet reliably know the clinical history, the precise ECG pattern, the genetic basis, the patho-physiology, the risk stratification and least but not last, the electrical and anatomic substrate.

Historical Notes

In 1953 Osher and Wolff reported a dynamic ECG abnormality, simulating acute myocardial infarction, in a healthy man [7]. It is of interest that they wrote: "This is apparently due to prolongation of the depolarization process by right bundle block (RBBB) or possibly focal block with delayed activation of a portion of the right ventricle (RV): unusually early onset of repolarization may also play a role". In 1988 Nava, presented a new syndrome characterized by aborted sudden death in a middle aged man with elevated J point and coved ST in the precordial leads (called early repolarization), delayed conduction at the right ventricular outflow tract (RVOT), and minor structural abnormalities of the right ventricle [1], similar to those found in minor forms of Arrhythmogenic Right Ventricular Dysplasia/Cardiomyopathy (ARVC/D) [6]. Most of the clinical and ECG features later discussed nowadays in up to 2,500 papers were completely described in that single patient. This happens frequently in Medicine and in human history, and was well affirmed by Vergilius *"Ab uno disce omnis":* when you see one, you learn all. (Publius Vergilius Maro 70-19 B.C Georgicon II, 64-65)

One year later a full description of the syndrome was published in the American Heart Journal [2]. In that paper it is noteworthy that not only "the typical" but most of the electrocardiographic variations of the syndrome, namely dynamic or isolated ST abnormalities, incomplete or complete right bundle branch block (RBBB), sometime associated with A-V and fascicular conduction impairment, and prolonged HV intervals were described. Prolonged PR interval, left axis deviation, incomplete RBBB and minor ST elevation, was present in patient 4 who had sudden death. The same patient was republished by Corrado, (Figure 1 of reference 8), and that ECG is an example of the dynamic ECG behavior, sometime seen in this syndrome. Despite the typical functional ECG behavior, and a SCN5A genetic anomaly in his family, this patient had anatomical evidence of ARVD/C, with fibrosis of the conduction system [8, 9].

Complete RBBB morphology was present in patient 1, with only a slight ST elevation in V1 and V2. Isolated slight ST/T anomalies/ elevation as seen in patients 2 and 5 of our paper [2] may very well have been a potential marker of the syndrome. Drug testing was not performed at that time.

The presence of late potentials, corresponding to ST segment elevation were proven both by intra-cavitary recordings [1] and by signal averaged ECG [4].

The second description of the syndrome was presented by Aihara [3] in patients without apparent heart disease, and the third by the Brugada brothers [5], five years after the initial Italian description. These authors are indeed deserved to be the first who confirmed that the discussed ECG pattern belonged to a new syndrome.

Further improvements in the evidence-based knowledge of this entity came from Naccarella [10] who demonstrated that the typical ECG can occasionally be recorded at a higher precordial level, by Brugada who introduced the class 1c drug challenge [11], by Yan who investigated laboratory models [12], by Chen who reported the first possible genetic abnormalities [13], by Gonzalez-Rebollo who reported the appearance of the ECG during fever [14].

Ablative intervention has been shown to cure this abnormality [15], and as a definitive conclusion of the patho-physiological debate, Shah and Nademanee [16, 17] eliminated the ST elevation by direct ablation of endocardial and epicardial late potentials.

In the future the major challenges will be the identification of the cause of the disease, and more importantly the correct epidemiological and risk stratification of this condition, in order to avoid the indiscriminate abuse of invasive diagnosis and therapies in healthy asymptomatic people.

Definition of Terms

A "Syndrome" (from Greek Σύνδρομή: σύν = together, δρόμοσ = run) is the association of several clinically recognizable features, signs (observed by someone other than the patient), symptoms (reported by the patient), phenomena or characteristics that often occur together. Ibn Sina (Avicenna, 980-1037), in "*The Canon of Medicine*", pioneered the idea of a syndrome in the diagnosis of specific diseases.

Some confusion, however, still exists even in recent consensus statement [5]. A "Disease" is the pathological condition of a part, organ, or system of an organism resulting from evidence-based patho-physiologic causes, such as infection, genetic defect, degenerative abnormalities etc., and characterized by an identifiable group of signs or symptoms.

For example the isolate detection of the Parkinson sign: tremor, is neither a syndrome, nor a disease. Parkinson syndrome is any of a group of nervous system signs and symptoms similar to Parkinson disease, marked by muscular rigidity, tremor, and impaired motor control and often having a specific secondary cause, such as the use of certain drugs or frequent exposure to toxic chemicals etc. Parkinson disease is a primary progressive neurologic disorder occurring most often after the age of 50, associated with the destruction of brain cells that produce dopamine., The same occurs for the isolated detection of the ECG "sign" of an atypical right bundle branch block (RBBB) and ST elevation in the precordial leads of an asymptomatic healthy subject. When "symptoms" like syncope or aborted sudden death are absent, a diagnosis of Brugada syndrome based only on an ECG finding is a relevant mistake, with deleterious medical and psychological consequences, often related to a Google rather than a Cardiologist consultation [18-20]. Moreover, at present, a diagnosis of disease for this entity is not possible, as the patho-physiology of the syndrome is still the topic of many interesting but inconclusive studies.

The purpose of this paper is to analyze some evidence based data, on the ECG, clinical, laboratory and patho-physiology underlying the syndrome.

The "Symptoms" of the Syndrome

Sudden or aborted sudden death, usually typically occurs between ages 35 and 50 years, in a male individual with a similar family history. This event is unfortunately "the gold standard" for an accurate diagnosis of the syndrome. The circumstances of death are usually unrelated to effort or stress, and may occur during sleep, particularly in Asians [21]. Syncope is another major symptom, and is probably due to self-limited episodes of PVT. It is of interest that several studies have confirmed a high frequency (35%) of vaso-vagal syncope in individuals with type 1 ECG [22], which indicates a limited accuracy of these symptoms during risk stratification. Palpitations and chest discomfort before syncope are rare but specific symptoms for the syndrome while vagal prodroms indicate a low risk group for the syndrome [23]. There is a high recurrence rate of ventricular fibrillation and unfortunately this lethal arrhythmia can be easily induced both in symptomatic and asymptomatic people with the discussed ECG, thus limiting its specificity. Symptoms and spontaneous type 1 ECG are the only evidence based predictors of arrhythmic events, whereas gender, familial history of sudden cardiac death (SCD), inducibility of ventricular tachy-arrhythmias during electrophysiological study, and the presence of an *SCN5A* mutation were not predictive of arrhythmic events. [24]. In Finger study, during follow-up, 22 of 62 patients (35%) from the cardiac arrest group, 19 of 313 patients (6%) from the syncope group, and 10 of 654 (1.5%) patients from the asymptomatic group had an arrhythmic event. The mean event rate per year was 7.7%, 1.9%, and 0.5% [24].

The "Signs" of the Syndrome

The Basal ECG

Since 2002 a new non-evidence-based classification has divided the ECG pattern of the syndrome in three types [25], based on the QRS-T morphology in the first three precordial leads, without any detail for the remaining nine leads. After a "decade of copy and paste" articles very few scientists remember that this classification is simply a case report that described the dynamic precordial ECG-leads of a single resuscitated patient. It has nothing to do with a scientific study that should have analyzed the prevalence of this sign in a relevant series of true patients. Unfortunately this classification has been severely abused, and asymptomatic healthy individuals incidentally found to have one of these three patterns have been submitted to invasive studies and therapies. A new classification has recently been proposed [26], and type 3 has been fortunately erased.

New criteria have however been proposed using "angles and index" that should require a more severe validation according to scientific principles.

At present time, the only serious way to discuss this topic is go back to the analysis of the published pathological cases that provide the following evidences:

1. The vast majority of the true patients show in the precordial leads QRST patterns resembling a right bundle branch block (RBBB) [1-5] and a coved ST elevation (Figure 1, 2). Differently from RBBB an S wave is reduced or absent in V6 [27], leading to a longer QRS duration in the precordial leads with a mismatch between V1 and V6 QRS duration. When this S wave is present and pronounced in V6 the QRS morphology and duration in V1 becomes similar to a RBBB pattern. A prolonged PR, HV interval and left axis deviation is not so rare in the true patients [1-5]; all indicate a conduction disturbance underlying the ECG. The most typical (type 1) ECG shows an high take-off coved ST pattern in V1 (the so called precordial early repolarization described by Wassenburg [28] with an occasional small sharp notch wave at the J point (the QRS-ST junction). This ECG pattern is, erroneously called but better known as a J wave, forgetting that is however so different from the true J wave described by Osborn [29-31].
2. The most typical ST segment has a coved ST morphology that continues with asymmetric inverted T waves in V1-V2, rarely in V3. Increased ST elevation can rarely precede the arrhythmic events [32], and spontaneous ECG alterations may predict VF recurrence [33]. Type 1 morphology induction at drug testing is retained a necessary condition to make a diagnosis of BS, but this assumption is controversial [18-20].

In occasional cases [34-36] the J point can be fragmented, both spontaneously and after ajmaline infusion [37], (Figure 5), which closely resemble the epsilon waves described by Guy Fontaine [38, 39].

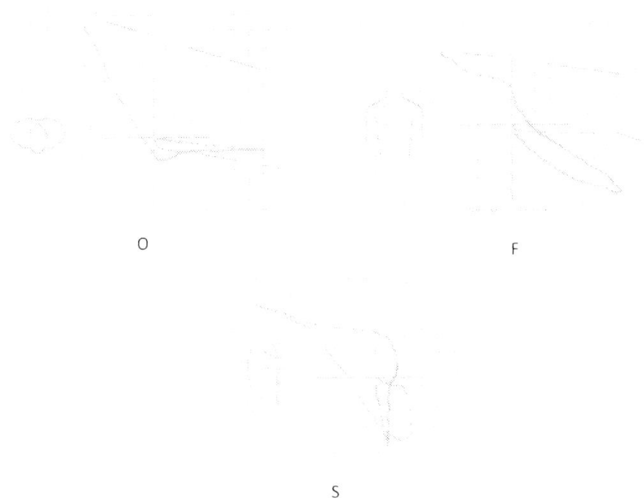

Figure 2. Vectorcardiographic analysis of terminal (amplified) QRS of the same patient (type 1 pattern) : The end of the QRS loop does not coincide with its beginning, and its distance depends on the degree of ST elevation. There is right superior and posterior conduction delay that probably suggests a partial block of fibers that approach the right ventricular outflow tract.

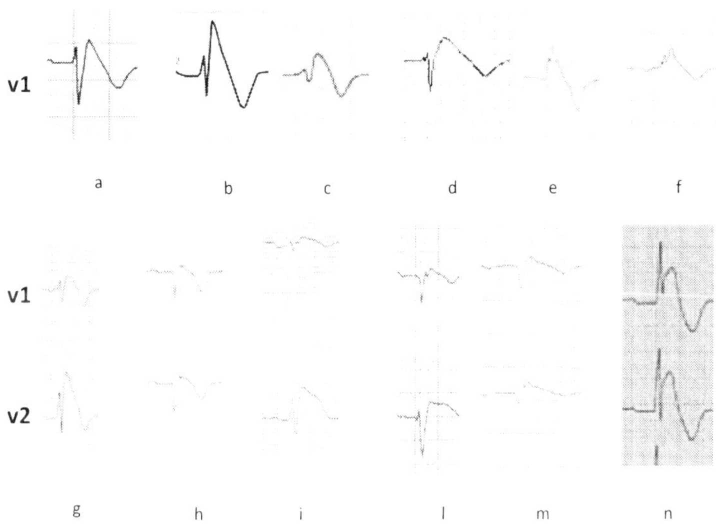

Figure 3. Precordial ECG traces in 12 different cases. In the first six cases (a-f), only V1 is showed. These cases a-f shows a progressive 1) disappearance of S wave 2) slowing of the final QRS and 3) smoothing of the J point that becomes fractionated. Similar progressive fractioning of J point is present in g-m, leading to typical epsilon waves. Fractioning can be present in lead V1 (g,i,l), or better seen in lead V2 (h and m). Case n is a rare example of a true J wave so similar to the one described by Osborn. It belongs to a patient treated with amiodarone intra-venously.

A fragmented terminal QRS (f-QRS) can be documented in up to 43% [40, 41] of individuals, more frequently in those with type 1, and in those with prolonged HV intervals and in those with VF. The fragmentation (both isolated and multiple), can be recorded all around the end of the QRS [40] (Figure 3). An f-QRS can be better recorded at higher intercostals spaces. A similar f-QRS can be recorded in the isolated canine RV tissue model of the syndrome, obtaining a large phase 1 notch of the action potential in epicardium and a local activation delay in the epicardium [40]. Increasing the cutoff frequency of the low-pass filter from 35 to 150 Hz, more spikes are visible [42]. Magnetocardiographic recordings increase the detection of f-QRS [43].

3. The ST segment elevation may also show a saddle-back configuration (so called type 2 and 3). These patterns un-rarely spontaneously change to type 1 in serial observations of the true patients, while have very limited relevance in the asymptomatic population. A "dome shaped" or up-looping ST elevation, without a high ST-QRS takeoff is unusual in the syndrome, and is a typical pattern in healthy athletes [44, 45].

   This spontaneous change between saddle-back to coved ST elevation, unfortunately also occurs in asymptomatic individuals not rarely inducing the J-ICD reflex. This change can be elicited by positioning the precordial leads in the third intercostals spaces, by the class 1c drug challenge, by antidepressant drugs, etc.

   Recently, Holst has reported a 4.7% non-specific prevalence of type 2 and 9.4% of type 3, by recording at different intercostal spaces among 340 healthy European individuals [46]. These data were also confirmed in Turkey [47].

   A Saddle back but also coved ST elevation in inferior and lateral leads has been described in patients with major cardiac event especially when there is a fragmentation of the terminal QRS [48-50]. Up to 11% of subjects with precordial type 1-2 ECG have an infero-lateral J point elevation [51]. Recently the presence of a J wave in multiple leads and horizontal ST-segment morphology after J wave may indicate a highly arrhythmogenic substrate in patients with BS [253]. It has not been demonstrated yet, that these ECG pattern truly belongs to the same syndrome. The proposed new groups of "J wave syndromes" or "early repolarization syndromes", share some limited ECG abnormalities but do not have yet any common evidence-based genetic and patho-physiologic substrate [50-52].

4. A febrile state of different etiologies can induce a type 1 pattern [14], and laboratory experiments confirmed a relationship between the discussed ECG and temperature [53, 54]. Many reports have been published on this topic raising the question if the ECG pattern is related to the body temperature or to the syndrome. In a highly selected group [55], fever was the cause of inducible type 1 ECG in 16 of 47 subjects.

   In another series 18% of patients with the true syndrome [56], had symptoms associated with fever. SCN5A and other different genetic abnormalities of the ion channels may concur to heart arrhythmias during fever [57, 58]. In healthy people with the ECG abnormality only during a febrile state the data are still controversial, but usually the prognosis is favorable [59].

   Healthy subjects with fever-inducible type 1, should however be clinically followed, as the phenomenon is not usual. Erdogan recently conducted an important survey on

2011 male subjects with fever ≥38 °C. This study demonstrated that when the ECG was recorded at the fourth intercostals level, no subject developed type 1 pattern, whereas almost 10% revealed type 2 or 3 pattern at higher intercostals level [60].
ECG variations may also related to food-consumption: Nogami [61] demonstrated that glucose and insulin infusion or an oral glucose tolerance test augments morphologic changes in ST-T waves in patients with syndrome but in none of the patients in the control group. Patients who showed coved-type ST elevation before the glucose load exhibited positive ECG changes more frequently than patients with saddleback-type elevation or transiently normalized ST.
A full stomach test has been proposed [62] as a test to identify high risk patients, but is rarely applied.

Prevalence of the ECG Pattern and of the Syndrome in Different Populations

Male predominance is an evident character of the syndrome, accounting for more than 80% of cases. Although the mechanism for the male predominance is not fully understood, it is believed that testosterone is also involved. A study suggests that higher testosterone level associated with lower visceral fat may have a significant role in the male predominance in Brugada syndrome [63].

Since the pioneer paper of Tohyu [64], the true prevalence both of the ECG and of the true syndrome is still controversial. In a large series, approximately 16 out 10,000 European individuals older than 18 years might have a spontaneous type 1 pattern [65]. Holst in a recent Danish registry has collected 1.1 true patients /100,000 inhabitants (67% had a type 1 pattern) [66]. However, other large series in northern Europe [67-69] did not find any type 1 ECG in non-selected populations, whereas type 2 and 3 were also rare (0.6%).

Interestingly, despite the rare finding of the typical ECGs in these European populations, many papers have described a relevant number of patients with the syndrome in this geographic area.

In south-east Asian population the isolated prevalence of the ECG was retained to be higher but controversial data are described, probably due to a limited availability of the health system for most of the people. In Korea [70], type 1 was not found in soldiers (0.9% had type 2-3). In the Philippines a 0.2% of type 1 and 1.8% of type 2-3 ECG has been reported [71]. Recently type 1-3 ECG was found in 0.1% of 18,476 young male conscripts [72]. Black people with the syndrome, both living in Africa or in western countries are only anecdotally reported [73, 74].

In Japanese infants [75] the prevalence is very low for type 1 (0.005%), and an age dependence of the discussed ECG has been shown [76]. When serial ECG are taken during a long term follow up to these individuals, 56% shows normalization or fluctuation between type 1-2 and 3 [76].

For what concern the prevalence of the true syndrome (symptoms+signs), Wilde and Brugada reported that the syndrome affects 3-5 in 10,000 people [77] while Ackermann [78] established a prevalence of 1 in 5,000 to 10,000. A possible relevant problem was anecdotally reported in Southeast Asia (up to 66 patients per 10,000 inhabitants) where it may be the cause of the nocturnal sudden unexplained death syndrome in young males (Pokkurry death,

Bangucut disease). The data are, however, controversial [79], because of the limited availability of clinical and necropsy studies. A recent large study in Southeast Asian refugees has shown a high prevalence of sleep disorder, paralysis and apnea [80], that might be the cause of nocturnal sudden death or a concurrence in Brugada syndrome [81]. These data need serious epidemiological reconsideration, as probably 1.1 true cases in 100,000 people is a more convincing prevalence [66], at least in Caucasians.

Class 1c Drugs Challenge

The use of ajmaline introduced by Brugada [11], and all class 1c drugs, to elicit a syndrome in an asymptomatic or mildly symptomatic cohort has a very poor predictive value. A type 1 pattern can be elicited in up to 50% of Italian and in 85% of German-French healthy, asymptomatic individuals with a type 2 or 3 pattern [82-84].

It is interesting to note that there was more positive tests in asymptomatic subjects than in symptomatic or familial cases, which raises scientific, ethical and legal questions on these, sometime unsafe, challenges [85-87].

In these and other published studies, severe limitations are noted because of the low prevalence of the true syndrome, the low event rate and the short follow up period [83].

A correlation of the drug challenges with genetic abnormalities has no evidence: Brugada [11] initially proposed a 100% correlation between SCN5A carriers and the spontaneous or drug inducible ECG pattern, but this assumption was not confirmed [88]. Priori demonstrated, that the test might be negative in as many as 80% of asymptomatic gene carriers [89-90]. These drugs are not specific for the syndrome, as normal subjects, and patients with right ventricular cardiomyopathy may show similar ECG changes [27, 91-92].

A simpler explanation for the effects of Flecainide does not involve repolarization or ionic channels but drug-induced conduction abnormalities, as documented in an old study[93]. When Flecainide is injected in these subjects with a possible latent conduction disturbance, the first thing to be expected is a maximal deterioration of depolarization with conduction delays, and not a repolarization abnormality. This is simply and well demonstrable by recording late potentials after the drug is given. [27, 94].

In four true patients with type 1 ECG, Miyazaki [95] demonstrated that ST elevation was augmented by selective stimulation of alpha adrenoceptors or muscarinic receptors or by class 1A drugs, but was mitigated by beta-adrenoceptor stimulation or alpha-adrenoceptor blockade. Other limited experiences with adrenergic drugs have partially confirmed these data [96].

The ECG during Effort

Sumiyoshi [21] reported syncope after effort in a female patient with the syndrome, with late VF during sleep. Since the historical paper by Douard [97], little interest has been devoted to the study of effort-related symptoms and the syndrome. At present time there is not a single published report of sudden death during effort in a patient with the syndrome.

One athlete had sustained monomorphic ventricular tachycardia during sport activity [98] but no symptoms during exercise stress test in hospital, where the J-ST pattern increased significantly during recovery. Another athlete with type 1 ECG had syncope and palpitation during cycling [99], but nothing during exercise test.

Also in non-athlete, symptoms are almost never related to efforts, and ventricular tachycardia during stress test has been only anecdotally reported [100]. Despite these limited evidences all guidelines and consensus paper discourage people with the discussed ECG to practice sports [101].

For what concern the ECG pattern (both in patients and asymptomatic subjects), Nademanee observed that during exercise stress test the ECG normalized in 25% of type 1 ECG, and then reappeared at the recovery phase [102]. Guevara Valdivia [103], observed a similar pattern with normalization during the effort, and reappearance of the ST elevation during the recovery phase. In another subject, the ST anomaly occurred during effort and disappeared at the recovery phase. Amin [104] evidentiated that QRS duration and both J point and coved ECG were enhanced during peak exercise (representing a stress induced conduction abnormality) and further during recovery in subjects with spontaneous or induced ECG; this pattern was not related to SCN5A abnormalities. No arrhythmias were induced in this population. Another conspicuous series confirmed that in 37% of type 1 ECG, this pattern is augmented at early recovery, and might have some negative predictor for future events [105]. Unmasking of type I Brugada ECG only in the recovery phase of exercise and during vaso-vagal reaction, has been described [106]. It is however of relevant interest that patients with right ventricular cardiomyopathy may also show ST elevation during exercise stress test [107].

Similar ECG in Different Situations

A recent review summarized the same or similar ECG patterns that have been recognized in different pathological, physiological or drug induced conditions [108]. In this and other review it is of relevant interest that the same ECG patterns are not so rare in patients with a definite diagnosis of ARVD/C [109-111].

These patients may also show similar ST modification after ajmaline [92].

Further Non-Invasive and Invasive ECG Evaluations

Since its first presentation [1], vectorcardiographic analysis is rarely performed but it shows some interesting features: The end of the QRS loop does not coincide with its beginning, and its distance depends on the degree of ST elevation. There is right superior and posterior conduction delay that probably suggests a partial block of fibers that approach the right ventricular outflow tract (Figure 2). This nowadays forgotten cultural approach to the electrical activity of the heart, helps to differentiate type 1 ECG from incomplete RBBB [4, 112]. Vectorcardiography provides informations on the terminal QRS, and indicates the presence of delayed depolarizations or late potentials (LP) caused by an organic heart disease. LP are however better recorded at signal averaged ECG study, where they are frequently positive (up to 70%) [113] (Figure 4). Late potentials may also be recorded at right ventricular outflow tract (RVOT) level during endocavitary recording, at body surface mapping, and at direct epicardial recordings [114-116]. Positive late potentials are more frequently found in patients with subsequent arrhythmic events [117].

As a rule, they can be recorded after Flecainide challenge [27], demonstrating that this drug could induce a late depolarization rather than an early repolarization abnormality. Late potentials are less frequent in type 2 and 3 ECG patterns that might indicate a true functional origin of these ST abnormalities. Nademanee [17] has highly enhanced the role of late potentials by simply demonstrating that the ablation of late depolarization waves (obviously linked to an organic substrate), at the epicardial surface of RVOT, eliminated the ST segment elevation. Thus the initial hypothesis by Osher [7] that the delayed repolarization at the RVOT level was responsible for an unusual ECG pattern has been confirmed after 50 years of heavy discussions. T Wave Alternans (TWA), indicating a repolarization abnormality, is positive only in 16% [118]. T wave alternans (both spontaneous or drugs/fever induced) and random T wave changes have been described in the syndrome, and their origin has been attributed to heterogeneity of infundibular action potentials [119, 120] not excluding a local conduction disturbance. A controversial exist on their clinical usefulness [121].

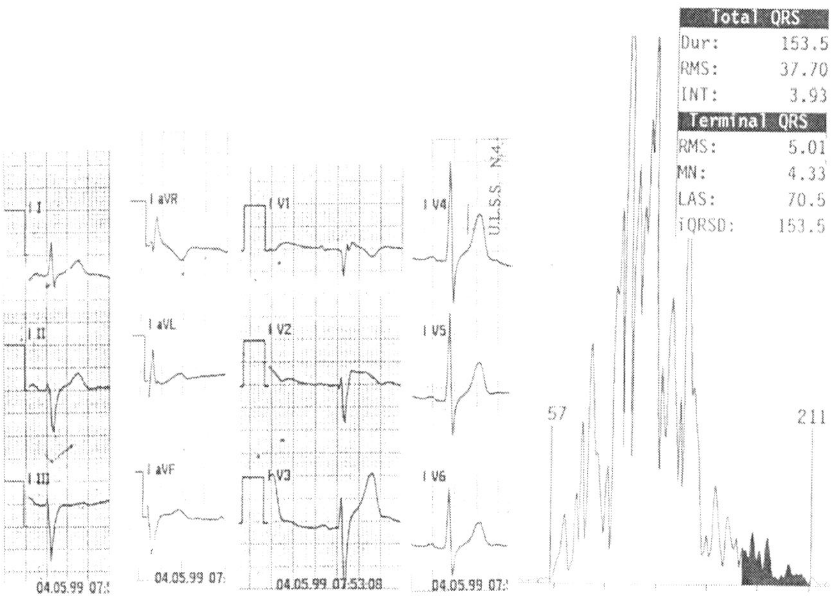

Figure 4. Basal ECG and Late Potentials study in a familial case of the syndrome associated to SCN5A homozigotic abnormality and structural heart disease. The ECG trace shows a prolonged PR interval, left axis deviation and a fragmented J point very similar to an epsilon wave and ST elevation. At signal averaged ECG study, there is a marked prolongation of depolarization, coincident with J point fragmentation.

Arrhythmias Linked to the Syndrome

Patients with the true syndrome develop VF or polymorphic VT. Repetitive monomorphic premature ventricular contractions (PVCs), mostly of LBBB morphology (with superior or inferior axis) are observed initiating ventricular tachyarrhythmias in more than 2/3 of cases [32]. Before the onset of VF, these PVC increase their intensity, and this is sometime associated also with increased ST segment elevation. There were no seasonal differences in cardiac arrest in the patients but a higher incidence of this event can be observed from midnight to 6:00 AM at least in Asian population [122]. In this population however, serious sleep disorders can be recorded, that indicate that the sudden nocturnal death syndrome has not yet a clarified mechanism [80, 81]. The long coupling interval (usually 300-380 milliseconds) of triggers, or their Purkinje origin, does not support epicardial phase 2 reentry [32]. These PVC, are usually abolished during exercise, or with adrenergic stimulation. Endocardial mapping of these PVCs can detect the earliest ventricular activation within the right Purkinje system or from the right ventricular outflow tract. Ablation of these PVCs can successfully abolish recurrences [15]. Severe arrhythmic storms are a rare but dramatic occurrence [123], and seems to well respond both to isoproterenol and quinidine [96, 97,124]. Cardiac Transplant is the last resource [125].

Sustained VT is a rare but well described arrhythmia [126] in this syndrome, clearly associated to a structural reentry circuit. Most of the cases show a LBBB morphology, and different axis [34]. RBBB morphology is not so rare [127].

The patients with major ventricle arrhythmias may have few premature contractions during Holter monitoring. The morphology of these ectopics is usually LBBB, mainly with an inferior axis, but RBBB morphology may also be recorded, with some correlations with genetic abnormalities [128].

Atrial arrhythmias [130] can be encountered in up to 20% of the true patients [130-131], and can be simply associated with a more advanced disease andto common genetic abnormalities[132]. It is not proven that patients with persistent atrial fibrillation and in whom a type 1 or 2 ECG pattern is induced after class 1C therapy have the syndrome [133]. Recent series still however include these patients in the syndrome [134].

Intra-Cavitary ECG Recordings and Stimulation Studies

Investigations evidentiated a prolonged HV interval as a frequent finding, mostly in the cases with major conduction abnormalities [1-3]. Prolonged HV interval is always a pattern of organic heart disease of the conduction system. Marked fibrosis of the conduction system has been shown to underlie this finding [8, 9]. Activation maps during stimulation from the AV nodal area in another patient with histological proven heart disease showed a normal rapid spread of activation of the left septal endocardium and of the LV; in the RVOT, crowding of isochrones indicated slowed conduction. The entire RV wall (endocardium and epicardium) was activated relatively late [125]. High resolution Electro- anatomic mapping, has further confirmed these underlying structural right heart diseases [135, 136], but this technique is unfortunately rarely used during routine electrophysiological study, which is mainly devoted to induce ventricular arrhythmias rather than understanding their origin and underlying mechanism (Figure 5).

Few but relevant studies have however indicated that this mapping reliably documents areas of slow conduction, particularly at the RVOT level [137-140] (Figure 5). In this area most of the isolated premature contractions have origin [128], and it is the best site to induce VF with premature electrical stimulation (PES) [2].

In this area radiofrequency ablation can be "curative" both experimentally [114, 140] and clinically [16, 17]. RVOT is a complex embryological structure [141], where different structures fuse together, creating a mixture of structural and physiological properties, uncommonin other myocardial regions.

From these area where depolarization and repolarization peculiarities can simultaneously be present [120, 142,] both benign [143] and lethal ventricular arrhythmias originate. VF and/or PVT are easily inducible both in symptomatic patients and asymptomatic subjects with the discussed ECG. Brugada could induce VF in 73% and 33% respectively [144], but some Japanese studies reported higher percentages of 92 and 64% [145].

The PES protocol and site of stimulation probably explain why the percentage of asymptomatic individuals with inducible VF was (much) higher in the Japanese studies.

Significantly more patients and subjects with inducible VF have their arrhythmia induced from the RVOT [145]. A prolonged HV interval is more frequent in inducible patients.

At present time the value of EP-studies, particularly in asymptomatic patients, is not robust enough to guide therapy. It is unclear why PES has only prognostic value in asymptomatic patients with a spontaneous type 1 in the hands of the Brugada brothers [146].

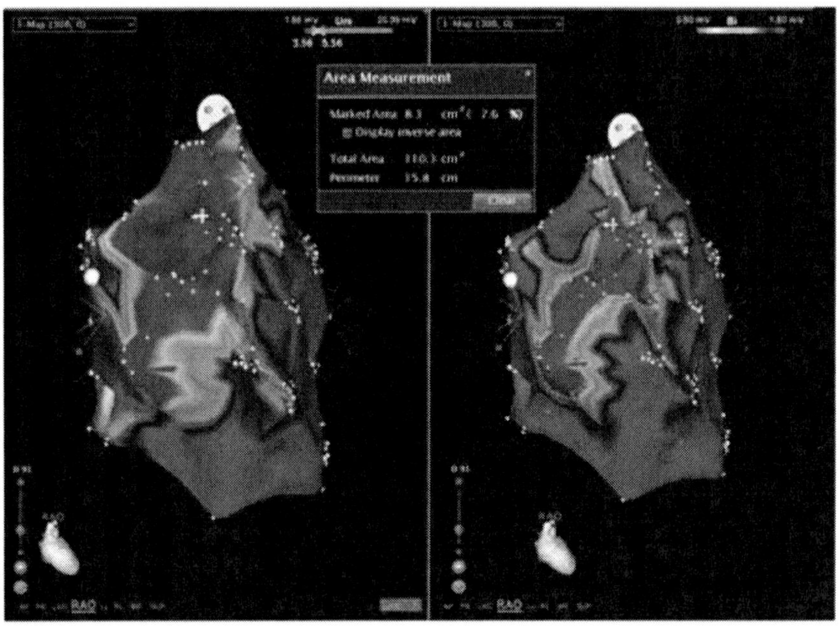

Figure 5. Electroanatomic mapping of the RV (RAO view, unipolar and bipolar recordings), show significant scares at the RVOT, consistent with a structural abnormality that underlies a conduction disturbance. (Courtesy of Dr. Marras, Corò and Delise).

2D Echocardiogram, Nuclear Magnetic Echocardiography, Resonance Studies (NMR), Radionuclide Angiography and Electron Beam Tomography

2D echocardiography usually excludes a structural heart disease in almost all series, but the accuracy of this investigation in the detection of subtle abnormalities is operator dependent [147]. A very careful analysis [148, 149] can however detects subtles abnormalities. A cardiac NMR study was firstly reported by D'Onofrio [150], who documented a fatty replacement of the RVOT in one patient with a true syndrome. Nine years later Papavassiliu confirmed an enlargement of the right ventricle, particularly of the RVOT and localized fatty replacement. These findings however did not reached significance in the first paper, but were relevant in the second study where only type 1 patients were enrolled [151], similarly to what found by Catalano [152] and Van Hoorn [153]. Other series [154] recently reached different conclusions, but these latter included subjects with a limited probability of having the true syndrome (females and drug induced ECG). According to Santangeli [155] however, Late Gadolinium Enhancement is significantly less sensitive than Electro Anatomic Mapping in identifying RV cardiomyopathic substrates (small scars), particularly at the RVOT level. Electron beam tomography has also been rarely used to study the RV in this population by Tada [156] and Takagi [157], and again RVOT and RV abnormalities were detected. At Radionuclide Angiographic study, Rouzet [158] assessed that RVOT contraction was delayed in patients with BS, and RV contraction heterogeneity increased according to the pattern of ST-segment elevation, without impairment of the amplitude of contraction.

RV volumes were greater in patients with BS compared with control subjects, without impairment of the ejection fraction, whatever the ST-segment elevation pattern or the magnitude of contraction heterogeneity.

Cardiac Angiography

Despite the extensive use of invasive electrophysiologic study in these subjects, limited data are available regarding the angiographic study of the left, and especially the RV, where some minor abnormalities were initially described [1-2], and recently confirmed by Durthoit [159]. A diagnosis of normal versus abnormal right angiography is often controversial in those frequent cases in which the anomaly is much localized.

A relevant role in the study of the RV is the operator experience and to the protocols utilized [160]. The first published image of a diagnostic angiography by Proclemer [161] was highly criticized by Brugada [162]. It is of notice that in the report by Remme [163] RV was retained normal in patients with a subsequent diagnosis of ARVD/C at necropsy study. As suggested by high experience colleagues, [159, 160], a single postero-anterior view has a limited accuracy in detecting minor abnormalities of the right ventricle, and multiple views, are required for a correct diagnosis. A correlation between any detected anomaly and electro-anatomic mapping, highly increases the accuracy [135-139].

Genetic Studies

The disease is clearly an autosomic dominant entity with variable expression, mainly affecting males, and possibly more frequent in Asia [1, 5, 164]. After the paper from Chen [13], a rush in the genetic studies has described hundreds SCN5A abnormalities, leading to authoritative classification of the syndrome among the channellopathy, without any clear evidence-based data. Specific genetic mutations of ion channels are not yet part of the diagnostic criteria of the Syndrome according to fair admission by leading authorities.

According to Hoogendick [165], and despite biologist, geneticist-cardiologist and industry pressure, a causative role of genes in the patho-physiology of the syndrome is still a hypothesis. The disorder and/or the ECG are clearly familial in a relevant number of patients but a Mendelian autosomal dominant pattern of transmission cannot explain the syndrome. Chen in 1998 identified SCN5A missense mutations in three out of six families with idiopathic ventricular fibrillation and the abnormal spontaneous or drug- induced ECG in some members [13].

Thus far, more than 300 mutations in 12 genes have been associated with the syndrome [165, 166]. Most of these mutations reduce the cardiac sodium current (I_{Na}) and are located in *SCN5A* [13], the gene encoding the cardiac sodium channel, its β-subunits *SCN1B* and *SCN3B* or in *GPD1L* and *MOG1,* which are thought to impair trafficking of the cardiac sodium channel to the cell membrane [167-170]. Other mutations associated with the Brugada syndrome reduce the L-type calcium current (I_{CaL}) and are located in *CACNA1C*, *CACNB2b* and *CACNA2D1,* which encode the α1-, β2b-, and α2δ-subunit of the L-type calcium channel [171, 172].

Lastly, mutations in *KCNE3* which encodes MiRP2, a β-subunit of several potassium channels, in *KCNJ8* encoding the ATP-sensitive potassium channel, and HCN4 that cause a reduction of pacemaker current, have been associated with the Brugada syndrome [173, 174].

What is evidenced from the published studies is that SCN5A-related patients (especially the younger [17, 177] have greater defects in impulse propagation (longer PR, HV, QRS duration), more severe QRS fragmentation and late potentials [40, 178-180]. Patients and relatives with a truncated protein might have a more severe phenotype. It is relevant that 2-5% of healthy individuals host missense SCN5A variants, leading to a potential conundrum in the interpretation of genetic results [181-183]. In blacks (that are so rarely affected by the syndrome), SCN5A variation are common [183], and can be related to PR prolongation [184]. Mutations of SCN5A genes have been found in patients with Long and short QT Syndromes [185-186], Early Repolarization Syndrome, Lev-Lenegre Disease, Idiopathic Ventricular Fibrillation, in dilated cardiomyopathy, in sinus node dysfunction and in atrial fibrillation [187-189].

Van Hoorn [153] reported that mutations were associated with increased cardiac dimensions and reduced contractility. Interestingly, the patient submitted to necropsy study in our initial report [2, 9] had both ARVD/C and SCN5A abnormalities present in his family. Frustaci [190] reported one more case. In the presence of an anatomic substrate (an area with slow conduction in RVOT), SCN5A abnormalities could have a strong role [77].

Only one family has been reported with a novel SCN5A missense mutation, R814Q, in homozygous, and this was associated with a coved ST, epsilon waves, sustained ventricular tachycardia of left bundle branch block morphology and structural right ventricular abnormalities [34]. A homozygous mutation has also been reported in a severe, recessive type of cardiac conduction disease [191], but without the discussed ECG. SCN5A mutations accounts for 75% of global anomalies [78], while the calcium channel mutations account for 10-15% of the published papers.

These mutations have been suggested to increase repolarizing currents activated early during the action potential, but clinical and laboratory role that these mutations play in the syndrome is subject of debate. Nine of the 11 genes other than SCN5A currently believed to be associated with the syndrome have been identified by the candidate gene approach, in the absence of linkage-analysis and definitive familial segregation and their disease-causation, suggested by the absence of the specific rare variants from control.

Patch-clamp studies could not clarify how SCN5A mutations can be responsible for such a large spectrum of disease and genetically modified mice are proposed as an interesting but still promising and non-specific tool [192]. This scientific mess caused by geneticist-cardiologists needs new evidence based rules. The major problem is that data are so lacking in the population with the true syndrome (spontaneous type 1 ECG and severe symptoms), as most of the reported series deals with unselected populations including true patients and healthy individuals with overt, masked and induced similar ECGs. In Kapplinger's report [182], the most common (missense) mutations, which possible pathological significance are poor [193], are located in *SCN5A and* can be identified in approximately 21% of people "accepted for genetic testing simply if the referring physician had made a clinical diagnosis of either possible or definite syndrome, and also if "an ECG was not always available" [182]. In this poorly selected population, positive genotype alone is not an independent risk factor for lethal events.

Roden [194] asked in an editorial note: What causes the syndrome in the remaining 79 %? In a more selected high risk (Japanese) population, an anomaly was found in 15% (195). Also Probst [196] in his series utilized a spontaneous or induced ECG as major diagnostic criteria, and found SCN5A anomalies in 26% of type 1 ECG. Thirteen of them belonged to 13 families with 115 carriers.

Eight individuals had type 1 ECG but not mutations. Type 1 ECG was spontaneous only in 18% of these, reaching 61% after drug challenge.

A family history of sudden death was present only in 3/12 families, and the probands did not have a severe clinical history. With this unclear selection the results created confusion between positive and negative phenotype and genotype; the only possible conclusion is that 26% of individuals (not syndromes!) with a spontaneous or induced ST elevation have some SCN5A abnormality.

As pointed out by Marian [197]: "by definition, the causal mutation cannot be absent in family members with the phenotype.

Expression of the Brugada phenotype in family members without the index *SCN5A* mutation, nonetheless, necessitates considering the possibility of another causal gene". In a following paper, Probst [24] increased his series to 808 individuals with spontaneous (43%) or induced type 1 ECG. He reported SCN5A mutations in 24% of survivors of cardiac arrest (spontaneous type 1 only in 50%), in 26% of syncope group (spontaneous type 1 in 54%), and 30% of asymptomatic individuals (spontaneous type 1 in 41%). In the screened families the prevalence of the gene abnormalities (not associated with the syndrome or the ECG) was 52%.

Hermida [198] and Santos [199] recently respectively reported a 43% and 40% familial prevalence of the gene anomalies (not the syndrome!!), with more pronounced conduction abnormalities in the carriers. In another, mostly ECG-based study Bai [176] had a positive genotype only in 13%. This author calculated that the cost per one positive genotyping was US $ 21,441. This should discourage indiscriminate use of this test, until evidence based data on its utility are available.

According to the hypothesis that the syndrome could be the cause of otherwise unexplained cases of sudden death, a "molecular autopsy" has been proposed, but cardiac channelopathies associated with structurally normal hearts such as long QT syndrome, catecholaminergic polymorphic ventricular tachycardia, and BS, leave no major evidence to be found at autopsy [200].

Thus, despite the term channellopathy to classify the syndrome is so popular, and it has been admitted that SCN5A gene abnormalities may be found only in a small proportion of patients [201], genetic testing however is still a Class I recommendation for family members and appropriate relatives following the identification of the BS-causative mutation in an index case [78], while it is a Class IIa recommendation (limited to SCN5A genes mutations) for any patient in whom a cardiologist has established a clinical index of suspicion for BS based on examination of the patient's clinical history, family history, and expressed electrocardiographic (resting 12-lead ECGs and/or provocative drug challenge testing) phenotype. Genetic testing is not indicated in the setting of an isolated type 2 or type 3 Brugada ECG patterns [78].

The rush for new SCN5A gene abnormalities has forgotten other genetic abnormalities, including isolated demonstration of mapping in the same loci of right ventricular cardiomyopathy [91, 202]. Thus, the genetic analysis of the disease must be considered as an on-going process.

Experimental Findings

The pioneer experimental study of Yan and Antzelevitch [13, 203], proposed to ascertain the lacking patho-physiologic basis of the syndrome, and completing the pathway to the promotion of a "syndrome" to a "disease" status. These outstanding studies derived from their research to explain the J wave of early repolarization in the "precordial leads" on a "left" ventricular wedge. As left J wave was similar to right precordial elevated J point, their subsequent studies were mainly devoted to this pattern, assuming that the two entities belonged to the same patho-physiologic pattern. The theory of impaired repolarization proposed in 1999 [203] was based on a non-homogeneous expression of the transient outward potassium current (I_{to}) between epicardium and endocardium. I_{to}, which is responsible for the early repolarization phase (phase 1 notch) during action potential (AP), is more strongly expressed in the epicardium, contributing to a "spike and dome" in AP. The phase 1 notch deepens in the presence of a loss or reduced function of the sodium channels. Progressive deepening of the phase 1 notch can first delay the activation of I_{CaL}, leading to a prominent dome and late repolarization. Further deepening of the phase 1 notch can prevent the activation of I_{CaL}, abbreviating AP. These effects on AP are more evident in the epicardium layer of RVOT, where the I_{to} is the strongest, resulting in simultaneous presence of APs with and without a phase 2 dome and long and short AP duration in the epicardium and across the wall of RVOT [118, 141]. A discrepancy in the AP shape between the endocardium and epicardium result in the surface BS ECG patterns. Abnormalities in the surface ECG are proportional to the discrepancy in the AP, creating slight ECG alterations (saddle-back ST elevation, J point <0.2 mv) or marked ECG alterations (cove type, J point >0.2 mv) according to the degree of sodium channel damage and the different I_{to} expression. Male hormones enhance I_{to}, thus, contributing to a male prominence of BS. Temperature modulates the shape and duration of AP, promoting the expression of BS type ECG at hypothermia and occurrence of arrhythmias at hyperthermia [54]. The conduction of the AP dome from sites where it is maintained to sites where it is lost provokes local re-excitation via a phase 2 reentry mechanism with a closely coupled extrasystole occurring during the vulnerable period. These PVC may then trigger malignant ventricular arrhythmias. Despite the well-known assumption that a "wedge is not a heart" this theory has become very popular among scientists, leading to a so relevant number of correlated experiments that have not been confirmed in the entire heart [125], .

Embryologic Studies

Elizari has recently conducted an outstanding embryologic study on the RVOT, and has proposed a theory, based on the abnormal expression of the neural crest on myocardial development of the RVOT and surrounding structures [141].

During embryogenesis, the cardiac neural crest plays a critical role in morphogenesis of the RVOT, which comprises the free wall and the aorto-pulmonary septum, and the great arteries.

A population of cardiac neural crest cells migrates toward the arterial pole of the embryonic heart leading to myocardial cell proliferation, differentiation and RVOT myocardialization. A second population of migratory cardiac neural crest cells enters the heart via the venous pole and plays a crucial role in the formation of the AV node, the His bundle, the beginning of the bundle branches, and atrial tissue. This pivotal study is very important as it enhance the embryological complexity of the RVOT that could lead to different structural abnormalities and to many different ventricular arrhythmias originating from this area [143, 204-207]. A detailed analysis of this structure [207] will limit in the future the so called cases of "idiopathic" ventricular arrhythmias.

Bioptic Studies and Autopsy

The "gold standard" investigation, to make a correct diagnosis and to quantify both the specificity and sensitivity of other different investigations is still necropsy study, while biopsy seems less important due to the impossibility or to dangerousness to examine only pathological localized areas of the right ventricle, namely the RVOT. Nowadays there are very few cases of autopsy in these patients (Table 1), and all have evidentiated both fibro-fatty substitution mainly of the RVOT and some conduction system disease [8, 9, 125, 156, 163, 208-210]. Biopsy study (Table 1) has been reported more frequently, with controversial results [2112-219]. Anecdotal studies by Gotoh and Kirshner [220-221] evidentiated significant histological lesions of the conduction system in the vast majority of Asians died suddenly at night (in whom the syndrome could retrospectively been suspected). Nowadays a normal heart belonging to a patient with the syndrome has never been reported. Our first reported patient with the syndrome had atrophy, fibrosis and adiposis of the right free wall [8, 9]; this patient also had an unusual lesion of the conduction system characterized by sclerotic interruption of the right bundle branch and by severe fibrosis of the bifurcating bundle. The right ventricular free wall showed bundles of viable myocardium. According to these findings, the conduction disturbance fit well with a septal and parietal conduction abnormality. The free wall lesions, particularly at the infundibular level, are compatible with a second conduction disturbance, at the end of ventricular depolarization.

Thus the right bundle branch block (in our hypothesis), might be explained by a His an Right bundle lesions, and the ST segment elevation by late depolarization of the RVOT. It was not easy until recently to accept that the ST elevation in this syndrome is a depolarization abnormality of the RVOT, but the presence of epsilon waves, f-QRS and late potentials could be ascribed to nothing else.

Table 1. Patients with the syndrome and some structural abnormality at biopsy, autopsy

Author	Number of patients/sex	Ecg type	Biopsy	Autopsy
Martini [2]	2 M,1 F	2 type 1, 1 type 3	2 Fibro/fatty susbstitution	1 ARVC/D
Sumyoshi [21]	1 F	Type 1	Fibrosis	
Brugada [211]	16	Type 1-2	"non specific abn."	
Tada [118]	2 M	Type 1	6/6 EMB negative but ARVD in one direct biopsy during open heart surgery	1 ARVD/C
Morgera[212]	1 M	Type 1	Fibro-fatty replacement	
Izumi [213]	1 M	Type 1	Fibrosis	
Remme [163]	9	Incomplete RBB + inverted t wave V1	All negative	1 ARVD/C: 1 pt with incomplete RBBB and inverted t waves
Corrado [8]	13 M, 1 F	ST segment elevation		all patients had ARVC predominant fatty replacement of the right ventricular anterior wall (92%) except one, who had no evidence of structural heart disease
Morimoto [208]	22+3	?	8/22 byopsy: Fatty infiltration in. Minor abnormalities in the remaining	3 autopsy: marked fatty infiltration (2 in the RVOT)
Buob [214]	1	Type 1		
Coronel [125]	1	Type 1 (drug 1c)		Right ventricular hypertrophy and fibrosis with epicardial fatty infiltration
Frustaci [215]	15 M, 3	Type 1-2	right ventricular myocarditis in 14 patients, viral genomes in 4; ARVD/C in 1; and cardiomyopathic changes in 3	
Morimoto [209]	1 M	Type 1		fatty replacement of the rvot. FF of sinus node
Kim [216]	14	Type 1	7/14 had fibro-fatty sustitution	
Fontaine [210]	1 M	?		1 ARVD/C
Marras [217]	1 M	Type 2	fibro-fatty replacement	
Zumhagen [218]	16 M, 5 F	type 1 (11 only after ajmaline)	Fibro-fatty replacement in 75%	
Ohkubo [219]	24 M, 1F	Type 1-2	Fatty replacement in 47.6%	

We have never been sure if the diseased right ventricle was a typical right ventricular cardiomyopathy, as most of the patients do not have the other typical features, including genetic profile. At the present time only one of our patients with the typical ECG, had a family history of right ventricular cardiomyopathy associated with an ARVD/ C chromosome 14 involvement [91].

It must be admitted however that the detailed and authoritative pathologic examination of a heart is not the rule, and some relevant different opinions between pathologists may exist according to their experience [210]. As written before, biopsy is an interesting but a very controversial investigation that has led to so different findings (Table I), possibly due to different population examined, but also to different techniques.

Biopsy does not seem so relevant for the detection of some structural heart disease, as noninvasive investigations like late potentials, electro-anatomic mapping and nuclear magnetic study can probably provide accurate data [157], also if different opinion on their significance has been proposed [222].

Other Clinical Features of the Syndrome: Role of the Autonomic Tone

Autonomic tone plays a role in this syndrome, and might be responsible for the dynamic behavior of the ECG, and for the high prevalence of event at rest or at night time, that highly suggested a functional abnormality [21, 73, 223, 224]. Further confirmation derives from ST segment elevation after effort of drug challenge and after meals, and in response to autonomic drugs, as being previously discussed. Differently from Miyazaki [9], an abnormal 123I-MIBG uptake can be found in patients with Brugada syndrome, indicating presynaptic sympathetic dysfunction of the heart [225-228]; he also demonstrated with heart rate variability study that high vagal tone and low sympathetic tone are specific properties of symptomatic BS. Yokokawa [22] recently confirmed that 35% of patients with type 1-2 ECG showed vaso-vagal responses during the Head Up Tilt Test. This should discourage to include syncope (unless a neuro-mediated reaction can be clearly excluded), in the risk stratification of the syndrome.

Risk Stratification and Therapy

Annual rate of lethal event ranges from 4.1% in Brugada series [229, 230], to 1.1-1.6% in recent series (0.5% event per year for both spontaneous and induced type 1 ECG (in 60%), in the Finger and other studies, [24, 41, 231].

The peak incidence of symptoms is in the third and fourth decades of life [232]. Indicators of high relative risk of sudden death associated with the syndrome include a personal history of aborted SCD or syncope (RR 3.51), the spontaneous presence of a type 1 ECG pattern (as opposed to a drug-induced type 1 pattern) (RR4.65), male gender (RR 3.47), and South-East Asian origin. A family history of sudden death and SCN5A mutation status do not carry an increased risk of sudden death. Many asymptomatic subjects have been and are still submitted to ICD implantation only because of a spontaneous or drug induced type 1 ECG, because of doubtful symptoms, family history, abnormal cardiac stimulation study, genetic abnormalities, etc., with very low consideration of the high rate of procedure related-complications [233]. After a relevant metanalysis [234], this asymptomatic healthy population has been deserved of major attention, and most of the authors now agree that ICD implantation should be a class 1A indication only for aborted sudden death or arrhythmic related syncope, in patients with a spontaneous type 1 ECG [235]. The electrophysiologic study, particularly, has not more a relevant predictive value for most of the authors, although different respectable opinions still consider this test as highly necessary. Registries and not personal series are needed to clarify the problem. Interesting results have been recently seen with quinidine [124] and with ablation [15, 17]. Some anecdotal patients treated with beta-blockers or amiodarone did not have however any relapse [1, 27]. A limited number of cases with electrical storms have been successfully treated with isoproterenol infusion [236].

Conclusion

This rare and sometime lethal syndrome is still in search of its identity, after having lost his paternity soon after birth [1, 5]. The initial theory that this new familial syndrome was related to a conduction disorder mainly at the RVOT level [1, 2, 9], after two decades of heavy discussions and criticism [237-241] has received recently authorital confirmations [114, 137, 138, 242-248]. Surface ECG, late potentials, HV interval, endocavitary recordings and mapping clearly indicated this electrical abnormality. The rare but increasing number of evidence based data confirms that the conduction delay may predominantly be related to a structural fibro-fatty substitution of the RVOT, histologically similar to ARVD/C, but mainly localized to the RVOT and the conduction system, and with a different genetic substrate. It is well known that different heart diseases can affect the RV, and that these different entities can produce similar structural lesions. The research in this syndrome should be addressed to the identification of minor structural abnormalities rather than to defend aggressively the theory of an idiopathic syndrome, only because some functional factors, the autonomic system, fever and drugs undoubtedly concur to the clinical picture. The future evidence-based definition of the cause of these structural abnormalities will be the last frontier that will transform a syndrome into a disease [249]. The oncoming studies should clarify the role of embryology [141, 250], the similarity with ARVD, the importance of new genetic abnormalities different from those well-known (SCN5A), but inconclusive. The roles of geneticist-cardiologist and that of wedge preparations will maintain importance, but they should not prevaricate the clinical work. A wedge is not a heart. Well controlled clinical and epidemiological surveys must clarify the true prevalence of a strange ECG and its role in inducing a so rare lethal event. The ECG interpretation should not start from a classification in types, angles, index etc. , but should review all the true published clinical case, avoiding those drug induced. We all are so ignorant on this rare but now popular "Media" syndrome, but we cannot passively accept the statements of hundreds of published papers where some authors apply a "copy and paste" procedure rather than trying to think with their own mind and give personal experience and contribution.

This common ignorance (mine first!)does not further justify the extensive use of drugs challenge, invasive investigations and consequent invasive therapies [251, 252]. The J-ICD reflex must be abandoned, and asymptomatic people must let live a normal life, do their sport activity, avoid the frightening consultations provided by Google and to see from time to time their wise cardiologist who is in charge to reassure these healthy individuals and not to terrify them, passively accepting the suggestions of the last published uncontrolled paper. A clinical follow up and noninvasive risk stratification is the only serious approach suggested at present time. We need to learn more before to cure a healthy individual, who so rarely needs a therapeutic intervention that can be at induced higher risk [234] than the estimated 0.5% per year risk of a spontaneous serious clinical event [24].

References

[1] Nava, A., Canciani, B., Schiavinato, M. L., Martini, B.: La repolarisation precoce dans le precordiales droites: trouble de la conduction intraventriculaire droite? Correlations de l'electrocardiographie- vectorcardiographie avec l'electro-physiologie. *Mises a Jour Cardiologiques* 1988;17:157-159

[2] Martini, B., Nava, A., Thiene, G., et al: Ventricular fibrillation without apparent heart disease: description Of six cases. *Am. Heart J.* 1989; 118: 1203-1209

[3] Aihara, N., Ohe, T., Kamakura, S., et al: Clinical and electro physiologic characteristics of idiopathic ventricular fibrillation. *Shinzo* 1990;22 (suppl. 2). 80-83

[4] Nava, A., Canciani, B., Buja, G. F., Martini, B.: El electrocardiograma y el vectorcardiograma en la dysplasia arritmogénica del ventriculo derecho. *Rev. Lat. Cardiol.* 1992;15:276-283

[5] Brugada, P., Brugada, J. Right bundle branch block, persistent ST segment elevation and sudden cardiac death: A distinct clinical and electrocardiographic syndrome. *J. Am. Coll. Cardiol.* 1992, 20:1391-1396

[6] Marcus FI, Fontaine GH, Guiraudon G. Right ventricular dysplasia: A report of 26 Adult cases. Circulation 1982;65:384-397

[7] Osher, H. L., Wolff, L. Electrocardiographic pattern simulating acute myocardial injury. *Am. Med. Sci.* 1953;226:541-5

[8] Corrado, D., Basso, C., Buja, G. F., Nava, A., Rossi, L., Thiene, G. Right bundle branch block, ST-segment elevation, and sudden death in young people. *Circulation* 2001; 103; 710-17

[9] Martini B., Corrado D., Nava A., Thiene G. Syndrome of Right bundle branch block, ST segment elevation and sudden death. Evidence of an organic substrate. In: Nava, A., Rossi L. and Thiene G. editors: *Arrhythmogenic right ventricular cardiomyopathy/ dysplasia*. Elsevier 1997: 438-53

[10] Naccarella F.: Malignant ventricular arrhythmias in patients with a right bundle branch block and persistent St segment elevation in V1-V3: A probable arrhythmogenic cardiomyopathy of the right ventricle. *G Ital. Cardiol.* 1993, 23: 1219-1222

[11] Brugada, J., Brugada, P., Brugada, R. Ajmaline unmasks right bundle branch block-like and ST segment elevation in V1-V3 in patients with idiopathic ventricular fibrillation. *PACE* (abstract) 1996, 19: 599

[12] Yan G. X., Antzelevitch C.: Cellular basis for the electrocardiographic J wave. *Circulation* 1996;93:372-379

[13] Chen, Q., Kirsch, G. E., Zhang, D., et al.: Genetic basis and al. Molecular mechanisms for idiopathic ventricular fibrillation. *Nature* 1998, 392; 293-296

[14] González-Rebollo, J. M., Hernández Madrid, A., García, A., García de Castro, A., Mejías, A., Moro, C. Recurrent ventricular fibrillation during a febrile illness in a patient with the Brugada syndrome. *Rev. Esp. Cardiol.* 2000;53:755-7
[15] Haïssaguerre M., MD; Extramiana, F., MD; Hocini, M., MD et al. Mapping and Ablation of Ventricular Fibrillation Associated With Long-QT and Brugada Syndromes. *Circulation* 2003;108:925.928
[16] Shah, A. J., Hocini, M., Lamaison, D., Sacher, F., Derval, N., Haïssaguerre, M. Regional substrate ablation abolishes syndrome. *J. Cardiovasc. Electrophysiol.* 2011 Nov.; 22(11):1290-1
[17] Nademanee, K., Veerakul, G., Chandanamattha, P., et al. Prevention of ventricular fibrillation episodes in syndrome by catheter ablation over the anterior right ventricular outflow tract epicardium. *Circulation*. 2011; 123:1270-9.
[18] Farre, J. The Brugada syndrome: do we need more than the 12-lead ECG? *Eur. Heart J.* 2000 Feb.;21(4):264-5
[19] Surawicz, B. Brugada syndrome: manifest, concealed, "asymptomatic," suspected and simulated. *J. Am. Coll. Cardiol.* 2001;38:775-7
[20] Ahn, J., Hurst, J. W. Worrisome thoughts about the diagnosis and treatment of patients with Brugada waves and the Brugada syndrome. *Circulation*. 2004;109:1463-7
[21] Sumiyoshi, M., Nakata, Y., Hisaoka, T. A case of idiopathic ventricular fibrillation with incomplete right bundle branch block and persistent ST segment elevation. *Jpn. Heart J.* 1993, 34: 661-663
[22] Yokokawa, M., Okamura, H., Noda, T., et al. Neurally mediated syncope as a cause of syncope in patients with Brugada electrocardiogram. *J. Cardiovasc. Electrophysiol.* 2010; 21:186-92
[23] Take, Y., Morita, H., Nishii, N., et al. Identification oh high-risk syncope related to ventricular fibrillation in patients with Brugada syndrome. *Heart Rhythm*. 2012;9:752-9
[24] Probst, V., Veltmann, C., Eckardt, L., et al. Long-term prognosis of patients diagnosed with Brugada syndrome: Results from the FINGER Brugada Syndrome Registry. *Circulation*. 2010;121:635-43
[25] Wilde, A. A. M., Antzelevitch, C., Borggrefe, M., et al. Proposed diagnostic criteria for the Brugada syndrome. *Eur. Heart J.* 2002; 23: 1648-1654
[26] Bayés de Luna, A., Brugada, J., Baranchuk, A., et al. Current electrocardiographic criteria for diagnosis of pattern: a consensus report. *J. Electrocardiol.* 2012;45:433-42
[27] Martini, B., Nava, A., Ruzza, L., Cannas, S., Bauce, B., Muriago, A. La sindrome “Morte improvvisa giovanile, blocco di branca destra e sopraslivellamento del tratto ST. *Giornale Italiano di Aritmologia e Cardiostimolazione* 1999;2:157-77
[28] Wasserburger, H., Alt, W. J., Lloyd, C. J. The normal RS-T segment elevation variant. *Am. J. Cardiol.* 1961; 8: 184-191.
[29] Osborn, J. J. Experimental hypothermia: respiratory and blood pH changes in relation to cardiac function. *Am. J. Physiol.* 1953;175:389-98.
[30] RuDuskj, B. M. The Osborn J Wave Revisited With Reference to the Brugada Syndrome. *Angiology*. 2013;64:161-2
[31] Perez, M., Friday, K., Froelicher, V. Semantic confusion: The case of early repolarization and the J point. *Am. J. Med.* 2012;125:843-4

[32] Kakishita, M., Kurita, T., Matsuo, K., et al. Mode of Onset of Ventricular Fibrillation in Patients With Brugada Syndrome Detected by Implantable Cardioverter Defibrillator Therapy. *J. Am. Coll Cardiol.* 2000; 36:1646 –53

[33] Take, Y., Morita, H., Wu, J., et al. Spontaneous ECG alterations predict ventricular fibrillation in Brugada Syndrome. *Heart Rhythm.* 2011;8: 1014-21

[34] Frigo, G., Rampazzo, A., Danieli, G. A., Nava, A., Martini, B. Homozygous SCN5A mutation in Brugada syndrome with monomorphic ventricular tachycardia and structural heart abnormalities. *Europace.* 2007;9:391-7

[35] Martini, B., Nava, A., A long lasting electrocardiographic history. *Heart Rhythm.* 2010; 10:1521

[36] Letsas, K. P., Efremidis, M., Weber, R., et al. Epsilon-like waves and ventricular conduction abnormalities in subjects with type 1 ECG pattern of Brugada syndrome. *Heart Rhythm.* 2011;8:874-8.

[37] Brugada, R., Brugada, J., Antzelevitch, C., et al. Sodium Channel Blockers Identify Risk for Sudden Death in Patients With ST-Segment Elevation and Right Bundle Branch Block but Structurally Normal Hearts. *Circulation* 2000;101;510-15

[38] Fontaine, G., Frank, R., Gallais-Hamonno, F., Allali, I., Phan-Thuc, H., Grosgogeat, Y. Electrocardiography of delayed potentials in post-excitation syndrome. *Arch. Mal. Coeur Vaiss.* 1978;71:854-64

[39] Bjerregaard, P., Molgaard, H. A Patient With Biventricular Dysplasia. *Journal of Electrocardiology* 2002;35:289-91

[40] Morita, H., Kusano, K. F., Miura, D., et al. Fragmented QRS as a marker of conduction abnormality and a predictor of prognosis of syndrome. *Circulation* 2008;118:1697-704

[41] Priori, S. G., Gasparini, M., Napolitano, C., et al. Risk stratification in syndrome: results of the PRELUDE (PRogrammed ELectrical stimUlation preDictive valuE) registry. *J. Am. Coll. Cardiol.* 2012;59: 37-45

[42] Take, Y., Morita, H. Fragmented QRS: What Is The Meaning? *Indian Pacing Electrophysiol. J.* 2012;12:213-25

[43] Korhonen, P., Husa, T., Tierala, I., et al. Increased intra-QRS fragmentation in magnetocardiography as a predictor of arrhythmic events and mortality in patients with cardiac dysfunction after myocardial infarction. *J. Cardiovasc. Electrophysiol.* 2006;17: 396-401

[44] Bianco, M., Bria, S., Gianfelici, A., Sanna, N., Palmieri, V., Zeppilli, P. Does early repolarization in the athlete have analogies with the Brugada syndrome? *Eur. Heart J.* 2001; 22:504-10

[45] Corrado, D., Pelliccia, A., Heidbuch, et al: Recommendations for interpretation of 12-lead electrocardiogram in the athlete. *Eur. Heart J.* 2010;31:243

[46] Holst, A., Tango, M., Batchvarov, V., et al. Specificity of elevated intercostals space ECG recording for the type 1 Brugada ECG pattern. *Ann. Noninvasive electrocardiol.* 2012; 17:108-112

[47] Hunuk, B., Kepez, A., Erdogan, O. Prevalence of Brugada-type electrocardiogram pattern by recording right precordial leads at higher intercostals spaces. *Europace* 2012 in press

[48] Takagi, M., Aihara, N., Takaki, H., et al. Clinical characteristics of patients with spontaneous or inducible ventricular fibrillation without apparent heart disease

presenting with and ST segment elevation in inferior leads. *J. Cardiovasc. Electrophysiol.* 2000;11:844-8

[49] Riera, A., Ferreira, C., Schapachnik, E., Sanches, C., Moffa, Riera P. G. Brugada Syndrome With Atypical ECG: Downsloping ST-Segment Elevation in Inferior Leads. *Journal of Electrocardiology* 2004;37:101-104

[50] Haïssaguerre, M., Derval, N., Sacher, F., Jesel, L., Deisenhofer, I., et al. Sudden cardiac arrest associated with early repolarization. *N Engl. J. Med.* 2008;358:2016-23

[51] Hoogendick, M. G., Coronel, R. The J-wave conundrum: Early repolarization and Brugada syndrome. *Heart Rhythm* 2013 in press

[52] Antzelevitch, C. Genetic, molecular and cellular mechanisms underlying the J wave syndromes. *Circ. J.* 2012;76:1054-65

[53] Dumaine, R., Towbin, J. A., Brugada, P. Ionic mechanisms responsible for the electrocardiographic phenotype of the Brugada syndrome are temperature dependent. *Circ. Res.* 1999;85:803-9.

[54] Morita, H., Zipes, D. P., Morita, S. T., Wu, J. Temperature modulation of ventricular arrhythmogenicity in a canine tissue model of Brugada syndrome. *Heart Rhythm.* 2007; 4:188-97

[55] Juntilla, M. J., Gonzalez, M., Lizotte, E., et al. Induced Brugada-type electrocardiogram, a sign for imminent malignant arrhythmias. *Circulation.* 2008;117: 1890–1893

[56] Amin, A. S., Meregalli, P. G., Bardai, A., Wilde, A. A., Tan, H. L. Fever increases the risk for cardiac arrest in the Brugada syndrome. *Ann. Intern. Med.* 2008;149:216-8

[57] Samani, K., Wu, G., Tohomohiko, A., et al. A novel SCN5A mutation V1340I in Brugada syndrome augmenting arrhythmias during febrile illness. *Heart and Rhythm* 2009;6:1318-26

[58] Egri, C., Ruben, P. C. A hot topic: temperature sensitive sodium channelopathies. *Channels* (Austin) 2012;6:75-85

[59] Guo, J., Sun, X., Martini, B., et al. Brugada Syndrome Unmasked by Fever - Is There Always a Need for Implantable Cardiac Defibrillator Placement? *Proceeding of the Heart and Rhythm society* 2009 Abstract P002-65

[60] Erdogan, O., Hunuk, B. Frequency of Brugada type ECG pattern in male subjects with fever. *Int. J. Cardiol.* 2012 in press

[61] Nogami, A., Nakao, M., Kubota, S., et al. Enhancement of J-ST-segment elevation by the glucose and insulin test in Brugada syndrome. *Pacing Clin. Electrophysiol.* 2003; 26: 332-7

[62] Ikeda, T., Abe, A., Yusu, S., et al. The full stomach test as a novel diagnostic technique for identifying patients at risk of Brugada syndrome. *J. Cardiovasc. Electrophysiol.* 2006;17:602-7

[63] Shimizu, W., Matsuo, K., Kokubo, Y., et al. Sex hormone and gender difference-role on male predominance in Brugada syndrome. *J. Cardiovasc. Electrophysiol.* 2007;18:415-21

[64] Tohyou, Y., Nakazawa, K., Ozawa, A., et al. A survey in the incidence of right bundle brunch block with ST segment elevation among normal population. *Jpn. J. Electrocardiol.* 1995;15:223–6

[65] Blangy, H., Seoul, N., Coutelour, J. M., et al. Prevalence of Brugada syndrome among 35,309 inhabitants of Lorraine screened at preventive medicine centre. *Arch. Mal. Coeur Vaiss.* 2005;98:175-80

[66] Holst, A. G., Jensen, H. K., Eschen, O., et al. Low disease prevalence and inappropriate implantable cardioverter defibrillator shock rate in Brugada syndrome: a nationwide study. *Europace* 2012;14:1025-9

[67] Junttila, M. J., Raatikainen, M. J., Karjalainen, J., Kauma, H., Kesäniemi, Y. A., Huikuri, H. V. Prevalence and prognosis of subjects with Brugada-type ECG pattern in a young and middle-aged Finnish population. *Eur. Heart J.* 2004;25:874-8

[68] Sinner, M. F., Pfeufer, A., Perz, S., et al. Spontaneous Brugada electrocardiogram patterns are rare in the German general population: results from the KORA study. *Europace.* 2009;11:1338-44

[69] Pecini, R., Cedergreen, P., Theilade, S., Haunsø, S., Theilade, J., Jensen, G. B. The prevalence and relevance of the Brugada-type electrocardiogram in the Danish general population: data from the Copenhagen City Heart Study. *Europace.* 2010;12:982-6

[70] Uhm, J. S., Hwang, I. U., Oh, Y. S., et al. Prevalence of electrocardiographic findings suggestive of sudden cardiac death risk in 10,867 apparently healthy young Korean men. *Pacing Clin. Electrophysiol.* 2011;34:717-23

[71] Gervacio-Domingo, G., Isidro, J., Tirona, J., et al. The Brugada type 1 electro cardiographic pattern is common among Filipinos. *J. Clin. Epidemiol.* 2008;61: 1067-72

[72] Ng, C. T., Ong, H. Y., Cheok, C., Chua, T. S., Ching, C. K. Prevalence of electrocardiographic abnormalities in an unselected young male multi-ethnic South-East Asian population undergoing pre-participation cardiovascular screening: results of the Singapore Armed Forces Electrocardiogram and Echocardiogram screening protocol. *Europace.* 2012;14:1018-24.

[73] Bjerregaard, P., Gussak, I., Kotar, S. L., Gessler, J. E., Janosik, D. Recurrent syncope in a patient with prominent J wave. *Am. Heart J.* 1994;127:1426-30

[74] Bonny, A., Tonet, J., Fontaine, G., et al. Brugada syndrome in pure black Africans. *J. Cardiovasc. Electrophysiol.* 2008;19:421-6

[75] Oe, H., Takagi, M., Tanaka, A., et al. Prevalence and clinical course of the juveniles with Brugada-type ECG in Japanese population. *Pacing Clin. Electrophysiol.* 2005;28: 549-54

[76] Sakabe, M., Fujiki, A., Tani, M., Nishida, K., Mizumaki, K., Inoue, H. Proportion and prognosis of healthy people with coved or saddle-back type ST segment elevation in the right precordial leads during 10 years follow-up. *Eur. Heart J.* 2003;24:1488-93

[77] Wilde, A. A., Brugada, R. Phenotypical manifestations of mutations in the genes encoding subunits of the cardiac sodium channel. *Circ. Res.* 2011; 108:884-97

[78] Ackerman, M. J., Priori, S. G., Willems, S., Berul, C., et al. HRS/EHRA expert consensus statement on the state of genetic testing for the channelopathies and cardiomyopathies this document was developed as a partnership between the Heart Rhythm Society (HRS) and the European Heart Rhythm Association (EHRA). *Heart Rhythm.* 2011; 8: 1308-39

[79] Littmann, L., Monroe, M. H. The Brugada numbers. *Circulation.* 2003 May 13;107 (18):e122

[80] Young, E., Xiong, S., Fin, L., Young, T. Unique sleep disorder of a population-based sample of 747 Hmong immigrants in Wisconsin. *Social Science Medicine* 2012, in press.
[81] Macedo, P., Brugada, J., Leinveber, P., et al. Sleep-Disordered Breathing in Patients With the Brugada Syndrome. *Am. J. Cardiol.* 2011; 107: 709-13
[82] Veltmann, C., Wolpert, C., Sacher, F., et al. Response to intravenous ajmaline: a retrospective analysis of 677 ajmaline challenges. *Europace* 2009;11:1345-52
[83] Zorzi, A., Migliore, F., Marras, E., et al: Should all individuals with a no diagnostic Brugada-electrocardiogram undergo sodium-channel block test? *Heart Rhythm* 2012:9: 909-16
[84] Gasparini, M., Priori, S. G., Mantica, M., et al. Flecainide test in Brugada syndrome: A reproducible but risky tool. *Pacing Clin. Electrophysiol.* 2003;26: 338–341.
[85] Joshi, S., Raiszadeh, F., Pierce, W., Steinberg, J. S. Antiarrhythmic induced electrical storm in Brugada syndrome: a case report. *Ann. Noninvasive Electrocardiol.* 2007; 12: 274–8
[86] Morita,H., Morita, S. T., Nagase, S., et al. Ventricular arrhythmia induced by sodium channel blocker in patients with Brugada syndrome. *J. Am. Coll. Cardiol.* 2003;42: 1624–31
[87] Antzelevitch, C. Brugada, P., Brugada, J., Brugada, R., Towbin, J. A., Nademanee, K. Brugada syndrome 1992- 2002 A historical perspective. *J. Am. Coll. Cardiol.* 2003;41: 1665-71
[88] Priori, S. G., Napolitano, C., Schwartz, P. J., Bloise, R., Crotti, L., Ronchetti, E. The Elusive Link Between LQT3 and Brugada Syndrome. The role of Flecainide challenge. *Circulation.* 2000;102:945-947
[89] Priori, S. G., Napolitano, C., Gasparini, M. Clinical and genetic heterogeneity of right bundle branch block and ST-Segment elevation syndrome. A Prospective Evaluation of 52 Families *Circulation* 2000; 102:2509-2515
[90] Priori, S. G., Napolitano, C., Gasparini, M., et al. Natural History of Brugada syndrome. Insight for risk stratification and management. *Circulation* 2002;105:1342-1357
[91] Nava, A., Bauce, B., Rampazzo, A. Further evidence that "Brugada syndrome" can be due to arrhythmogenic right ventricular cardiomyopathy with disease locus in chromosome 14q24.4. *G. Ital. Cardiol.* 1999;29 (suppl. 5) 366-9
[92] Peters, S., Trummel, M., Denecke, S., Koehler, B. Results of ajmaline testing in patients with arrhythmogenic right ventricular dysplasia-cardiomyopathy. *Int. J. Cardiol.* 2004;95:207-10
[93] Brugada, J. Mechanisms of the pro-arrhythmic effects of Flecainide and related anti arrhythmic drugs. *The New Frontiers of Arrhythmias*. 1992; 7: 353-6
[94] Martini, B., Cannas, S., Ruzza, L. The syndrome of right bundle branch block, ST segment elevation and sudden death: Nava-Martini and/or Brugada syndrome. In: *Cardiac Arrhythmias: How to improve the reality in the third millennium?* Luigi Pozzi ed. Rome. 2000:206–15
[95] Miyazaki, T., Mitamura, H., Miyoshi, S., et al. Autonomic and anti-arrhythmic drug modulation of ST segment elevation in patients with Brugada syndrome. *J. Am. Coll. Cardiol.* 1996;27:1061–1070

[96] Omiya, T., Shimizu, A., Ueyama, T., et al. Effects of isoproterenol and propanolol on the inducibility and frequency of ventricular fibrillation in patients with Brugada syndrome. *J. Cardiol.* 2012 Jul.;60(1):47-54
[97] Douard, H., Sagardiluz, J., Chevalier, L., Labbé, L., Broustet, J. P. Fortuitous discovery of Brugada syndrome in an asymptomatic 70-year-old sportsman. *Ann. Cardiol. Angeiol.* 1996;45:577-80
[98] García-Borbolla, M., García-Borbolla, R., Valenzuela, L. F., Trujillo, F. Ventricular tachycardia induced by exercise testing in a patient with Brugada syndrome. *Rev. Esp. Cardiol.* 2007;60:993-4
[99] Esperer, H., Hoos, O., Hottenrott, K. Syncope due to Brugada syndrome in a young athlete. *Br. J. Sports Med.* 2007;41:180-1
[100] Ozeke, O., Cağli, K. E., Aras, D., Ilkay, E. Exercise-induced ventricular tachycardia associated with asymptomatic syndrome in a patient with urinary bladder stone. *Turk. Kardiyol. Dern. Ars.* 2009;37:128-31
[101] Sarquella-Brugada, G., Campuzano, O., Iglesias, A., Genetics of sudden cardiac death in children and young athletes. *Cardiology in the Young.* 2012 in press
[102] Nademanee, K., Veerakul, G., Nimmannit, S., et al. Arrhythmogenic marker for the sudden unexplained death syndrome in Thai men. *Circulation.* 1997;96:2595-600
[103] Guevara-Valdivia, M. E., Iturralde Torres, P., De Micheli, A., Colín Lizalde, L., Medeiros Domingo, A., González-Hermosillo, J. A. Electrocardiographic changes during stress test in a patient with "syndrome". *Arch.* 2001;71:66-72
[104] Amin, A., Fe Groos, E., Ruijter, J., Wilde, A., Tan, H. Exercise induced changes in Brugada syndrome. *Circ. Arrhythmia Electrophysiol.* 2009; 2: 531-9
[105] Makimoto, H., Nakagawa, E., Takaki, H., et al. Augmented ST-Segment elevation during recovery from exercise predicts cardiac event in patients with Brugada syndrome. *J. Am. Coll. Cardiol.* 2010;56:1576-84
[106] Gimster, A., Segal, O. R., Behr, E. R. Type I Brugada electrocardiogram pattern during the recovery phase of exercise testing. *Europace* 2008; 10:897-8
[107] Toyofuku, M., Takaki, H., Sunagawa, K., et al: Exercise induced ST elevation in patients with arrhythmogenic right ventricular dysplasia. *J. Electrocardiol.* 1999;32:1-5
[108] Baranchuk, A., Nguyen, T., Ryu, M. H., et al. Brugada phenocopy: new terminology and proposed classification. *Ann. Noninvasive Electrocardiol.* 2012;17:299-314
[109] Sheinman, M. M. Right bundle branch block and ST Elevation is not a distinct syndrome identifying patients at risk for sudden cardiac death. *European Journal of Cardiac Pacing and Electrophysiology* 1996;6:7 (abstract)
[110] Scheinman, M. M. Is the Brugada syndrome a distinct clinical entity? *J. Cardiovasc. Electrophysiol.* 1997;8:332-6
[111] Fontaine, G., Piot, O., Sohal, P., et el. Dérivations en précordiales droites et mort subite. *Arch. Mal. Coeur.* 1996, 89: 1323-1329
[112] Riera, A. P., Filho, C. F., De Abreu, L. C., et al. Do patients with electrocardiographic Brugada type 1 pattern have associated right bundle branch block? A Comparative vectorcardiographic study. *Europace* 2012 in press
[113] Ikeda, T., Sakurada, H., Sakabe, K., et al. Assessment of noninvasive markers in identifying patients at risk in the Brugada syndrome: insight into risk stratification. *J. Am. Coll. Cardiol.* 2001;37:1628-34

[114] Nagase, S., Kusano, K. F., Morita, H., et al. Epicardial electrocardiogram of the right ventricular outflow tract in patients with Brugada syndrome using the epicardial lead. *J. Am. Coll. Cardiol.* 2002; 39:1992–5
[115] Takami, M., Ikeda, T., Enjoji, Y., Sugi, K. Relationship between ST-segment morphology and conduction disturbances detected by signal-averaged electrocardiography in Brugada syndrome. *Ann. Noninvasive Electrocardiol.* 2003;8: 30-6
[116] Hisamatsu, K., Kusano, K. F., Morita, H., et al. Relationships between depolarization abnormality and repolarization abnormality in patients with Brugada syndrome: using body surface signal-averaged electrocardiography and body surface maps. *J. Cardiovasc. Electrophysiol.* 2004;15:870-6
[117] Huang, Z., Patel, C., Li, W., et al. Role of signal-averaged electrocardiograms in arrhythmic risk stratification of patients with Brugada syndrome: a prospective study. *Heart Rhythm.* 2009;6:1156-62
[118] Tada, H., Nogami, A., Shimizu, W. ST Segment and T Wave Alternans in a Patient with Brugada Syndrome. *PACE* 2000; 23:413-415
[119] Morita, H., Zipes, D. P., Wu, J. Brugada syndrome: Insights of ST elevation, arrhythmogenicity, and risk stratification from experimental observations. *Heart Rhythm* 2009;6:S34–S43
[120] Morita, H., Zipes, D., Lopshire, J., Morita, S. T., Wu, J. T wave alternans in an in vitro tissue model of Brugada syndrome. *Am. J. Physiol. Heart Circ. Physiol.* 2006;291:421-428
[121] Kirchhof, P., Eckardt, L., Rolf, S., Esperer, H. D. T wave alternans does not assess arrhythmic risk in patients with Brugada syndrome. 2004; 9: 162-5
[122] Kim, S. H., Nam, G. B., Baek, S., Choi, H. O., et al. Circadian and seasonal variations of ventricular tachyarrhythmias in patients with early repolarization syndrome and syndrome: analysis of patients with implantable cardioverter defibrillator. *J. Cardiovasc. Electrophysiol.* 2012;23:757-63
[123] Suzuki, H., Torigoe, K., Numata, O., Yazaki, S. Infant case with a malignant form of Brugada syndrome. *J. Cardiovasc. Electrophysiol.* 2000;11:1277e80
[124] Belhassen, B., Glick, A., Viskin, S. Efficacy of quinidine in high-risk patients with Brugada syndrome. *Circulation.* 2004;110:1731-7
[125] Coronel, R., Casini, S., Koopmann, T. T., et al. Right ventricular fibrosis and conduction delay in a patient with clinical signs of Brugada syndrome: a combined electrophysiological, genetic, histopathologic, and computational study. *Circulation.* 2005; 112:2769-77
[126] Shimada, M., Miyazaki, T., Miyoshi, S., Soejima, K., Hori, S., Mitamura, H., Ogawa, S. Sustained monomorphic ventricular tachycardia in a patient with Brugada syndrome. *Jpn. Circ. J.* 1996; 60: 364–370
[127] G. Proclemer, A., Nucifora, G., Dall'Armellina, E., Rebellato, L. Monomorphic ventricular tachycardia in 'Brugada syndrome': clinical case and literature review. *J. Cardiovasc. Med.* 2008;9:842–846
[128] Morita, H., Nagase, S., Miura, D. Differential effects of cardiac sodium channel mutations on initiation and termination of ventricular arrhythmias in Brugada syndrome. *Heart Rhythm* 2009;6:487-492

[129] Brugada, J., Brugada, P., Brugada, R.: The syndrome of right bundle branch block ST segment elevation in V1 to V3 and sudden death: The Brugada syndrome. *Europace* 1999;1:156-166
[130] Eckardt, L., Kirchhof, P., Loh, P., et al. Brugada syndrome and supraventricular tachyarrhythmias: a novel association? *J. Cardiovasc. Electrophysiol.* 2001;12:680-5
[131] Letsas, K. P., Sideris, A., Efremidis, M., et al. Prevalence of paroxysmal atrial fibrillation in Brugada syndrome : a case series and a review of the literature. *Journal of Cardiovascular Medicine* 2007, 8:803–806
[132] Olesen, M. S., Holst, A. G., Svendsen, J. H., Haunsø, S., Tfelt-Hansen, J. SCN1Bb R214Q found in 3 patients: 1 with Brugada syndrome and 2 with lone Atrial Fibrillation. *Heart Rhythm*. 2012;9:770-3
[133] Krishnan, S. C., Josephson, M. E. ST segment elevation induced by class IC antiarrhythmic agents: underlying electrophysiologic mechanisms and insights into drug-induced proarrhythmia. *J. Cardiovasc. Electrophysiol.* 1998;9:1167-72
[134] Rodríguez-Mañero, M., Namdar, M., Sarkozy, A., Prevalence, Clinical Characteristics and Management of Atrial Fibrillation in Patients With Brugada Syndrome. *Am. J. Cardiol.* 2013;111:362-7
[135] Corrado, D., Basso, C., Leoni, L., et al. Three-Dimensional Electroanatomic Voltage Mapping Increases Accuracy of Diagnosing Arrhythmogenic Right Ventricular Cardiomyopathy/Dysplasia. *Circulation*. 2005;111:3042-50
[136] Sciarra, L., Marras, E., De Ruvo, E., et al. Results of right ventricular endocardial mapping in patients with Brugada Syndrome: not always an electrical disease in normal hearts. *Europace* 2007; 50:PW_105
[137] Postema, P. G., van Dessel, P. F., de Bakker, J. M., et al. Slow and Discontinuous Conduction Conspire in Brugada Syndrome. A Right Ventricular Mapping and Stimulation Study. *Circ. Arrhythm. Electrophysiol.* 2008;1:379-86
[138] Lambiase, A. K. Ahmed, E. J. Ciaccio, R. High-Density Substrate Mapping in Brugada Syndrome: Combined Role of Conduction and Repolarization Heterogeneities in Arrhythmogenesis. *Circulation*. 2009; 120:2 106-117
[139] Kofune, M., Watanabe, I., Ohkubo, K., et al. Clarifying the arrhythmogenic substrate for Brugada syndrome. *Int. Heart J.* 2011; 52:290-4
[140] Morita, H., Zipes, D., Morita, S. T., Lopshire, J., Wu, J. Epicardial ablation eliminates ventricular arrhythmias in an experimental model of Brugada syndrome. *Heart Rhythm* 2009; 6:665-671
[141] Elizari, M. V., Levi, R., Acunzo, R. S., Chiale, P. A., Civetta, M. M., Ferreiro, M., Sicuri, S. Abnormal expression of cardiac neural crest cells in heart development: A different hypothesis for the etiopathogenesis of Brugada syndrome. *Heart Rhythm*. 2007; 4:359-65
[142] Morita, H., Zipes, D. P., Morita, S. T., Wu, J. Differences in arrhythmogenicity between the canine right ventricular outflow tract and anteroinferior right ventricle in a model of Brugada syndrome. *Heart Rhythm*. 2007;4:66-74
[143] Martini, B., Nava, A., Thiene, G., et al. Monomorphic repetitive rhythms originating from the right ventricular outflow tract in patients with minor forms of right ventricular cardiomyopathy. *Intern. J. Cardiol.* 1990; 27: 211-21
[144] Brugada, J., Brugada, J., Antzelevitch, C., Towbin, J., Nademanee, K., Brugada, P. Long-Term Follow-Up of Individuals With the Electrocardiographic Pattern of Right

Bundle-Branch Block and ST-Segment Elevation in Precordial Leads V1 to V3. *Circulation.* 2002; 105:73-78

[145] Ohkubo, K., Watanabe, I., Okumura, Y. Surface ECG characteristics of ventricular tachyarrhythmias before degeneration into ventricular fibrillation in patients with Brugada-type ECG. *Int. Heart J.* 2009;50: 477-

[146] Wilde, A. A., Viskin, S. EP testing does not predict cardiac events in Brugada syndrome. *Heart Rhythm.* 2011;8:1598-600

[147] Scognamiglio, R., Fasoli, G., Nava, A., Miraglia, G., Valentina, D., Thiene, G., Dalla Volta, S. Relevance of subtle echocardiographic findings in the early diagnosis of the concealed form of right ventricular dysplasia. *Eur. Heart J.* 1989;10 Suppl. D:27-8.

[148] Murata, K., Ueyama, T., Tanaka, T., Nose, Y., Wada, Y., Matsuzaki, M. Right ventricular dysfunction in patients with Brugada-like electrocardiography: a two dimensional strain imaging study. *Cardiovasc. Ultrasound.* 2011,9:30

[149] Jacoviello, M., Forleo, C., Puzzovivo, A., et al. Altered two-dimensional strain measures of the right ventricle in patients with Brugada syndrome and arrhythmogenic right ventricular dysplasia/cardiomyopathy. *European Journal of Echocardiography.* 2011;12:773-81.

[150] D'Onofrio, A., Cuomo, S., Musto, B., Boccalattc, A. Right bundle branch block, persistent ST segment elevation in V1-V3 and sudden cardiac death: always a distinct syndrome? *G Ital. Cardiol.* 1995;25: 1171-1175

[151] Papavassiliu, T., Veltmann, C., Doesch, C., et al. Spontaneous type 1 electrocardiographic pattern is associated with cardiovascular magnetic resonance imaging changes in Brugada syndrome. *Heart Rhythm.* 2010; 7:1790-6

[152] Catalano, O., Antonaci, S., Moro, G., Mussida, M., et al. Magnetic resonance investigations in Brugada syndrome reveal unexpectedly high rate of structural abnormalities. *Eur. Heart J.* 2009;30:2241-8

[153] Van Hoorn, F., Campian, M. E., Spijkerboer, A., et al. SCN5A mutations in Brugada syndrome are associated with increased cardiac dimensions and reduced contractility. *PLoS One.* 2012;7:e42037

[154] Tessa, C., Del Meglio, J., Ghidini Ottonelli, A., et al. Evaluation of Brugada syndrome by cardiac magnetic resonance. *Int. J. Cardiovasc. Imaging.* 2012;28:1961-70

[155] Santangeli, P., Hamilton-Craig, C., Dello Russo, A.: Imaging of Scar in Patients with Ventricular Arrhythmias of Right Ventricular Origin: Cardiac Magnetic Resonance Versus Electroanatomic Mapping. *J. Cardiovasc. Electrophysiol.*, 2011: 22:1359-1366

[156] Tada, H., Aihara, N., Ohe, T., Yutani, C., Hamada, S., Miyanuma, H., Takamiya, M., Kamakura, S. Arrhythmogenic right ventricular cardiomyopathy underlies syndrome of right bundle branch block, ST-segment elevation, and sudden death. *Am. J. Cardiol.* 1998; 81:519-22.

[157] Takagi, M., Aihara, N., Kuribayashi, S., Taguchi, A., Shimizu, W., Kurita, T., Suyama, K., Kamakura, S., Hamada, S., Takamiya, M. Localized right ventricular morphological abnormalities detected by electron-beam computed tomography represent arrhythmogenic substrates in patients with the Brugada syndrome. *Eur. Heart J.* 2001; 22: 1032-41

[158] Rouzet, F., Algalarrondo, V., Burg, S., et al. Contraction delay of the RV outflow tract in patients with Brugada syndrome is dependent on the spontaneous ST-segment elevation pattern. *Heart Rhythm.* 2011;8:1905-12

[159] Duthoit, G., Fressart, V., Hidden-Lucet, F., Simon, F., et al. Brugada ECG pattern: a physiopathological prospective study based on clinical, electrophysiological, angiographic, and genetic findings. *Front Physiol.* 2012;3:474

[160] Daliento, L., Rizzoli, G., Thiene, G., Nava, A., Rinuncini, M., Chioin, R., Dalla Volta, S. Diagnostic accuracy of right ventriculography in arrhythmogenic right ventricular cardiomyopathy. *Am. J. Cardiol.* 1990; 66:741-5

[161] Proclemer, A., Facchin, D., Feruglio, G. A., Nucifora, R. Fibrillazione ventricolare recidivante, blocco di branca destra, persistent sopraslivellamento del tratto ST in V1-V3: una nuova sindrome aritmica? Descrizione di un caso clinico. *G Ital. Cardiol.* 1993; 23:1211-1218.

[162] Brugada, P., Brugada, J. Let us do not get confused, please! *G Ital. Cardiol.* 1994; 24:797-800

[163] Remme, C. A., Wever, E. F., Wilde, A. A., Derksen, R., Hauer, R. N. Diagnosis and long-term follow-up of the Brugada syndrome in patients with idiopathic ventricular fibrillation. *Eur. Heart J.* 2001;22:400-9.

[164] Corrado, D., Nava, A., Buja, G. F., et al. Familial cardiomyopathy underlies syndrome of right bundle branch block, ST segment elevation and sudden death. *J. Am. Coll. Cardiol.* 1996;27:443-8

[165] Hoogendick, M. G.: Diagnostic dilemmas: overlapping features of Brugada syndrome and arrhythmogenic right ventricular cardiomyopathy. *Frontiers in Physiology*. 2012;3: 144

[166] Misuzawa, Y., Wilde, A. A. Brugada syndrome. *Circ. Arrhythm. Electrophysiol.* 2012; 5; 606-616

[167] Watanabe, H., Koopmann, T. T., Le Scouarnec, S., et al. Sodium channel β1 subunit mutations associated with Brugada syndrome and cardiac conduction disease in humans. *J. Clin. Invest.* 2008;118:2260-8

[168] Hu, D., Barajas-Martinez, H., Burashnikov, E., et al. A mutation in the beta 3 subunit of the cardiac sodium channel associated with Brugada ECG phenotype. *Circ. Cardiovasc. Genet.* 2009;2:270-8

[169] London, B., Michalec, M., Mehdi, H., et al. Mutation in glycerol-3-phosphate dehydrogenase 1 like gene (GPD1-L) decreases cardiac Na+ current and causes inherited arrhythmias. *Circulation.* 2007;116:2260-8

[170] Kattygnarath, D., Maugenre, S., Neyroud, N., et al. MOG1: a new susceptibility gene for Brugada syndrome. *Circ. Cardiovasc. Genet.* 2011;4:261-8

[171] Antzelevitch, C., Pollevick, G. D., Cordeiro, J. M., et al. Loss-of-function mutations in the cardiac calcium channel underlies a new clinical entity characterized by ST-segment elevation, short QT intervals, and sudden cardiac death. *Circulation.* 2007;115:442-9

[172] Burashnikov, E., Pfeiffer, R., Barajas-Martinez, H., et al. Mutations in the cardiac L-type calcium channel associated with inherited J-wave syndromes and sudden cardiac death. *Heart Rhythm.* 2010;7:1872-82

[173] Delpón, E., Cordeiro, J. M., Núñez, L., et al. Functional effects of KCNE3 mutation and its role in the development of Brugada syndrome. *Circ. Arrhythm. Electrophysiol.* 2008; 1:209-18

[174] Barajas-Martínez, H., Hu, D., Ferrer, T., et al. Molecular genetic and functional association of Brugada and early repolarization syndromes with S422L missense mutation in KCNJ8. *Heart Rhythm.* 2012;9:548-55

[175] Crotti, L., Marcou, C. A., Tester, D. J.,et al. Spectrum and prevalence of mutations involving BrS1- through BrS12-susceptibility genes in a cohort of unrelated patients referred for Brugada syndrome genetic testing: implications for genetic testing. *J. Am. Coll Cardiol.* 2012;60: 1410-8

[176] Bai, R., Napolitano, C., Bloise, R., Monteforte, N., Priori, S. G. Yield of genetic screening in inherited cardiac channelopathies: how to prioritize access to genetic testing. *Circ. Arrhythm. Electrophysiol.* 2009;2:6-15

[177] Chockalingam, P., Clur, S. A., Breur, J. M., et al. The diagnostic and therapeutic aspects of loss-of-function cardiac sodium channelopathies in children. *Heart Rhythm.* 2012;9:1986-92

[178] Meregalli, P. G., Tan, H. L., Probst, V., et al. Type of SCN5A mutation determines clinical severity and degree of conduction slowing in loss-of-function sodium channelopathies. *Heart Rhythm.* 2009;6:341-8

[179] Smits, J. P., Eckardt, L., Probst, V., et al. Genotype-phenotype relationship in Brugada syndrome: electrocardiographic features differentiate SCN5A-related patients from non-SCN5A-related patients. *J. Am. Coll. Cardiol.* 200;40:350-6

[180] Mizusawa, Y., Wilde, A. A. Brugada syndrome. *Circ. Arrhythm. Electrophysiol.* 2012; 5:606-16

[181] Ackerman, M. J., Splawski, I., Makielski, J. C., et al. Spectrum and prevalence of cardiac sodium channel variants among black, white, Asian, and Hispanic individuals: implications for arrhythmogenic susceptibility and Brugada/long QT syndrome genetic testing. *Heart Rhythm.* 2004;1:600-7.

[182] Kapplinger, J. D., Tester, D. J., Alders, M., et al. An international compendium of mutations in the SCN5A-encoded cardiac sodium channel in patients referred for Brugada syndrome genetic testing. *Heart Rhythm.* 2010;7:33-46

[183] Splawski, I., Timothy, K. W., Tateyama, M., et al. Variant of SCN5A sodium channel implicated in risk of cardiac arrhythmia. *Science.* 2002; 297:1333-6

[184] Jeff, J. M., Brown-Gentry, K., Buxbaum, S. G., et al. SCN5A Variation Is Associated With electrocardiographic Traits in the Jackson Heart Study. *Circ. Cardiovasc. Genet.* 2011; 4:139-44

[185] Bezzina, C., Veldkamp, M. W., van Den Berg, M. P., et al. A single Na(+) channel mutation causing both long-QT and Brugada syndromes. *Circ. Res.* 1999;85:1206-13

[186] Hong, K., Bjerregaard, P., Gussak, I., Brugada, R. Short QT syndrome and atrial fibrillation caused by mutation in KCNH2. *J. Cardiovasc. Electrophysiol.* 2005;16:394-6

[187] Watanabe, H., Nogami, A., Ohkubo, K., et al. Electrocardiographic characteristics and SCN5A mutations in idiopathic ventricular fibrillation associated with early repolarization. *Circ. Arrhythm. Electrophysiol.* 2011;4:874-81

[188] Kyndt, F., Probst, V., Potet, F., et al. Novel SCN5A mutation leading either to isolated cardiac conduction defect or Brugada syndrome in a large French family. *Circulation.* 2001;104:3081-6

[189] Akai, J., Makita, N., Sakurada, H., Shirai, N., et al. A novel SCN5A mutation associated with idiopathic ventricular fibrillation without typical ECG findings of Brugada syndrome. *FEBS Lett.* 2000;479:29-34

[190] Frustaci, A., Russo, M. A., Chimenti, C. Structural myocardial abnormalities in asymptomatic family members with Brugada syndrome and SCN5A gene mutation. *Eur. Heart J.* 2009;30:1763
[191] Neu, A., Eiselt, M., Paul, M., Sauter, K., Stallmeyer, B., Isbrandt, D., Schulze-Bahr, E. A homozygous SCN5A mutation in a severe, recessive type of cardiac conduction disease. *Hum. Mutat.* 2010;31:E1609-21
[192] Derangeon, M., Montnach, J., Baró, I., Charpentier, F. Mouse Models of SCN5A-Related Cardiac Arrhythmias. *Front Physiol.* 2012;3:210
[193] Skinner, J. R., Love, D. R. The SCN5A gene in Brugada syndrome: mutations, variants, missense and nonsense. What's a clinician to do? *Heart Rhythm.* 2010;7:50-1.
[194] Roden, D. M. Brugada syndrome: lots of questions, some answers. *Heart Rhythm.* 2010; 7:47-9
[195] Nishii, N., Ogawa, M., Morita, H., et al. SCN5A mutation is associated with early and frequent recurrence of ventricular fibrillation in patients with Brugada syndrome. *Circ. J.* 2010;74:2572-8
[196] Probst, V., Wilde, A. A., Barc, J., et al. SCN5A mutations and the role of genetic background in the pathophysiology of Brugada syndrome. *Circ. Cardiovasc. Genet.* 2009; 2:552-7
[197] Marian, A. J. Nature's Genetic Gradients and the Clinical Phenotype. *Circ. Cardiovasc. Genet.* 2009;2;537-539.
[198] Hermida, J. S., Dassonvalle, E., Six, I., et al. Prospective evaluation of the familial prevalence of the Brugada syndrome. *Am. J. Cardiol.* 2010; 106:1758-62
[199] Santos, L. F., Rodrigues, B., Moreira, D., et al. Criteria to predict carriers of a novel SCN5A mutation in a large Portuguese family affected by the Brugada syndrome. *Europace.* 2012;14:882
[200] Boczek, N. J., Tester, D. J., Ackerman, M. J. The molecular autopsy: an indispensable step following sudden cardiac death in the young? *Herzschrittmacherther Elektrophysiol.* 2012;23:167-73
[201] Priori, S. G. The Brugada Syndrome: The Path toward Complexity. *Hellenic J. Cardiol.* 2003; 44: 95-101
[202] Weiss, R., Barmada, M., Nguyen, B. A., et al. Clinical and molecular Heterogeneity in the Brugada syndrome. A Novel locus on chromosome 3. *Circulation* 2002;105:707-713
[203] Yan, G. X. C Antzelevitch: Cellular basis for the Brugada syndrome and other mechanism of Arrhythmogenesis associated with ST segment elevation. *Circulation* 1999; 100:1660-1666
[204] John Gomes, Malcolm Finlay, Akbar K. Ahmed et al. Electrophysiological abnormalities precede overt structural changes in arrhythmogenic right ventricular cardiomyopathy due to mutations in desmoplakin-A combined murine and human study. *Eur. Heart J.* 2012; 33:1942-53
[205] Igarashi, M., Tada, H., Kurosaki, K., Yamasaki, H., et al. Electrocardiographic determinants of the polymorphic QRS morphology in idiopathic right ventricular outflow tract tachycardia. *J. Cardiovasc. Electrophysiol.* 2012;23:521-6
[206] Maury, P. Why is the right ventricular outflow tract so arrhythmogenic? (... or is it really?...). *Heart.* 2011;97:1631-3

[207] Furushima, H., Chinushi, M., Iijima, K., Izumi, D., Hosaka, Y., Aizawa, Y. Relationship between electroanatomical voltage mapping characteristics and breakout site of ventricular activation in idiopathic ventricular tachyarrhythmia originating from the right ventricular outflow tract septum. *J. Interv. Card. Electrophysiol.* 2012;33:135-41.

[208] Morimoto, S. A multicenter histological study of autopsied and biopsied specimens in BS. *Eur. Heart J.* 2003;24 (suppl.):147 poster n.888

[209] Morimoto, S., Uemura, A., Hishida, H. An autopsy case of Brugada syndrome with significant lesions in the sinus node. *J. Cardiovasc. Electrophysiol.* 2005;16:345-7

[210] Fontaine, G. H. *La mort subite du jeune et de l'athlète*. SFEM éditions, Paris 2010; pag. 271-2

[211] Brugada, J., Brugada, P. What to do in patients with no structural heart disease and sudden arrhythmic death? *Am. J. Cardiol.* 1996;78(5A):69-75

[212] Morgera, T., Sinagra, G. F., Viel, E., Ricci, C., Bussani, R., Camerini, F. The syndrome of right bundle branch block, persistent ST segment elevation and sudden cardiac death. Which is the histological substrate? *Eur. Heart J.* (letter) 1997, 18: 1190-1191.

[213] Izumi, T., Ajiki, K., Nozaki, A., Takahashi, S., Tabei, F., Hayakawa, H., Sugimoto, T. Right ventricular cardiomyopathy showing right bundle branch block and right precordial ST segment elevation. *Intern. Med.* 2000;39:28-33

[214] Buob, A., Siaplaouras, S., Janzen, I., et al. Focal parvovirus B19 myocarditis in a patient with Brugada syndrome. *Cardiol. Rev.* 2003;11

[215] Frustaci, A., Priori, S. G., Pieroni, M., et al. Cardiac histological substrate in patients with clinical phenotype of Brugada syndrome. *Circulation.* 2005;112:3680-7

[216] Kim, H., Cho, Y., Parkkim, Y. Underlying Cardiomyopathy in Patients With ST-Segment Elevation in the Right Precordial Leads. *Circ. J.* 2006; 70: 719 –725

[217] Marras, E., Basso, C., Sciarra, L., Delise, P. Unexplained syncope, Brugada-like ECG and minimal structural right ventricular abnormalities: which is the right diagnosis? *J. Cardiovasc. Med.* (Hagerstown). 2009;10:273-5

[218] Zumhagen, S., Spieker, T., Rolinck, J., et al. Absence of pathognomonic or inflammatory patterns in cardiac biopsies from patients with Brugada syndrome. *Circ. Arrhythm. Electrophysiol.* 2009;2:16-23

[219] Ohkubo, K., Watanabe, I., Okumura, Y., et al. Right ventricular histological substrate and conduction delay in patients with Brugada syndrome. *Int. Heart J.* 2010;51:17-23

[220] Gotoh, K. A histopathological study on the conduction system of the so called "Pokkurri disease" (sudden unexpected cardiac death of unknown origin in Japan). *Jpn. Circ. J.* 1976;40:753-6

[221] Kirschner, R. H., Echner, F. A. O., Baron, R. C. The cardiac pathology of sudden unexplained nocturnal death in Southeast Asian refugees. *JAMA* 1986; 256: 2700-2705

[222] Brugada, P., Brugada, J., Brugada, R. 'Localized' right ventricular morphological abnormalities in patients with the Brugada syndrome: What is their significance? *Eur. Heart J.* 2001; 22: 982 – 984

[223] Nomura, M., Nada, T., Endo, J., et al. Brugada syndrome associated with an autonomic disorder. *Heart.* 1998;80:194-6

[224] Matsuo, K., Kurita, T., Inagaki, M., et al. The circadian pattern of the development of ventricular fibrillation in patients with Brugada syndrome. *Eur. Heart J.* 1999;20:465-70.

[225] Oyama, N., Oyama, N., Yokoshiki, H., et al. Iodine-123-metaiodobenzylguanidine scintigraphy of total cardiac adrenergic denervation in Brugada syndrome. *Jpn. Heart J.* 2002; 43:183-6
[226] Wichter, T., Matheja, P., Eckardt, L., et al. Cardiac autonomic dysfunction in Brugada syndrome. *Circulation.* 2002;105:702-6
[227] Krittayaphong, R., Veerakul, G., Nademanee, K., Kangkagated, C. Heart rate variability in patients with Brugada syndrome in Thailand. *Eur. Heart Jl.* 2003; 24:1771–1778
[228] Nakazawa, K., Sakurai, T., Takagi, A., et al. Autonomic imbalance as a property of symptomatic Brugada syndrome. *Circ. J.* 2003;67:511-4
[229] Brugada, P., Brugada, R., Mont, L., Rivero, M., Geelen, P., Brugada, J. Natural history of Brugada syndrome: the prognostic value of programmed electrical stimulation of the heart. *J. Cardiovasc. Electrophysiol.* 2003;14:455-7
[230] Brugada, J., Brugada, R., Brugada, P. Determinants of sudden cardiac death in individuals with the electrocardiographic pattern of Brugada syndrome and no previous cardiac arrest. *Circulation.* 2003;23; 108: 3092-6
[231] Delise, P., Allocca, G., Marras, E., et al. Risk stratification in individuals with the Brugada type 1 ECG pattern without previous cardiac arrest: usefulness of a combined clinical and electrophysiologic approach. *Eur. Heart J.* 2011;32:169-76
[232] Napolitano, C., Bloise, R., Monteforte, N., Priori, S. Sudden Cardiac Death and Genetic Ion Channelopathies Long QT, Brugada, Short QT, Catecholaminergic Polymorphic Ventricular Tachycardia, and Idiopathic Ventricular Fibrillation. *Circulation* 2012;125: 2027-2034
[233] Sarkozy, A., Boussy, T., Kourgiannides, G., et al. Long-term follow-up of primary prophylactic implantable cardioverter-defibrillator therapy in Brugada syndrome. *Eur. Heart J.* 2007;28:334-44
[234] Gehi, A. K., Duong, T. D., Metz, L. D., Gomes, J. A., Mehta, D. Risk stratification of individuals with the Brugada electrocardiogram: a meta-analysis. *J. Cardiovasc. Electrophysiol.* 2006;17:577-83
[235] Garratt, C. J., Elliott, P., Behr, E., et al. Heart Rhythm UK position statement on clinical indications for implantable cardioverter defibrillators in adult patients with familial sudden cardiac death syndromes. *Europace* 2010;12:1156-75
[236] Tanaka, H., Kinoshita, O., Uchikawa, S., et al. Successful prevention of recurrent ventricular fibrillation by intravenous isoproterenol in a patient with Brugada syndrome. *Pacing Clin. Electrophysiol.* 2001;24:1293-4
[237] Martini, B. Case 37-2005: a man with cardiac arrest while sleeping. *N Engl. J. Med.* 2006; 354:1432-3; author reply 1432-3.
[238] Martini, B., Nava, A. 1988-2003. Fifteen years after the first Italian description by Nava-Martini-Thiene and colleagues of a new syndrome (different from the Brugada syndrome?) in the Giornale Italiano di Cardiologia: do we really know everything on this entity? *Ital. Heart J.* 2004;5:53-60
[239] Martini, B. Brugada syndrome; an organic syndrome. *Iranian Cardiovascular Research Journal.* 2007;1:70
[240] Martini, B., Wilde, A. A., Wilde, A. A. M., Alings, A. M. W. Right bundle branch block, ST-segment elevation, and sudden death. (Letter and Response). *Circulation.* 2000; 101: e176

[241] Wilde, A. A. M., Antzelevitch, C. The continuing story: The aetiology of Brugada syndrome: functional or structural basis? *Eur. Heart J.* 2003; 24: 2073

[242] Tukkie, R., Sogaard, P., Vleugels, J., de Groot, I. K., Wilde, A. A., Tan, H. L. Delay in right ventricular activation contributes to Brugada syndrome. *Circulation.* 2004; 109: 1272-7

[243] Meregalli, P. G., Wilde, A. A., Tan, H. L. Pathophysiological mechanisms of Brugada syndrome: depolarization disorder, repolarization disorder, or more? *Cardiovasc. Res.* 2005;67:367-78

[244] Wilde, A. A., Postema, P. G., Di Diego, J. M., et al. The pathophysiological mechanism underlying Brugada syndrome: depolarization versus repolarization. *J. Mol. Cell. Cardiol.* 2010;49:543-53

[245] Postema, P. G., van Dessel, P. F., Kors, J. A., et al. Local depolarization abnormalities are the dominant pathophysiologic mechanism for type 1 electrocardiogram in brugada syndrome a study of electrocardiograms, vectorcardiograms, and body surface potential maps during ajmaline provocation. *J. Am. Coll. Cardiol.* 2010;55:789-97

[246] Hoogendijk, M. G., Opthof, T., Postema, P. G., Wilde, A. A., de Bakker, J. M., Coronel, R. The Brugada ECG pattern: a marker of channelopathy, structural heart disease, or neither? Toward a unifying mechanism of the Brugada syndrome. *Circ. Arrhythm. Electrophysiol.* 2010;3:283-90

[247] Postema, P. G. Brugada syndrome and right ventricular conduction delay: what else? *Heart Rhythm.* 2011;8:1913-4

[248] Postema, P. G., Mosterd, A., Hofman, N., Alders, M., Wilde, A. A. Sodium channelopathies: do we really understand what's going on? *J. Cardiovasc. Electrophysiol.* 2011;22:590-3

[249] Coronel, R., Berecki, G., Opthof, T. Why the Brugada syndrome is not yet a disease: syndromes, diseases, and genetic causality. *Cardiovasc. Res.* 2006;72:361-3

[250] Boukens, B. J., Christoffels, V. M., Coronel, R., Moorman, A. F. Developmental basis for electrophysiological heterogeneity in the ventricular and outflow tract myocardium as a substrate for life-threatening ventricular arrhythmias. *Circ. Res.* 2009;104:19-31

[251] Priori, S. G., Napolitano, C. Should patients with an asymptomatic Brugada electrocardiogram undergo pharmacological and electrophysiological testing? *Circulation.* 2005;112:279-92

[252] Martini, B. The Ajmaline challenge and a strange ECG. *Europace.* 2009; 11:1406

[253] Takagi, M., Aonuma, K., Sekiguchi, Y., Yokoyama, Y., Aihara, N., Hiraoka, M. The prognostic value of early repolarization (J wave) and ST-segment morphology after J wave in Brugada syndrome: Multicenter study in Japan. *Heart Rhythm.* 2013 in press.

In: Sudden Death
Editors: Jiashin Wu and Jessica Wu
ISBN: 978-1-62618-825-9

Chapter II

Experimental Mechanisms of Arrhythmias in Brugada Syndrome

Hiroshi Morita,[1] Douglas P. Zipes[2] and Jiashin Wu[3,*]
[1]Department of Cardiovascular Medicine, Okayama University Graduate School of Medicine, Dentistry and Pharmaceutical Sciences, Okayama, Japan
[2]Krannert Institute of Cardiology, Indiana University School of Medicine, Indianapolis, IN, US
[3]University of South Florida, Tampa, FL, US

Abstract

This chapter reviewed the mechanisms of Brugada syndrome (BS) as we explored in experimental models created with drug-induced channelopathies in isolated, arterially perfused canine right ventricular tissues. These experimental studies revealed the mechanisms of arrhythmogenicity in terms of repolarization heterogeneity both inside the epicardium and across the right ventricular outflow tract and mechanisms of its sensitivity to temperature, rate dependency, T wave alternans, and fragmented QRS. These experimental models also illustrated the origins of the characteristic features of the typical BS electrocardiograms and the genotype-phenotype relationships in BS with Na^+ or Ca^{2+} channelopathies.

We also explored the effects of blocking the transient outward current, I_{to}, and of treatments with quinidine or isoproterenol on the electrophysiologic heterogeneity and arrhythmias in these models. Ablation and body surface mapping in patients with BS supported these experimental findings.

* Corresponding author: Jiashin Wu, University of South Florida, Tampa, FL 33612; E-mail: jiashinwu@alumni.duke.edu.

Abbreviations

AP	action potential
APD	action potential duration
BS	Brugada syndrome
BSM	body surface mapping
ECG	electrocardiogram
f-QRS	fragmented QRS
$I_{Ca\text{-}L}$	the L-type Ca^{2+} current
I_{Na}	the Na^+ current
I_{K1}	the inward rectifier K^+ current
I_{Kr} and I_{Ks}	the rapid and slow delayed rectifier K^+ currents
I_{to}	the transient outward K^+ current
ICD	implantable cardioverter defibrillator
PVC	premature ventricular complexes
RFCA	radiofrequency catheter ablation
RV	right ventricle
RVAI	right ventricular anteroinferior
RVOT	right ventricular outflow tract
TWA	T wave alternans
VA	ventricular arrhythmia
VF	ventricular fibrillation
VT	ventricular tachycardia

Introduction

Brugada syndrome (BS) is the most common cause of non-traumatic sudden death in young men in some Asian countries [1]. It is associated with genetic defects in membrane ion channels and is characterized clinically by coved ST elevation and negative T waves in the right precordial leads. The electrophysiological phenotypes of BS occur predominantly in male adults and can be affected by heart rate, autonomic nervous activity, fever, and drugs [1-6].

In patients with BS, polymorphic ventricular tachycardia (VT) and fibrillation (VF) have been reported to occur spontaneously at night [1, 4], can be triggered by programmed electrical stimulation in some instances [7], by pharmacological blockade of the sodium channel [3], or by administration of acetylcholine [1], and have been associated with T wave alternans (TWAs) and QRS fragmentation [3, 31]. Excessive ST elevation is a major prognostic risk factor of BS [8, 9].

Recent experimental [13-17] and clinical [18-20] studies have illustrated electrophysiological mechanisms responsible for the ECG characteristics and arrhythmogenesis of BS. This review updates our previous review on the same topic [60] with two of our recent publications [61, 62] to discuss the current understanding of the electrophysiological mechanisms in BS, with special emphasis on the mechanisms of temperature sensitivity, TWAs, the RVOT origin of arrhythmia, the fragmented QRS (f-

QRS), and genotype-phenotype correlations (with permissions from the Heart Rhythm Journal).

Ion Currents and Action Potentials in Brugada Syndrome

Transmembrane ionic fluxes generate an action potential [AP, 33]. A rapid inward Na^+ current, I_{Na}, depolarizes the cell membrane, produces the phase 0 of the AP, and subsequently activates other slower ion currents.

Activation of the transient outward K^+ current, I_{to}, when overwhelming the late phase of the inward I_{Na} and the early phase of the L-type Ca^{2+} current, $I_{Ca\text{-}L}$, causes a phase 1 notch in the AP [37]. Activation of the $I_{Ca\text{-}L}$, rapid and slow delayed rectifier K^+ currents, I_{Kr} and I_{Ks}, and inward rectifier K^+ current, I_{K1}, etc, produce the phase 2 dome and phase 3 repolarization of the AP.

The phase 1 notch of the AP plays a pivotal role in arrhythmogenesis in BS. The membrane density of I_{to}, which is the major contributor of the phase 1 notch, is higher in the right than left ventricles, in the epicardium than endocardium, and near the base than near the apex of the ventricles [57].

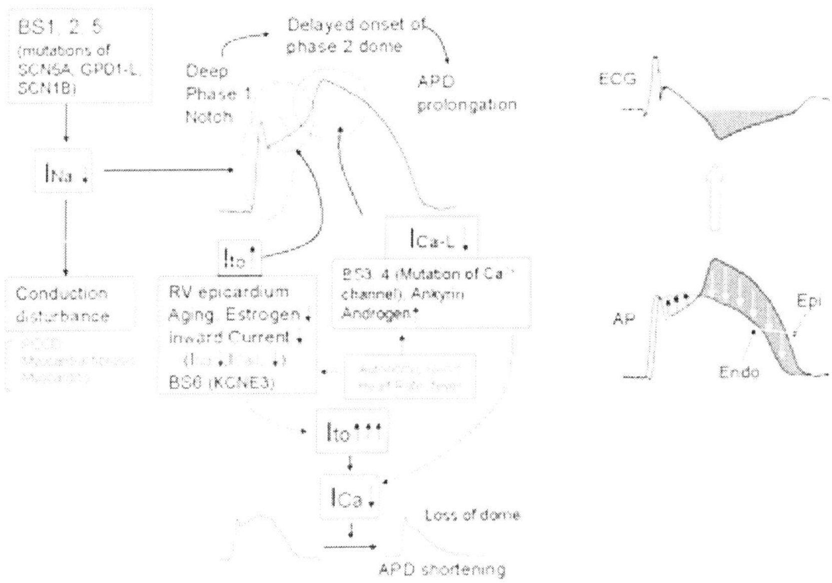

A B

Figure 1. Ion channel mutation and Brugada syndrome (BS). A. A reduced Na^+ current (SCN5A, GPD1-L or SCN1B mutations) slows conduction and enables the transient outward current (I_{to}) to deepen the phase 1 notch of the action potential (AP). A prominent phase 1 notch delays activation of the calcium current (I_{Ca}) and causes a delayed but prominent phase 2 dome. Excessively deepened phase 1 notch eliminates the phase 2 dome. I_{to} enhancement can be produced by mutation of KCNE3, which encodes the β subunit of the I_{to} channel. I_{Ca} reduction can be caused by mutated calcium channel gene. These AP changes occur predominantly in the epicardium of the right ventricular outflow tract (RVOT). B. Transmural gradient of AP causes ST elevation and deep negative T waves in the electrocardiogram (ECG).

The heterogeneic distribution of I_{to} causes the deepest phase 1 notch to appear in the epicardium of the RVOT (Figure 1A).

In patients with BS, the RVOT is a critical area associated with prominent spike-and-dome in the monophasic AP, depolarization and repolarization abnormalities, J-ST elevation in the ECG, and is a frequent origin of VT and VF [7, 18, 19, 41].

The phase 1 notch modulates the kinetics of slower activating ion currents, and consequently, the later phases of the AP. Initial enhancement of the phase 1 notch promotes the phase 2 dome and delays repolarization, presumably by delaying the peak of $I_{Ca\text{-}L}$. However, further enhancement of the phase 1 notch prevents the rising of the phase 2 dome and abbreviates the AP duration (APD), presumably by deactivation or voltage-modulation that reduces $I_{Ca\text{-}L}$ [15, 37]. Thus, progressive deepening of the phase 1 notch can cause initial enhancement followed by sudden disappearance of the phase 2 dome and corresponding prolongation followed by abbreviation of the APD [13-17]. The phase 1 notch also affects the function of the Na-Ca exchanger, and subsequently, intracellular Ca^{2+} handling and Na^+ channel function [37]. Sex hormones modulate the phase 1 notch, thus contributing to the male predominance of BS [39]. I_{to} can be enhanced by aging, low sympathetic activity, high parasympathetic activity, bradycardia, hypothermia, estrogen reduction, and drugs [38]. Estrogen suppresses the expression of Kv4.3 channel, resulting in reduced I_{to} and a shallow phase 1 notch. Testosterone enhances the outward currents (I_{Kr}, I_{Ks}, I_{K1}) and reduces the inward current ($I_{Ca\text{-}L}$), thus, deepening the phase 1 notch [40].

Gene Mutations and Brugada Syndrome

Several gene mutations that affect Na^+, L-type Ca^{2+}, or transient outward K^+ channels are identified in patients with BS (Table 1). However, the relationships between genotype and phenotype are not always predictive. Mutations in different genes can lead to expression of similar BS phenotypes. Conversely, mutations in the same gene can also lead to different syndromes. Mutations in the gene encoding the α subunit of the Na^+ channel (SCN5A) [1, 22, 23] that hamper its opening (loss of function) have been identified in 18-30% of the patients with BS (BS1) [1, 9] and also in patients with progressive cardiac conduction system disease [22]. Mutated SCN5A can also impede the closure (gain of function) of the Na^+ channel, leading to type 3 long QT syndrome [58, 43]. It was reported that all three syndromes noted above occurred within a single family due to a single mutated SCN5A gene [24]. Mutations in the glycerol-3-phosphate dehydrogenase 1-like gene (GPD1L) on chromosome 3p22-25 (BS2) [25] and in SCN1B on chromosome 19q13.1, which encodes the β-subunit of Na^+ channel (BS5) [26], can also cause Na^+ channel dysfunction, reducing the I_{Na} and resulting in BS. These proteins are components of the macromolecular complex of the Na^+ channel, and thus, modulate Na^+ channel function [27]. Haplotype of the promoter region of SCN5A also prolongs the PR and QRS durations in the ECG of BS patients [28].

Although Na^+ channel mutations are most common, mutations in the α and β subunits of the Ca^{2+} channel gene were found in some patients with BS (BS3 and BS4, respectively).

These mutations cause loss-of-function of the Ca^{2+} channel, resulting in phenotypical expression of BS in combination with short QT intervals and familial sudden cardiac death

[29]. Mutation of KCNE3, which encodes the β-subunit of Kv4.3 channel, enhances the I_{to} and can also lead to BS (BS6, Table 1) [30].

On the other hand, the failure of identifying gene mutations in the majority of patients with BS suggests that either unknown mutations or patho-physiological cellular regulations (such as posttranslational modulations, phosphorylation, glycosylation, etc.) may also cause similar ion current defects and clinical manifestations.

Table 1. Gene mutations and Brugada syndrome

Type	Chromosome	Gene	Protein	Current	Function	Incidence
1	3p21	SCN5A	Nav1.5	I_{Na}	Loss of function	11-28%
2	3p24	GPD1-L	GPD1-L	I_{Na}	Loss of function	Rare
3	12p13.3	CACNA1c	Cav1.2	I_{Ca}	Loss of function	6.6%
4	10p12.33	CACNB2b	Cavβ2b	I_{Ca}	Loss of function	4.8%
5	19q13.1	SCN1B	Navβ1	I_{Na}	Loss of function	1.1%
6	11q13-14	KCNE3	MiRP2	I_{to}	Gain of function	Rare
7	11q23.3	SCN3B	Navβ3	I_{Na}	Loss of function	Rare
8	12p11.23	KCNJ8	Kir6.1	$I_{K\text{-}ATP}$	Gain of function	2%
9	7q21.11	CACNA2D1	Cavα2d	I_{Ca}	Loss of function	1.8%
10	1p13.1	KCND3	Kv4.3	I_{to}	Gain of function	Rare
11	17p13.1	MOG1	MOG1	I_{Na}	Loss of function	Rare
12	12p12.1	ABCC9	SUR2A	$I_{K\text{-}ATP}$	Gain of function	Rare

While gene mutations provide a proarrhythmic substrate, the adult male dominance of clinical manifestation suggests that gender and age related factors (e.g., sex hormones) are triggers for arrhythmia in BS [35, 40].

Although genotype-phenotype correlations have been well investigated in patients with long QT syndrome [54], only a few similar investigations have been reported in patients with BS. Compared to patients without SCN5A mutation, patients with SCN5A mutation had longer and progressive conduction delays (PQ, QRS, and HV intervals) [34-35], frequent occurrences of fragmented QRS complex (f-QRS) [21], and ventricular arrhythmias (VAs) of extra RVOT origin. In contrast, most (about 80%) of the BS patients without SCN5A mutation had ventricular arrhythmias of RVOT origin [36]. Patients with Ca^{2+} channel gene mutation had short QT interval [29].

Electrophysiological Abnormality and Heterogeneity in the Right Ventricular Outflow Tract of an Experimental Model of Brugada Syndrome

We induced an experimental model of BS using isolated canine right ventricular tissues treated with pilsicainide, pinacidil, and terfenadine [15-17]. Both pilsicainide and terfenadine reduce I_{Na}, and thus, mimicked the Na^+ channel dysfunction in BS. Terfenadine also reduces

$I_{Ca\text{-}L}$ [59], mimicking a mutated Ca^{2+} channel gene observed in some patients with BS and also an effect of testosterone. Pinacidil produced a deep phase 1 notch, consistent with the male predominance of BS [39-40]. This model of BS has successfully reproduced the ECG characteristics, TWA, RVOT origin of arrhythmia and the temperature sensitivity that were observed clinically in patients with BS. We have also confirmed the mechanistic insights revealed experimentally in this tissue model by using body surface mapping (BSM) in clinical patients with BS [20]. Therefore, this experimental model is an effective electrophysiological representation of clinical BS.

When being treated with low doses of the BS-inducing drugs, isolated RVOT tissues showed small J waves following the QRS and flat ST segments in the transmural ECG. Earlier repolarization in the epicardium than in the endocardium produced positive T waves in the ECG [15-17] (Figure 3A), indicating a mild abnormality in ion currents and low arrhythmogenicity. A small J wave with a positive T wave formed a saddle-back type of ST elevation, similar to the type II or III ECG morphology in clinical BS [1]. These ECG features were due to a relatively small and shallow phase 1 notch and small transmural gradient in the AP during phase 1 and minimal heterogeneity in the phase 2 dome.

Progressively higher doses of BS-inducing drugs caused the RVOT APs to have deeper phase 1 notch, larger phase 2 dome, and later phase 3 repolarization in the epicardium than in the endocardium, inverting the transmural gradient of repolarization and resulting in coved J-ST elevation and deep negative T waves in the ECG [15-17] (Figure 3B), similar to the type I ECG in the consensus report [1].

These experimental observations correlated well with clinical observations of prominent spike-and-dome in the monophasic APs recorded in the epicardium of RVOT and of later repolarization in the epicardium than in the endocardium in association with type I ST elevation and deep negative T wave [18, 19].

Exacerbation of BS with deeper phase 1 notch eliminated the phase 2 dome and abbreviated the APD in parts of the epicardium, but not in the midmyocardium and endocardium [16], resulting in large transmural dispersion of the phases 2 and 3 of the AP and prominent J-ST elevation without deep negative T waves in the corresponding transmural ECG (Figure 3C).

However, the heterogeneity in phase 1 notch permitted a prominent phase 2 dome and a prolonged APD in other regions of the RVOT epicardium. The simultaneous presence of neighboring regions with and without a phase 2 dome produced corresponding neighboring regions having reverse and normal transmural gradients of repolarization and different local ECGs (ST elevation with and without negative T wave) in the RVOT. The highly heterogeneic dispersion of repolarization also facilitated the initiation of premature ventricular complexes (PVC) and polymorphic ventricular tachycardias [20] (Figures 4B, 5A-C). In addition to affecting the shape of the AP, a reduced I_{Na} also contributed to an epicardial conduction delay, which further enhanced the J-ST elevation (Figure 4) and facilitated reentry in the RVOT model of BS.

Further exacerbation of BS (with higher doses of the drugs) eliminated the phase 2 dome of the AP in the entire epicardium, but not in the midmyocardium and endocardium, resulting in steep transmural gradient of repolarization, prominent J-ST elevation without deep negative T waves in the transmural ECG.

Similar ECGs were reported in association with frequent VF in patients with BS, especially after administration of Na^+ channel blocker, during febrile illness, autonomic modulation, or glucose overload [1-3, 42].

In contrast to the RVOT, paired right ventricular anteroinferior (RVAI) tissues (isolated from the same heart and treated identically) had much less heterogeneity, normal transmural gradient of APD, as well as a small J wave and positive T waves in the transmural ECG.

Compared to RVAI, RVOT tissues have a deeper phase 1 notch in the epicardial AP, a larger J wave in the ECG, greater arrhythmogenesis and an increased sensitivity to drugs that induced the Brugada ECG characteristics (Figure 2) [16, 20]. Therefore, the experimental studies also demonstrated a critical role of the RVOT in BS.

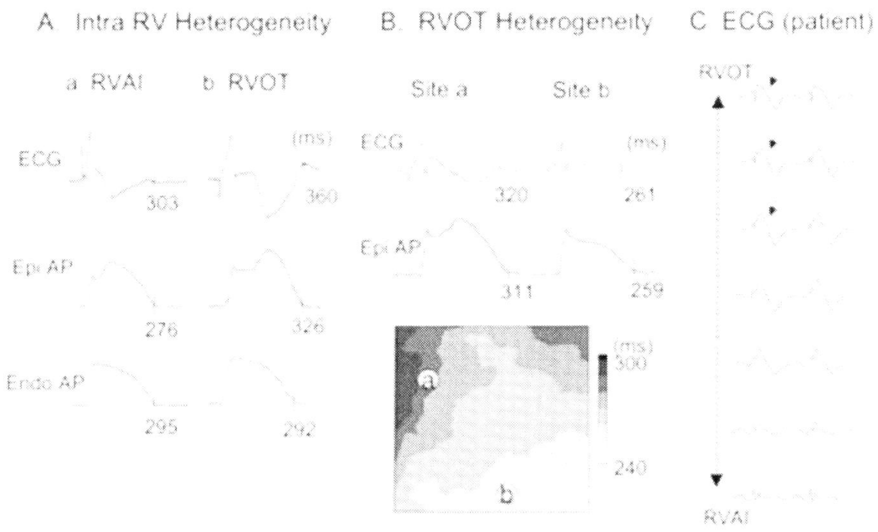

Figure 2. Electrophysiological heterogeneity in a canine tissue model of BS (A: intra-ventricular, B: intra-epicardial) and in a clinical patient with BS (C). A. Comparing to the right ventricular anteroinferior (RVAI) preparation (small J wave and positive T wave), the RVOT preparation [from the same heart and treated identically with (in μM) pilsicainide (7.5), pinacidil (5.0), and terfenadine (2.0)] had large J-ST elevation, negative T wave, and longer QT in ECG, and more prominent phase 1 notch and phase 2 dome in the epicardial AP. B. Significant heterogeneity of APD within the epicardium (in the map) of a RVOT model of BS (pilsicainide 10.0, pinacidil 7.5, and terfenadine 2.0). Comparing to site b, site a had a prominent dome, longer APD, and corresponding negative T wave and longer QT in ECG. C. Unipolar ECG leads in a patient. The RVOT (the upper 3 leads) had prominent J-ST elevation (arrows) with negative T wave, and the RVAI (the lower 2 leads) had saddle-back type ECG with small J wave.

In addition to reproducing major features of the clinical ECG, the experimental studies also provided mechanistic insights and causal relationships between abnormalities in the AP and the ECG. The experimental studies suggested that prominent J-ST elevation without deep negative T in the ECG indicates severe AP abbreviation in the epicardium, and that simultaneous presence of ECGs with and without negative T waves in association with ST elevation indicates significant dispersion of repolarization and presence of both APs with and without the phase 2 dome in the epicardium of RVOT, and thus, a high risk of VT.

Mechanism of Arrhythmogenesis in Brugada Syndrome

Experimental studies [13-17] suggested that excessive repolarization heterogeneity within the epicardium of the RVOT, especially with simultaneous regional presence and absence of the phase 2 dome, triggers PVCs, maintains a polymorphic VT, and contributes to the degeneration of VT to VF in BS. Traveling (by both electrotonic and induced ionic currents) of the dome caused phase 2 reentry, which, after initial conduction within the epicardium (from the region having a prominent dome to regions without a dome, and then reentering the region of its origin), conducted into mid- and endocardium following the recovery of local excitability [13-17]. Sustained VT occurred when the long APD region was reactivated repetitively by the reentrant wave front. A single premature activation [17] and bizarre T wave changes without a QRS complex in the transmural ECG [13, 15] (Figure 6A-C) occurred when a reentrant wave front was blocked returning to the long APD region that was still refractory.

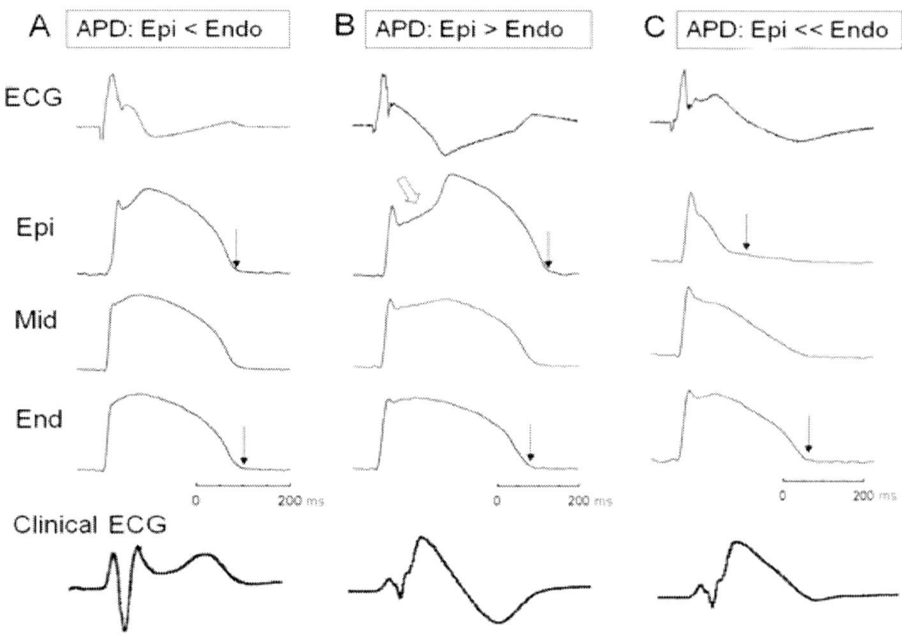

Figure 3. ECGs and APs in a canine RVOT tissue model of BS (the top and middle) and clinical ECGs with similar features in a patient with BS (the bottom). In the tissue model, Brugada-type ECG was induced with pilsicainide (in μM, 5.0), pinacidil (A: 2.5, B and C: 5.0), and terfenadine (A: 2.0, B and C: 2.5). A: Lower dose of pinacidil deepened mildly the phase 1 notch of the epicardial AP and elevated J-ST with positive T waves, similar to the saddle-back type clinical ECG. B: Initial perfusion of higher doses of pinacidil and terfenadine deepened the phase 1 notch (the large hollow arrow), delayed the phase 2 dome, resulted in later repolarization in the epicardium (Epi) than in the endocardium (Endo) and caused J-ST elevation, deep negative T wave, and long QT interval, similar to the coved-type ECG with deep negative T wave in the clinical ECG. C: Further perfusion of the higher doses of pinacidil and terfenadine abbreviated the epicardial AP, steepened the transmural gradient of repolarization, elevated J-ST, and generated small and shallow negative T waves. Arrows indicate repolarization. Clinical ECGs were recorded in a 45 year-old male with BS who was resuscitated from cardiac arrest.

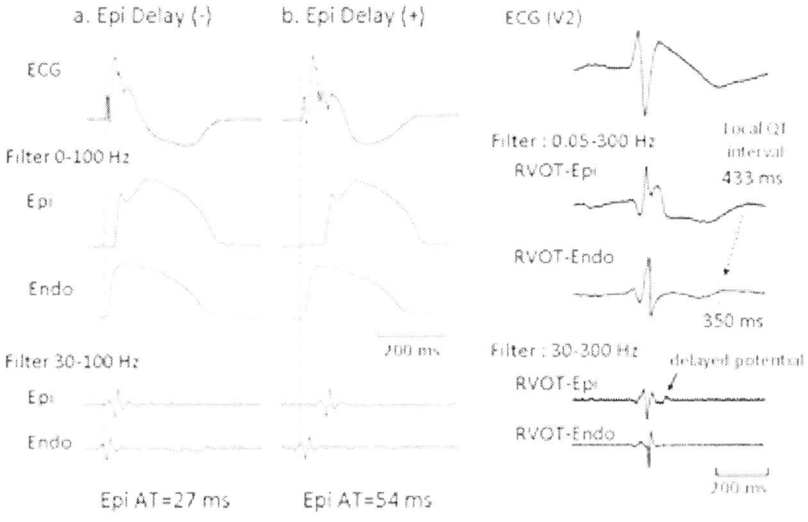

A B

Figure 4. Conduction disturbance enhances Brugada-type ECG. A. Epicardial conduction delay [from 27 ms (a) to 54 ms (b) after the endocardial stimulation] exaggerated J-ST elevation in a RVOT model of BS (in μM, pinacidil 7.5, terfenadine 2.0, pilsicainide 7.5). B. ECG and local electrograms in the RVOT in a patient with BS-type ECG. Prominent J-ST elevation in ECG associated with a delayed repolarization time and delayed potential in the epicardium but not in the endocardium of RVOT. Numbers show local QT intervals.

The long APD region in the epicardium of RVOT contributed to the arrhythmogenesis in BS by initiating phase 2 reentry, providing unidirectional block (refractoriness) and slowing conduction (partial recovery of excitability) [17]. The presence of abnormal AP restitution further facilitated the maintenance of polymorphic VT in BS [14]. Conduction disturbances also contribute to the development of VF.

Although the excessive heterogeneity promoted arrhythmogenesis within the RVOT, the presence of long APD regions also facilitated spontaneous termination of VT in the experimental model of BS.

Clinical observations have supported and validated the mechanisms of ECG characteristics and arrhythmogenesis discovered experimentally. Multisite unipolar ECGs and BSMs revealed significant repolarization heterogeneity within the RVOT in patients with BS [20].

These patients had longer QT intervals in the RVOT than in other areas and minimal QT heterogeneity at their basal state.

Administration of a Na^+ channel blocker exaggerated the J-ST elevation, increased repolarization heterogeneity with contiguous RVOT regions having prolonged and shortened QT intervals, increased QT dispersion, and caused spontaneous VAs [20] (Figures 6D-F).

Similar to our experimental observations, clinical observations also reported frequent spontaneous terminations of polymorphic VT in patients with BS who experienced recurrent syncope [1].

Both the repolarization heterogeneity and conduction abnormality in the RVOT contributed to the degeneration of VT into VF and sudden death in BS [14].

The experimental studies suggest that interventions of the functional substrates of repolarization heterogeneity can effectively control recurrent VF in BS.

Because of epicardial origin of the phase 2 reentry, epicardial ablation that disconnects regions with and without a phase 2 dome may eliminate reentry and VT, as has been demonstrated in the isolated RVOT model of BS [48].

Conduction Delay in the Epicardium of the Right Ventricular Outflow Tract and Fragmented QRS in Brugada Syndrome

Brugada syndrome is also associated with conduction abnormalities [10-12, 22, 41]. Reduction in I_{Na} not only deepens the phase 1 notch, but also slows conduction. Slowed transmural conduction contributes to J-ST elevation by delaying epicardial activation, thus increasing the transmural gradient of membrane potential (Figure 4A). Delayed epicardial activation in the RVOT region (e.g., Figure 4B) [19, 20, 47] was associated with late potentials and VF in BS [12].

Similar conduction slowing can also be caused by myocardial fibrosis secondary to myocardial degeneration or myocarditis [46]. Therefore, the BS characteristic ST elevation can be caused by reduced inward currents (e.g., I_{Na} and I_{Ca-L}), by increased outward currents (e.g., I_{to}), and by fibrosis. In patients with BS, intraventricular conduction abnormalities are often manifested as right bundle branch block and prolonged HV interval [1].

We reported recently [21] that f-QRS occurred frequently in BS patients having episodes of VF and/or SCN5A mutations.

We also established a causal relationship between the epicardial conduction delay and f-QRS in an experimental model of BS. Because epicardial conduction delay provides a proarrhythmic substrate, the clinical correlation between f-QRS and VF could be due to their common origin of epicardial conduction delay. Based on these findings, we suggested that f-QRS may be used as an indicator of high arrhythmic risk in patients with BS.

T Wave Alternans in Brugada Syndrome

T wave alternans (TWA, 55) and random T wave changes, characterized by beat-to-beat changes in the polarity, amplitude, and morphology of the T wave in the right precordial ECG leads, especially in the 2nd or 3rd intercostal spaces, have been reported in patients with BS [3, 20] (Figure 6A). TWA indicates repolarization instability and predicts the occurrence of serious VAs that can lead to sudden cardiac death.

In association with the deep and shallow negative T waves during TWA, the J-ST elevations also alternate between high and low amplitudes. TWA can be induced by sodium channel blocker, β-adrenergic blocker, vasospasm, febrile illness, glucose loading, heavy meal, sympathetic stimulation, long QT syndrome, as well as spontaneously [1, 3, 42].

In contrast to the TWA in the long QT syndrome, which has left ventricular midmyocardial origin and occurs during short cycle lengths [43], TWAs in BS is generated by alternating phase 2 dome of APs within the epicardium of the RVOT (Figure 5B), along with alternating APDs within a range of relatively long activation cycle lengths [15] (Table 2).

In association with TWA, unstable intraepicardial and transmural dispersion of APs facilitates arrhythmia induction.

In addition to alternating phase 2 dome, alternating occurrence of blocked phase 2 conduction can produce similar T wave changes in BS [13, 15].

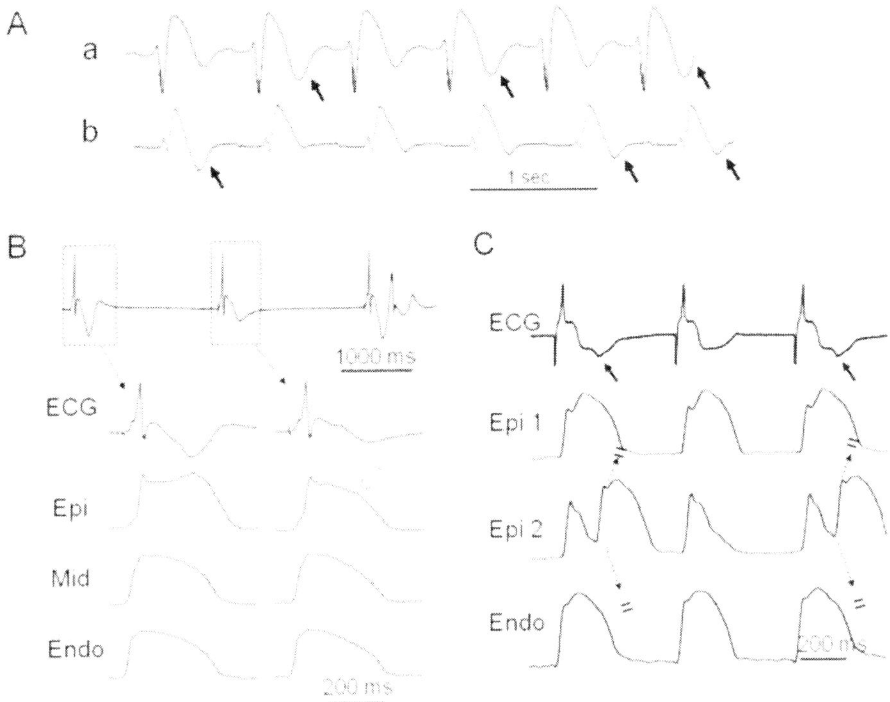

Figure 5. T wave alternans (TWA) and random T wave changes in BS. A. Patients with BS and TWAs (A-a, 75-year-old male) or random T wave changes (A-b, 45 year-old male). Arrows indicate the deep T waves. B. A canine RVOT model of BS (in μM, pinacidil 5.0, pilsicainide 8.0, terfenadine 2.0) having TWA (alternating ST level and T wave depth). Alternating appearance and disappearance (white arrow) of the phase 2 dome occurred only in the epicardium. C. APs with and without blocked premature ventricular complexes (PVCs) produced TWA-like ECG activity, in a RVOT model of BS (in μM, pinacidil 3.75, pilsicainide 7.5).

Temperature Sensitivity in Brugada Syndrome

Brugada syndrome is sensitive to body temperature. Febrile illness unmasks Brugada-type ECG, aggravates the ST elevation, and causes TWAs, PVCs, frequent VAs, and VF [1-2, 44, 52-53]. It was also reported that a hot bath elevated the ST segment and triggered VF [45]. Severe fever (>39°C) can increase the heart rate, elevate the J-ST segment, shorten the QT interval and diminish the negative T wave in the right precordial leads [44]. In addition to fever, hypothemia can also aggravate BS-type ECG [5, 39].

Temperature affects the heart rate, autonomic activity, and the kinetics of ion currents (especially I_{to}), transporters, and exchangers [2, 16]. It was reported that temperature elevation caused positive shift of steady state activation, acceleration of inactivation and slow recovery from inactivation in both wild and mutant Na^+ channels (F1344S in the SCN5A gene), resulting in I_{Na} reduction, deepening of the phase 1 notch of the AP, and aggravation of BS [2].

The fever-unmasked Brugada syndrome has also been linked to a single amino acid substitution (H681P) in the SCN5A gene that shifted both steady-state activation and inactivation, resulting in a 60% reduction of Na^+ window current [53].

Table 2. Risk stratification of Brugada syndrome

Clinical findings	Basic findings	Significance
Spontaneous type 1 ECG	Accentuation of phase 1 notch of APs at RVOT epicardium	Progressive deepening of phase 1 notch of AP lose AP dome and can cause repolarization heterogeneity, and it can occur spontaneously
Induced VF by PES	PES Induces of AP heterogeneity and restitution abnormality and conduction disturbance can be a substrate for VF	Prognostic value of induced VF is still controversial
Prolonged Tpeak-end interval	Transmural or spacial dispersion of repolarization at RVOT area	Accentuation of phase 1 notch induces londer AP at RVOT epicardium than endocardium
QT dispersion at RVOT area (simultaneous existence of both long and short QT interval at localized area)	Simultaneous existence of both long and short AP at RVOT epicardium	AP heterogeneity initiate premature ventricular complexes and polymorphic VT (phase 2 reentry)
T wave alternals	Alternating pase 2 dome in the epicardium at RVOT	Presence of unstable APs and enhances AP heterogeneity
QRS widening, fragmented QRS	Conduction disturbance of the right ventricle, especially at RVOT epicardium.	Conduction disturbance can degenerate non-sustained polymorphic VT (phase 1 reentry) into VF

AP: action potential, PES: programmed electrical stimulation, RVOT: right ventricular outflow tract.

In the isolated RVOT tissue model of BS [17], the combination of tachycardia and elevated temperature caused the epicardial AP to lose its phase 2 dome, resulting in J-ST elevation without deep negative T wave in the transmural ECG, resembling the ECG characteristics in patients having sinus tachycardia induced by severe fever.

High temperature also abbreviated APD and refractory period, facilitating the maintenance of reentry. In contrast, hypothermia prolonged APDs, enhanced the phase-1 notch of epicardial APs, and induced prominent phase-2 domes of APs that frequently led to spontaneous PVCs.

Therefore, fever aggravates the ECG characteristics and promotes arrhythmias in patients with BS by reducing I_{Na}, increasing the heart rate, and abbreviating the refractory period and hypothermia promotes spontaneous activation and arrhythmia by prolonging APDs and increasing the dispersion of APDs.

Spontaneous ECG Alterations Predict Ventricular Fibrillation in Brugada Syndrome

Patients with BS often have spontaneous changes in their ECG. To evaluate the significance of ECG alterations, a recent study [61] investigated the relationships between the ECG and the occurrence of VF in both patients and an experimental model of BS.

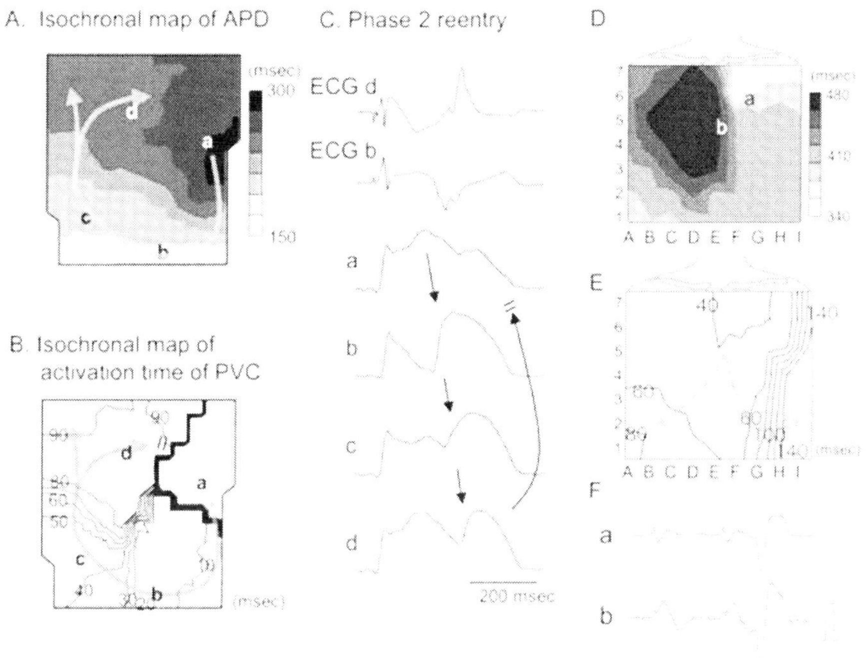

Figure 6. Ventricular arrhythmias induced by epicardial heterogeneity of AP in a canine RVOT model (A-C) and in a 48 year-old male with BS (D-F). Experiment (A: APD map; B: activation isochronal map; C: local ECGs and APs from the sites indicated in A and B): Large phase 2 dome conducted (along the arrows) from the long APD region (site a, black color in A) to the short APD region (sites b and c, light color), then reentered the long APD region (site d), and finally blocked by refractoriness (B and C). Local transmural ECGs (C) showed ST elevation with negative T wave in the long APD region (site d) and large ST elevation in the short APD region (site b). BS was induced by pinacidil (in μM, 10.0), terfenadine (2.0), and pilsicainide (12.5). Patient (87-lead body surface map): The distribution of QT intervals in the anterior chest (D) shows that the upper chest (the RVOT region) had simultaneous presences of both short and long QT intervals (a and b), resembling the APD heterogeneity in the epicardium of canine RVOT model of BS (A). The isochronal map (E) shows the RVOT origin of PVC. J-ST elevation occurred in the local ECGs at both sites a and b (F). Site a had a short QT interval without negative T wave.

In the clinical study, ECG alterations in BS patients with (VF+, n=33) and without (VF-, n=41) spontaneous VF were evaluated. Here, Type 0 ECG is defined as coved-type ST elevation without a negative T wave (representing the existence of loss-of-dome, LOD, type of APs). Changes in ST level $\geq$ 0.2 mV were more frequent in the VF+ group than in VF- group ($p<0.01$). Spontaneous ECG alterations and appearances of Types 1 and 0 ECGs were more frequent in the VF+ group than in the VF- group ($p<0.01$).

In comparison with the clinical study, we carried out an experimental study in 34 isolated canine right ventricular tissues with BS induced by combination of pinacidil and pilsicainide. We optically mapped epicardial APs and recorded transmural ECGs in the tissue model. BS-model with spike-and-dome (SAD) epicardial APs exhibited Type 1 ECG. Deepening of the phase 1 notch of the APs induced heterogeneous conversion of the APs (SAD→LOD) and resulted in ECG conversion from Type 1 to Type 0.

Significant AP heterogeneity often appeared during AP alterations and initiated phase 2 reentry. Alterations in APs and in ECG occurred more frequently in tissues having VT (n=20) than without VT (n=14) ($p<0.01$). Both the clinical and experimental studies demonstrated that ECG alterations, especially conversion between Types 0 and 1, are associated with significant AP heterogeneity that can initiate VF in BS.

Genotype-Phenotype Correlation in Brugada Syndrome

Genetic defects in the sodium channel (Na-Ch) or in the calcium channel (Ca-Ch) have been identified in patients having BS [32]. However, the differences in their genotype-phenotype correlations are still unclear. Brugada syndrome patients with Na^+ channelopathy are associated with conduction abnormalities, such as prolongation of PQ, QRS intervals, and HV interval [34], that progress with age [35]. Na^+ current dysfunction contributes to local conduction block in the epicardium, resulting in multiple spikes within the QRS complex and triggering of VF [21].

Although ST-elevation and occurrences of arrhythmias were similar between Brugada patients with and without SCN5A mutation, patients with SCN5A mutations had arrhythmias arising from both ventricles [36]. In contrast, patients with Ca^{2+} channel dysfunction were not associated with conduction slowing and exhibited Brugada type ECG after administration of ajmaline [29].

We evaluated the phenotypic differences and therapeutic effects between the Na-Ch and Ca-Ch abnormalities in vitro models of BS [62]. We used a Na^+ channel blocker, pilsicainide (2.5-12.5 μmol/l), and a K^+ channel opener, pinacidil (1.25-12.5 μmol/l), to create a Na^+ channel dysfunction model of Brugada syndrome (Na-model, n=11).

Because there are only a few reports about Ca^{2+} channel dysfunction in patients with Brugada syndrome and their disease progression and involvement of K^+ currents are still unclear, we chose to use only a Ca^{2+} channel blocker, verapamil (5-10μmol/l), to create a Ca^{2+} channel dysfunction model (Ca-model, n=7). Both models used the isolated and arterially-perfused canine right ventricular preparations.

We observed that at the cycle length (CL) of 1,000 ms, both models had coved-type ST elevation in the ECG, longer APD in the epicardium than in the endocardium and a similar incidence of spontaneous VAs.

However, the Ca-model had a higher incidence of TWAs than the Na-model. In contrast, at the CL of 2,000 ms, ECGs of the Ca-model converted to saddle-back type ST elevation with shorter APDs in the epicardium than in the endocardium, whereas the Na-model still had coved-type ST elevation and longer APDs in the EPI. None of the Ca-model preparations had VAs or TWA, although the Na-model had frequent VAs and TWA (Table 3).

Table 3. Summary of the experimental models of Na^+ and Ca^{2+} dysfunction

	Na model		Ca model	
Cycle Length (ms)	ECG morphology	VT	ECG morphology	VT
2000	Coved type with deep negative T wave	+++	Saddle back type with positive T wave	-
1000	Coved type with deep negative T wave	++	Coved type with TWA	++
500	Coved type without negative T wave	+	Coved type without negative T wave	-
Quinidine	QRS widening and no ST elevation	-	Coved type with TWA at CL 1000 ms	-
Isoproterenol	No ST elevation	-	No ST elevation	-

VT: ventricular tachycardia.

Further studies showed that, although both quinidine and isoproterenol restored the dome in the AP and abolished arrhythmias in both Na^+ and Ca^{2+} channelopathy models, quinidine did not prevent J-ST elevation and TWA at the CL of 1,000 ms in the Ca-model. We concluded that although both Na-Ch and Ca-Ch dysfunction produced similar BS ECGs and arrhythmogenesis at 60 bpm, Ca-Ch dysfunction was associated with a higher incidence of TWAs at 60 bpm, less ST elevation and fewer arrhythmias at 30 bpm compared to Na-Ch dysfunction.

Risk Stratification of Brugada Syndrome from Experiment Observations

Spontaneous type I J-ST elevation and a history of syncope can be powerful predictors of the outcome of patients with BS [8, 9]. Induction of VT/VF by programmed electrical stimulation may also predict prognosis [8].

However, its predictive accuracy is still controversial [9, 49].

Prominent J-ST elevation in the lead corresponding to the RVOT suggests an increased possibility of phase 2 reentry and VT [13, 16] and possible conduction abnormality in the epicardium of the RVOT [20]. The dispersion between the peak and end of the T wave (Tpeak-end) in the RVOT, which reflects transmural APD dispersion, can be an indicator of the abnormality in the epicardial AP [50]. The presence of both long and short QT intervals in the leads corresponding to the RVOT suggests a proarrhythmic substrate having heterogeneity in the phase 2 dome and in the duration of AP [13-17]. The occurrence of TWAs or spontaneous ST-T variation suggests the presence of unstable APs with alternating phase 2 dome in the epicardium of the RVOT, and of corresponding elevated heterogeneic and unstable dispersion of repolarization that can initiate phase 2 reentry [19, 20]. Abnormal depolarization, which is a substrate for VF, can be detected by QRS widening or f-QRS [21, 51]. Presence of f-QRS suggests elevated arrhythmic risk. Although the above indexes (Table 2) suggest the presence of underlying electrophysiological causes, because of frequent spontaneous changes in the Brugada-type ECG, the usefulness of these indexes should be evaluated prospectively in large number of patients with BS. Our experiments suggest that patients with Ca^{2+} channelopathy type Brugada syndrome are likely to have rate dependent changes of ST-T morphology and arrhythmogenesis. We observed that Ca^{2+} channelopathy had saddle-back type ST elevation, which is a low risk ECG sign, in association with reduced arrhythmogenicity during bradycardia (CL 2,000 ms), in contrast to the typical Brugada-type ECG and increased arrhythmogenicity in the Na-model during bradycardia. We observed coved-type J-ST elevation with negative T wave, TWA and ventricular arrhythmias during a more physiological heart rate (CL 1,000 ms) in the Ca-model. The rate dependent ECG responses and arrhythmogenicity in the Ca-model suggest that patients with Ca^{2+} channelopathy may have arrhythmic events during daytime, whereas cardiac events may be infrequent at night due to slower heart rates. Quinidine and isoproterenol can be effective in Brugada syndrome with either Na^{+} or Ca^{2+} channelopathies, but quinidine may not fully prevent arrhythmias in patients with Brugada syndrome caused by Ca^{2+} channelopathy.

Limitations

Extrapolating conclusions from animal studies and applying them to clinical situations must always be done carefully and with a certain amount of speculation.

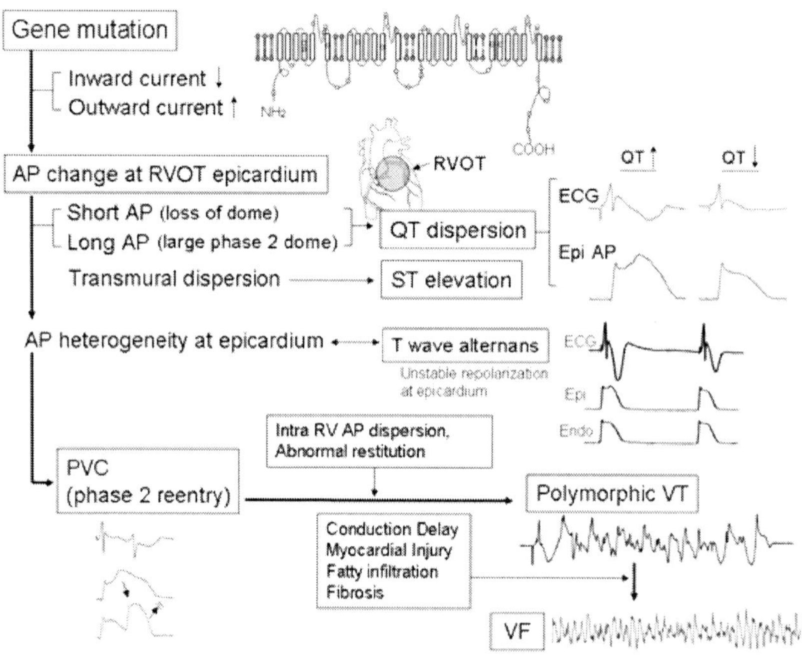

Figure 7. Pathophysiology of BS. Ion channel mutations (e.g., in SCN5A) deepen the phase 1 notch of the AP, especially in the epicardium of RVOT. The phase 1 notch modulates the phases 2 and 3 of the AP. Transmural difference in APs elevates J-ST and generates a negative T wave in ECG. Epicardial co-existence of APs with and without a dome produces QT dispersion. Instability in the dome exaggerates AP heterogeneity and causes TWAs. Conduction of the phase 2 dome generates PVCs, which can lead to VT and degenerate into VF.

That is why, when possible, we have directly compared experimental and clinical observations and have found striking similarities. However, that does not necessarily mean the mechanisms observed in the Brugada model are the same ones operating in patients with BS. Ultimately, the proof must be obtained from patients, but the animal model does provide a reasonable starting point and offers hypotheses to test clinically.

Summary

Brugada syndrome can be caused by a reduced I_{Na}, a reduced I_{Ca}, and/or an enhancement of I_{to}, and is mediated by the phase 1 notch of the AP. A high density of I_{to} causes the electrophysiological abnormality to manifest in the epicardium of the RVOT. A deepened phase 1 notch of the AP, enhanced by the effects of testosterone, is responsible for the male predominance of BS. The AP heterogeneity within the RVOT generates the ECG characteristics of BS. Excessive and dynamic AP heterogeneity in the epicardium of RVOT causes TWA and phase 2 reentry, which initiates VT (Figure 7). A reduced I_{Na} also slows conduction, which can result in activation delay in the epicardium of RVOT and f-QRS.

Notes

This chapter is partially supported by a NSF grant (1146882).

References

[1] Antzelevitch, C., Brugada, P., Borggrefe, M., et al. Brugada syndrome: report of the second consensus conference. *Heart Rhythm*. 2005;2:429-40.

[2] Keller, D. I., Huang, H., Zhao, J., et al. A novel SCN5A mutation, F1344S, identified in a patient with Brugada syndrome and fever-induced ventricular fibrillation. *Cardiovasc. Res*. 2006;70:521-9.

[3] Morita, H., Morita, S. T., Nagase, S., et al. Ventricular arrhythmia induced by sodium channel blocker in patients with Brugada syndrome. *J. Am. Coll. Cardiol*. 2003;42: 1624-31.

[4] Matsuo, K., Kurita, T., Inagaki, M., et al. The circadian pattern of the development of ventricular fibrillation in patients with Brugada syndrome. *Eur. Heart J*. 1999;20:465-70.

[5] Noda, T., Shimizu, W., Taguchi, A., et al. ST-segment elevation and ventricular fibrillation without coronary spasm by intracoronary injection of acetylcholine and/or ergonovine maleate in patients with Brugada syndrome. *J. Am. Coll. Cardiol*. 2002;40: 1841-7.

[6] Takigawa, M., Noda, T., Shimizu, W., et al. Seasonal and circadian distributions of ventricular fibrillation in patients with Brugada syndrome. *Heart Rhythm*. 2008;5:1523-7.

[7] Morita, H., Fukushima-Kusano, K., Nagase, S., et al. Site-specific arrhythmogenesis in patients with Brugada syndrome. *J. Cardiovasc. Electrophysiol.* 2003;14:373-9.
[8] Brugada, J., Brugada, R., Antzelevitch, C., et al. Long-term follow-up of individuals with the electrocardiographic pattern of right bundle-branch block and ST-segment elevation in precordial leads V1 to V3. *Circ.* 2002;105:73-8.
[9] Priori, S. G., Napolitano, C., Gasparini, M., et al. Natural history of Brugada syndrome: insights for risk stratification and management. *Circ.* 2002;105:1342-7.
[10] Brugada, P., Brugada, J. Right bundle branch block, persistent ST segment elevation and sudden cardiac death: A distinct clinical and electrocardiographic syndrome. *J. Am. Coll. Cardiol* 1992, 20: 1391-1396.
[11] Kanda, M., Shimizu, W., Matsuo, K., et al. Electorophysiologic characteristics and implication of induced ventricular fibrillation in symptomatic patients with Brugada syndrome. *J. Am. Coll. Cardiol.* 2002;39:1799-1805.
[12] Morita, H., Takenaka-Morita, S., Fukushima-Kusano, K., et al. Risk stratification for asymptomatic patients with Brugada syndrome. *Circ. J.* 2003;67:312-6.
[13] Fish, J. M., Antzelevitch, C. Role of sodium and calcium channel block in unmasking the Brugada syndrome. *Heart Rhythm.* 2004;1:210-7.
[14] Aiba, T., Shimizu, W., Hidaka, I., et al. Cellular basis for trigger and maintenance of ventricular fibrillation in the Brugada syndrome model: high-resolution optical mapping study. *J. Am. Coll. Cardiol.* 2006; 47: 2074-85.
[15] Morita, H., Zipes, D. P., Lopshire, J., et al. T wave alternans in an in vitro canine tissue model of Brugada syndrome. *Am. J. Physiol. Heart Circ. Physiol.* 2006;291:H421-8.
[16] Morita, H., Zipes, D. P., Morita, S. T., et al. Differences in arrhythmogenicity between the canine right ventricular outflow tract and anteroinferior right ventricle in a model of Brugada syndrome. *Heart Rhythm.* 2007;4:66-74.
[17] Morita, H., Zipes, D. P., Morita, S. T., et al. Temperature modulation of ventricular arrhythmogenicity in a canine tissue model of Brugada syndrome. *Heart Rhythm* 4:188-97, 2007.
[18] Kurita, T., Shimizu, W., Inagaki, M., et al. The electrophysiologic mechanism of ST-segment elevation in Brugada syndrome. *J. Am. Coll. Cardiol.* 2002;40:330-4.
[19] Nagase, S., Kusano, K. F., Morita, H., et al. Longer Repolarization in the Epicardium at the Right Ventricular Outflow Tract Causes Type 1 ECG in Patients with Brugada Syndrome. *J. Am. Coll. Cardiol.* 2008;51:1154-61.
[20] Morita, H., Zipes, D. P., Fukushima-Kusano, K., et al. Repolarization heterogeneity in the right ventricular outflow tract: Correlation with ventricular arrhythmias in Brugada patients and in an in vitro canine Brugada model. *Heart Rhythm*, 2008; 5:725-33,
[21] Morita, H., Fukushima, K. K., Miura, D., et al. Fragmented QRS as a marker of conduction abnormality and a predictor of prognosis of Brugada syndrome. *Circ.* 2008; 118:1697-704.
[22] Tan, H. L., Bezzina, C. R., Smits, J. P., et al. Genetic control of sodium channel function. *Cardiovasc. Res.* 2003;57:961-73.
[23] Chen, Q., Kirsch, G. E., Zhang, D., et al. Genetic basis and molecular mechanism for idiopathic ventricular fibrillation. *Nature.* 1998;392:293-6.
[24] Grant, A. O., Carboni, M. P., Neplioueva, V., et al. Long QT syndrome, Brugada syndrome, and conduction system disease are linked to a single sodium channel mutation. *J. Clin. Invest.* 2002;110:1201-1209.

[25] London, B., Michalec, M., Mehdi, H., et al. Mutation in glycerol-3-phosphate dehydrogenase 1 like gene (GPD1-L) decreases cardiac Na^+ current and causes inherited arrhythmias. *Circulation*. 2007;116:2260-8.

[26] Watanabe, H., Koopmann, T. T., Le Scouarnec, S., et al. Sodium channel beta1 subunit mutations associated with Brugada syndrome and cardiac conduction disease in humans. *J. Clin. Invest.* 2008;118:2260-8.

[27] Abriel, H. Roles and regulation of the cardiac sodium channel Nav1.5: recent insights from experimental studies. *Cardiovasc. Res.* 2007;76: 381-389.

[28] Bezzina, C. R., Shimizu, W., Yang, P., et al. Common sodium channel promoter haplotype in Asian subjects underlies variability in cardiac conduction. *Circulation*. 2006;113:338-44.

[29] Antzelevitch, C., Pollevick, G. D., Cordeiro, J. M., et al. Loss-of-function mutations in the cardiac calcium channel underlie a new clinical entity characterized by ST-segment elevation, short QT intervals, and sudden cardiac death. *Circulation* 2007;115:442-9.

[30] Delpón, E., Cordeiro, J. M., Núñez, L., et al. Functional Effects of KCNE3 Mutation and its Role in the Development of Brugada Syndrome. *Circ. Arrhythm. Electrophysiol.* 2008;1:209-218.

[31] Priori, S. G., Gasparini, M., Napolitano, C., Della Bella, P., Ottonelli, A. G., Sassone, B., Giordano, U., Pappone, C., Mascioli, G., Rossetti, G., De Nardis, R., Colombo, M. Risk stratification in Brugada syndrome: results of the PRELUDE (PRogrammed ELectrical stimUlation preDictive valuE) registry. *J. Am. Coll. Cardiol.* 2012;59:37-45.

[32] Morita, H., Nagase, S., Miura, D., et al. Differential effects of cardiac sodium channel mutations on initiation of ventricular arrhythmias in patients with Brugada syndrome. *Heart Rhythm* 2009;6:487-92.

[33] Yan, G. X., Antzelevitch, C. Cellular basis for the Brugada syndrome and other mechanisms of arrhythmogenesis associated with ST-segment elevation. *Circulation* 1999;100:1660-6.

[34] Smits, J. P., Eckardt, L., Probst, V., et al. Genotype-phenotype relationship in Brugada syndrome: electrocardiographic features differentiate SCN5A-related patients from non-SCN5A-related patients. *J. Am. Coll. Cardiol.* 2002;40:350-6.

[35] Yokokawa, M., Noda, T., Okamura, H., et al. Comparison of long-term follow-up of electrocardiographic features in Brugada syndrome between the SCN5A-positive probands and the SCN5A-negative probands. *Am. J. Cardiol.* 2007;100:649-55.

[36] Morita, H., Nagase, S., Miura, D., et al. Differential effects of cardiac sodium channel mutations on the initiation of ventricular arrhythmias in patients with Brugada syndrome. *Heart Rhythm*, 2009;.6:487-92.

[37] Sah, R., Ramirez, R. J., Oudit, G. Y., et al. Regulation of cardiac excitation-contraction coupling by action potential repolarization: role of the transient outward potassium current (I(to)). *J. Physiol.* 2003;546(Pt 1):5-18.

[38] Van der Heyden, M. A., Wijnhoven, T. J., et al. Molecular aspects of adrenergic modulation of the transient outward current. *Cardiovasc. Res.* 2006;71:430-42.

[39] Di Diego, J. M., Cordeiro, J. M., Goodrow, R. J., et al. Ionic and cellular basis for the predominance of the Brugada syndrome phenotype in males. *Circulation* 2002;106: 2004-2011.

[40] Shimizu, W., Matsuo, K., Kokubo, Y., et al. Sex hormone and gender difference--role of testosterone on male predominance in Brugada syndrome. *J. Cardiovasc. Electrophysiol.* 2007;18:415-21.

[41] Hisamatsu, K., Kusano, K. F., Morita, H., et al. Relationships between depolarization abnormality and repolarization abnormality in patients with Brugada syndrome: using body surface signal-averaged electrocardiography and body surface maps. *J. Cardiovasc. Electrophysiol.* 2004; 15:870-6.

[42] Nishizaki, M., Sakurada, H., Ashikaga, T., et al. Effects of glucose-induced insulin secretion on ST segment elevation in the Brugada syndrome. *J. Cardiovasc. Electrophysiol.* 2003;14:243-9.

[43] Morita, H., Wu, J., Zipes, P. D. The QT syndrome: long and short. *Lancet* 2008;372: 750-63.

[44] Saura, D., García-Alberola, A., Carrillo, P., et al. Brugada-like electrocardiographic pattern induced by fever. *Pacing Clin. Electrophysiol.* 2002;25:856-9.

[45] Mori, A., Kusano, K. F., Nagase, S., et al. Clinical impact of the hot-bath test in patients with Brugada syndrome. *Circulation.* 2008;118:S674 (abstract)

[46] Coronel, R., Casini, S., Koopmann, T. T., Wilms-Schopman, F. J., et al. Right ventricular fibrosis and conduction delay in a patient with clinical signs of Brugada syndrome: a combined electrophysiological, genetic, histopathologic, and computational study. *Circulation* 2005;112:2769-77.

[47] Nagase, S., Kusano, K. F., Morita, H., et al. Epicardial electrogram of the right ventricular outflow tract in patients with the Brugada syndrome: using the epicardial lead. *J. Am. Coll. Cardiol.* 2002;39:1992-5.

[48] Morita, H., Zipes, D. P., Morita, S. T., et al. Epicardial ablation eliminates ventricular arrhythmias in an experimental model of Brugada syndrome, *Heart Rhythm*, 2009; 6: 665-71.

[49] Paul, M., Gerss, J., Schulze-Bahr, E., Wichter, T., et al. Role of programmed ventricular stimulation in patients with Brugada syndrome: a meta-analysis of worldwide published data. *Eur. Heart J.* 2007;28: 2126-33.

[50] Castro Hevia, J., Antzelevitch, C., Tornes Barzaga, F., et al. Tpeak-Tend and Tpeak-Tend dispersion as risk factors for ventricular tachycardia/ ventricular fibrillation in patients with the Brugada syndrome. *J. Am. Coll. Cardiol.* 2006;47:1828-34.

[51] Takagi, M., Yokoyama, Y., Aonuma, K., et al. Clinical characteristics and risk stratification in symptomatic and asymptomatic patients with brugada syndrome: multicenter study in Japan. *J. Cardiovasc. Electrophysiol.* 2007;18:1244-51.

[52] Wakita, R., Watanabe, I., Okumura, Y., et al. Brugada-like electrocardiographic pattern unmasked by fever. *Jpn. Heart J.* 2004;45: 163-7.

[53] Mok, N. S., Priori, S. G., Napolitano, C., et al. A newly characterized SCN5A mutation underlying Brugada syndrome unmasked by hyperthermia. *J. Cardiovasc. Electrophysiol.* 2003;14:407-11.

[54] Schwartz, P. J., Priori, S. G., Spazzolini, C., et al. Genotype-phenotype correlation in the long QT syndrome. Gene-specific triggers for life-threatening arrhythmias. *Circ.* 2001;103:89-95.

[55] Schwartz, P. J., Malliani, A. Electrical alternation of the T wave. Clinical and experimental evidence of its relationship with the sympathetic nervous system and with the long QT syndrome. *Am. Heart J.* 1975;89:45-50.

[56] Calloe, K., Cordeiro, J. M., Di Diego, J. M., et al. A transient outward potassium current activator recapitulates the electrocardiographic manifestations of Brugada syndrome. *Cardiovasc. Res.* 2009;81:686-94.

[57] Boukens, B. J., Christoffels, V. M., Coronel, R., et al. Developmental basis for electrophysiological heterogeneity in the ventricular and outflow tract myocardium as a substrate for life-threatening ventricular arrhythmias. *Circ. Res.* 2009;104:19-31.

[58] Wang, Q., Shen, J., Splawski, I., et al. SCN5A mutations associated with an inherited cardiac arrhythmia, long QT syndrome. *Cell.* 1995;80:805-11.

[59] Liu, S., Melchert, R. B., Kennedy, R. H. Inhibition of L-type Ca2+ channel current in rat ventricular myocytes by terfenadine. *Circ. Res.* 1997; 81:202-10.

[60] Morita, H., Zipes, D. P., Wu, J. Brugada syndrome: insights of ST elevation, arrhythmogenicity, and risk stratification from experimental observations. *Heart Rhythm*, 2009;6:S34-S43.

[61] Take, Y., Morita, H., Wu, J., Nagase, S., Morita, S. T., Toh, N., Nishii, N., Nakamura, K., Kusano, K. F., Ohe, T., Ito, H., Zipes, D. P. Spontaneous electrocardiogram alterations predict ventricular fibrillation in Brugada syndrome. *Heart Rhythm*, 2011; 8: 1014-1021.

[62] Morita, H., Zipes, D. P., Morita, S. T., Wu, J. Genotype-phenotype correlation in tissue models of Brugada syndrome simulating patients with sodium and calcium channelopathies. *Heart Rhythm*, 2010;7:820-827.

In: Sudden Death
Editors: Jiashin Wu and Jessica Wu

ISBN: 978-1-62618-825-9

Chapter III

SCN5A Variants and Sudden Cardiac Death

Aijun Sun**, *Lei Xu, Cheng Shen and Junbo Ge
Shanghai Institute of Cardiovascular Diseases, Zhongshan Hospital,
Institutes of Biomedical Sciences, Fudan University, Shanghai, China

Abstract

Mutations in the gene encoding for the major sodium channel (Na(v)1.5) in the heart, SCN5A, has been shown to cause a number of arrhythmia syndromes (with or without structural changes in myocardia), most of which could cause sudden cardiac death, such as the long-QT syndrome (type 3), Brugada syndrome, progressive cardiac conduction disease, sinus node dysfunction, and dilated cardiomyopathy. We investigated 32 members of a Chinese family, and found a novel SCN5A mutation A1180V associated with familial progressive atrioventricular block of adult onset and dilated cardiomyopathy.

The mutation caused a rate-dependent sodium current reduction, and a moderate increase in late sodium current. In parallel, our clinical study revealed QRS widening at high heart rates and QTc prolongation at rest in unaffected carriers. The presence of rate-dependent phenotypes in ECG may provide opportunity for early diagnosis of the dilated cardiomyopathy-associated mutation even in the absence of a genetic test. In addition, in another Chinese family with cardiac conduction abnormalities and sudden cardiac death, we identified SCN5A R1193Q polymorphism which has a similar electrophysiological property to the mutations causing long-QT syndrome (type 3). Especially, the frequency of R1193Q polymorphism is 12% in the healthy Chinese population, much higher than the Caucasians and Japanese. In this chapter, the molecular and clinical characterizations of SCN5A A1180V mutation and R1193Q polymorphism would be elucidated in detail as our original research.

Keywords: Cardiac sodium channel, sudden cardiac death

* Corresponding Author address: Email: jbge@zs-hospital.sh.cn; sun.aijun@zs-hospital.sh.cn.

Introduction

Voltage-gated sodium (Na^+) channels are responsible for the rapid upstroke of the action potential in excitable tissues. The Na^+ channel isoform $Na_v1.5$, encoded by the SCN5A gene, is predominant in the heart and plays a key role for excitability of atrial and ventricular cardiomyocytes and for rapid impulse propagation through the specific conduction system. [1] Variants in SCN5A are associated with distinct cardiac excitation disorders often leading to sudden cardiac death. Mutations in SCN5A are linked to three distinct cardiac rhythm disorders: long QT syndrome subtype 3, Brugada syndrome, and cardiac conduction diseases. [1-2] In addition to the above arrhythmias, SCN5A variants can also cause sudden cardiac death by inducing structural disease, such as dilated cardiomyopathy (DCM), which is the most common form of heart muscle diseases and a leading cause of congestive heart failure.

We identified and studied 2 SCN5A variants in 2 Chinese families respectively. One is A1180V mutation in a family with DCM preceded by progressive atrioventricular block (AVB), and the other is R1193Q polymorphism in another family with progressive cardiac conduction defect (PCCD) and long QT syndrome. As our original studies, the characterizations of R1193Q and A1180V would be elucidated as follows.

Part One

A1180V and Dilated Cardiomyopathy

Previously, SCN5A mutations have been linked with arrhythmias and cardiac conduction defect, including AV conduction block, long QT syndrome, sick sinus syndrome, sudden infant death syndrome. [3-4] Recent evidence supported that cardiac Na^+ channel gene mutation might also associate with cardiac damage and dilation. [5] Olson et al. determined that cardiac Na^+ channel mutations could lead more susceptibility to early-onset DCM, heart failure and atrial fibrillation. [6] McNair et al. also reported that D1275N of SCN5A mutation implicated in cardiac dilation and dysfunction except some conduction disorder. [7] McNair et al. detected SCN5A mutations in several DCM families and suggested a shared mechanism of disruption of the voltage-sensing mechanism of this channel leading to DCM. [8] Evidence for SCN5A mutations resulting in myocardial damage and structural abnormalities have been studied extensively, however, there are still no agreement on common mechanisms.

We found a novel SCN5A mutation A1180V in a three-generation Chinese family with age-related DCM and progressive AVB. All patients were A1180V carriers and the mutant Na^+ channel displayed abnormal properties by electrophysiological experiments in vitro. Moreover, A1180V was absent in 200 control individuals. Clinical examinations also revealed differences between the carrier and non-carrier family members. Our studies suggest that systematic characterization of the A1180V phenotype both in vitro and in clinic can help to clarify whether and how this mutation causes structural cardiac disease, which is a risk factor for sudden cardiac death.

The proband (II-1 in Figure1) had palpitation for the first time and ECG showed a first-degree AVB when he was 37 years old in 1987. He developed third-degree AVB, atrial fibrillation (AF) and cardiac dilation in 1991. He died suddenly in 2005, although a pacemaker was implanted 8 years ago. His father (I-1) progressed to third-degree AVB and AF at age 47 and died suddenly 6 years later. In addition, the proband's grandmother died suddenly at age 52. However, detail clinical records of his father and grandmother had been lost. We examined and followed up on the other members of his family until 2012, and found the carriers exhibited analogous clinical characteristics. II-3, II-7 and III-1 originally displayed first-degree AVB at ages ranging from 31 to 37 years old.

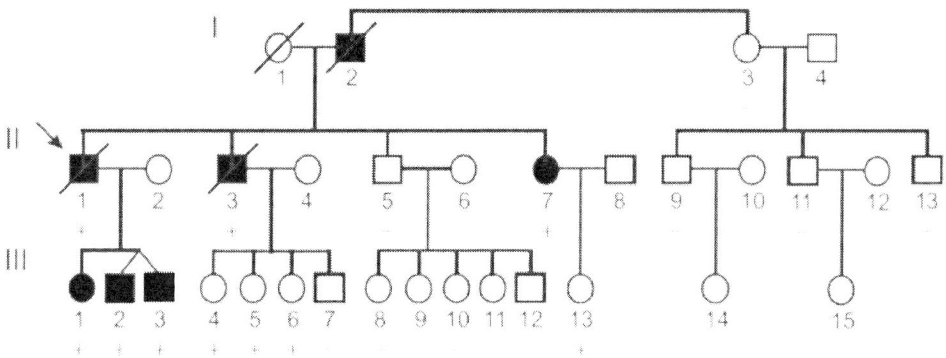

Figure 1. Pedigree of the affected family displaying the segregation of A1180V with cardiopathies in 2012. Family members are identified by represented by generations and numbers. Male and female members are respectively represented by squares and circles. Darkened symbols indicate individuals diagnosed with DCM and/or AVB. Deceased people are marked by a slash symbol. + indicates those who were proved as carriers of heterozygous A1180V mutation and - indicates noncarriers.

All of them developed third-degree AVB, cardiac dilation within 5 years after their initial onsets. II-3 died of serious heart failure in 2006, II-7 suffered severe cardiac dysfunction with a left ventricular ejection fraction of 36% as examined by echocardiography in March, 2012. In addition, III-2, III-3 were diagnosed with first-degree AVB at the ages of 31 to 33, but there had been no evidence of cardiac enlargement, conduction dysfunction, myopathy or other neuromuscular diseases at the followed-up in 2012.

We screened SCN5A mutations in all relevant members of the pedigree's family and identified several pathological regularities since 2008. To screen the encoding region of SCN5A, we isolated the participants' peripheral blood leucocytes (PBLs), and amplified genomic DNA by polymerase chain reaction using 28 pairs of intronic primers. We then compared the results with 200 unrelated healthy individuals. We identified one mutation, c.3539C>T, which results in an amino acid substitution of alanine to valine (A1180V) locating in exon 20 of SCN5A. Interestingly, A1180V was discovered in all patients and several unaffected members. In contrast, the mutation was not found among the 200 control samples. The results suggested that A1180V might be a functional mutation increasing susceptibility to cardiac dilation and progressive AVB. Figure 1 displays the distribution of A1180V in the family.

To further identify the function of A1180V mutation, we transiently transfected a wild-type cDNA and the mutated cDNA containing A1180V using an Effectene™ reagent into HEK293 cells stably expressing the β1-subunit of human Na^+ channel. Wild-type channels and A1180V channels had no differences between their maximal current densities and levels of Nav1.5 protein expression. Although without major alteration in activation, A1180V channels exhibited a moderate enhancement in the late Na^+ current and slower recovery than the wild-type channels. These changes contributed to the rate-dependency of Na^+ current, with less current at higher rate of activation.

We proposed that A1180V mutation might be a risk factor for familial DCM since it affects cardiac sodium channel function, especially at a faster rate. This could be the basis of a higher cardiac burden at faster heart rate in the A1180V carriers. To verify the hypothesis, we examined whether there were more differences between unaffected carriers and non-carriers when their heart rate was increased by exercise. On the basis of voluntary and security, all participants performed treadmill under ECG and blood pressure monitoring. 12-lead ECG and echocardiograms were recorded at different states, including resting and immediately after exercise when the heart rate was >150 bpm. There were no statistical differences in most parameters between the two groups, except the mean QRS duration, which was mildly lengthened in the unaffected carrier group while shorted in the non-carrier group with the increase of heart rate. In addition, the unaffected carrier group showed a statistically longer but normal QTc interval at rest, but the statistically discrepancy disappeared after treadmill exercise.

Our data suggested that A1180V carriers were more susceptible to DCM, especially in patients with chronic rapid heart rate. Recently, some databases showed that the prevalence rate of A1180V mutation among Asian was about 6%, suggesting that A1180V might be a common variant other than pathogenic mutations among Asians, in contrary to our previous findings. To reconcile the inconsistence, we screened A1180V among 460 healthy individuals and found the rate was 0%. In all, we concluded A1180V was likely a risk factor for familial DCM and progressive AVB, though additional genetic or environmental factors may also play roles in causing DCM.

We have identified A1180V as a major pathogenetic player in familial DCM with preceding AVB based on our basic researches and nearly 25 years of clinical follow-up of the Chinese family. Our studies found A1180V heterozygous inheritance only in this family and was absent in 660 unrelated healthy individuals. Furthermore, similar cardiovascular abnormalities and syndromes occurred only in the A1180V carriers, while absent in the non-carriers. The progression of the disease was age-dependent, with initial appearance of first-degree AVB at about 31 to 37 years old, and complete AVB and cardiac dilation nearly 5 years later in the carriers. It is well recognized that familial DCM has various modes of inheritance and phenotypic expressions depending on the defective gene. [5, 9-10] Some researchers considered DCM-related SCN5A mutations a likely initial cause of the DCM with conduction defects and arrhythmias. [6-7] Our studies suggest similar roles of A1180V in DCM, in addition to other known factors.

Because several SCN5A mutations have been linked to DCM, studies are needed to identify their mechanisms. SCN5A gene was indispensable for heart development and for maintenance of normal cardiac function. Thomas, et al. found $SCN5A^{-/-}$ mice died at the early embryos period with ventricular malformation.(11) Mutations of cardiac Na^+ channel were found to directly cause myocardial damage and structural abnormalities. So far, almost all of the reported DCM-related SCN5A mutations altered the Na^+ current, which would disturb Na^+ homeostasis, leading to dysfunction of the cellular pH and Ca^{2+} homeostasis.(12) Because Nav1.5 channels interact directly with cytoskeletal proteins, [13-14] SCN5A mutations can damage the interaction, and subsequently affect the cytoskeletal network, which is essential for the cellular structure and function.

Compared with the wild-type, A1180V channels exhibited a moderate increase in the late Na^+ current and slower recovery, which led to lower Na^+ current during tachycardia. Wagner et al. found that Ca^{2+}/calmodulin-dependent protein kinase IIδC (CaMKIIδC) could lead to the same sodium channel change as A1180V channels by direct reaction with phosphorylated cardiac Na^+ channels. [15] It was demonstrated that transgenic mice over-expressing CaMKIIδC developed DCM and heart failure. [16] Based on these, we hypothesize that A1180V might intricately result in cardiac dilation via the potential target protein CaMKIIδC. Further mechanistic insights will be available by studies on transgenic mice with A1180V mutation.

Although unveiled the roles of A1180V, we cannot rule out other possible genetic and/ or environment elements. We found that three A1180V carriers did not express any abnormalities in ECG and echocardiography even when they were almost 38 years old. The absence of abnormalities might be due to either long intervals between examinations that missed minor anomalies or due to the fact that these 3 unaffected carriers are sisters, who may share the same protective mechanisms from A1180V mutation.

Taken together, we conclude that SCN5A A1180V mutation can disturb cardiac Na^+ current and substantially contribute to the development of myocardial damage and, ultimately, to DCM.

Part Two

R1193Q and Long QT Syndrome

We have reported R1193Q polymorphism of SCN5A related to progressive cardiac conduction disease and long QT syndrome (LQTS) in a Chinese pedigree with syncope.(17) R1193Q, a single base substitution (G to A transition; 3578G→A) at the second nucleotide of codon R1193 of SCN5A, is considered as a risk factor of cardiac conduction disease, Brugada syndrome and LQTS, all of which can lead to sudden cardiac death. [2, 18-22] R1193 is located in the linker between domains II and III, several residues upstream from the proposed boundary of transmembrane segment DIIIS1. This residue is conserved among mammalian Na^+ channel isoforms, but the functional importance of the linker is still unclear and under active investigations. R1193Q can result in the neutralization of a highly conserved, positively charged side chain within the intracellular domain of the channel protein. [21] Wang et al. established R1193Q as a functional mutation using electrophysiological studies. The biophysical phenotype of the R1193Q channels markedly resembles that of well established mutations, N1325S and R1644H in SCN5A. All of them generated similar late inward currents via dispersed reopening, causing LQTS subtype 3. [21]

Interestingly, the prevalence of R1193Q differs greatly across ethnic groups. Of 281 healthy Han Chinese, we found that R1193Q was carried in 36 individuals, indicating a frequency of 12.8%, much higher than 0.2% in Whites and 2% in Japanese, but similar to 12% in Han Chinese in Taiwan. [21, 23-24] Thus, R1193Q is a common polymorphism in the Han Chinese population. However, Brugada syndrome and LQTS are very rare in Han Chinese, although R1193Q is a pathogenic mutation for Brugada syndrome and LQTS in patients of other ethnicities. Because of the differences, we speculate the presence of different characteristics of R1193Q between Han Chinese and other ethnic groups. This polymorphism might contribute to the incidence of LQTS with the presence of other co-factors, such as hypokalemia and administration of drugs lengthening QT interval. Whether this variant indeed carries an increased risk or a susceptible factor for arrhythmias in the Chinese population needs further investigations to determine.

Recently, we enrolled 128 healthy Han Chinese (77 males) volunteers who underwent R1193Q screening and standard 12-lead electrocardiograms. By direct DNA sequencing, their genotypes (R1193 or R1193Q) were identified. QT interval was measured by a technician unknown about the genotypes, and QTc was calculated by using the Bazett's formula. The result showed that among the 128 subjects, 21 were R1193Q carriers (16.4%). The average QTc of carriers was 428ms, compared with 417ms (p=0.13) of non-carriers. Furthermore, we divided the participants into 2 subgroups by gender, and found that in the female group, R1193Q carriers had a longer QTc duration (444ms) than non-carriers (422ms) with a statistical significance (p=0.03). Male carriers had a longer QTc (420ms) tendency than non-carriers (413ms) even though not reaching statistical significance (p=0.5).

Although the frequency (16.4%) of R1193Q is higher in this 128 cohorts than our previous study (12.8%), the two studies were not statistically different (p=0.33), revealing again that R1193Q is a common polymorphism in healthy Han Chinese. QTc was longer in the female group than the male group, and R1193Q is more susceptible to prolong female QTc. In addition to the genotype, acquired factors may also play a significant role in the manifestation of arrhythmias. For those female carriers, the necessity of electrocardiogram follow-ups and avoiding predisposing factors of acquired LQTS will need further investigations.

Several SCN5A mutations or polymorphisms have been associated with sudden death. For example, Winkel et al reported a SCN5A P1177L mutation by investigating the prevalence of SCN5A mutations among unselected sudden unexplained death individuals. [25] Lahtinen et al found that SCN5A rs41312391 were related to sudden cardiac death. [26] Our latest studies revealed that a novel SCN5A A1180V mutation and R1193Q polymorphism could lead to DCM, LQTS and AVB. In all, we studies suggested that SCN5A A1180V mutation could substantially contribute to cardiac injury, even though other genetic and/ or environmental factors such as rapid heart rate may also be involved in the process.

References

[1] Zimmer T, Surber R. SCN5A channelopathies--an update on mutations and mechanisms. *Prog. Biophys. Mol. Biol.* 2008 Oct-Nov;98(2-3):120-36.

[2] Morita H, Zipes DP, Wu J. Brugada syndrome: insights of ST elevation, arrhythmogenicity, and risk stratification from experimental observations. *Heart Rhythm.* 2009 Nov;6(11 Suppl):S34-43.

[3] Schott JJ, Alshinawi C, Kyndt F, Probst V, Hoorntje TM, Hulsbeek M, et al. Cardiac conduction defects associate with mutations in SCN5A. *Nature Genetics.* 1999 Sep;23(1):20-1.

[4] Tan HL, Bink-Boelkens MTE, Bezzina CR, Viswanathan PC, Beaufort-Krol GCM, van Tintelen PJ, et al. A sodium-channel mutation causes isolated cardiac conduction disease. *Nature*. 2001 Feb 22;409(6823):1043-7.

[5] Ge J, Sun A, Paajanen V, Wang S, Su C, Yang Z, et al. Molecular and Clinical Characterization of a Novel SCN5A Mutation Associated With Atrioventricular Block and Dilated Cardiomyopathy. *Circulation-Arrhythmia and Electrophysiology*. 2008 Jun;1(2):83-92.

[6] Olson TM, Michels VV, Ballew JD, Reyna SP, Karst ML, Herron KJ, et al. Sodium channel mutations and susceptibility to heart failure and atrial fibrillation. *Jama-Journal of the American Medical Association*. 2005 Jan 26;293(4):447-54.

[7] McNair WP, Ku L, Taylor MRG, Fain PR, Dao D, Wolfel E, et al. SCN5A mutation associated with dilated cardiomyopathy, conduction disorder, and arrhythmia. *Circulation*. 2004 Oct 12;110(15):2163-7.

[8] McNair WP, Sinagra G, Taylor MRG, Di Lenarda A, Ferguson DA, Salcedo EE, et al. SCN5A Mutations Associate With Arrhythmic Dilated Cardiomyopathy and Commonly Localize to the Voltage-Sensing Mechanism. *Journal of the American College of Cardiology*. 2011 May 24;57(21):2160-8.

[9] Towbin JA, Bowles NE. The failing heart. *Nature*. 2002 Jan 10;415(6868):227-33.

[10] Olson TM. What makes the heart fail? New insights from defective genes. *Acta Paediatrica*. 2006 Jul;95:17-21.

[11] Zimmer T, Bollensdorff C, Haufe V, Birch-Hirschfeld E, Benndorf K. Mouse heart Na+ channels: primary structure and function of two isoforms and alternatively spliced variants. *American Journal of Physiology-Heart and Circulatory Physiology*. 2002 Mar;282(3):H1007-H17.

[12] Frustaci A, Priori SG, Pieroni M, Chimenti C, Napolitano C, Rivolta I, et al. Cardiac histological substrate in patients with clinical phenotype of Brugada syndrome. *Circulation*. 2005 Dec 13;112(24):3680-7.

[13] Mohler PJ, Rivolta I, Napolitano C, LeMaillet G, Lambert S, Priori SG, et al. Na(v)1.5 E1053K mutation causing Brugada syndrome blocks binding to ankyrin-G and expression of Na(v)1.5 on the surface of cardiomyocytes. *Proceedings of the National Academy of Sciences of the United States of America*. 2004 Dec 14;101(50):17533-8.

[14] Gavillet B, Rougier J-S, Domenighetti AA, Behar R, Boixel C, Ruchat P, et al. Cardiac sodium channel Na(v)1.5 is regulated by a multiprotein complex composed of syntrophins and dystrophin. *Circulation Research*. 2006 Aug 18;99(4):407-14.

[15] Wagner S, Dybkova N, Rasenack ECL, Jacobshagen C, Fabritz L, Kirchhof P, et al. Ca2+/calmodulin-dependent protein kinase II regulates cardiac Na+ channels. *Journal of Clinical Investigation*. 2006 Dec;116(12):3127-38.

[16] Zhang T, Maier LS, Dalton ND, Miyamoto S, Ross J, Bers DM, et al. The delta(C) isoform of CaMKII is activated in cardiac hypertrophy and induces dilated cardiomyopathy and heart failure. *Circulation Research*. 2003 May 2;92(8):912-9.

[17] Sun A, Xu L, Wang S, Wang K, Huang W, Wang Y, et al. SCN5A R1193Q polymorphism associated with progressive cardiac conduction defects and long QT syndrome in a Chinese family. *J. Med. Genet.* 2008 Feb;45(2):127-8.

[18] Park HS, Kim YN, Lee YS, Jung BC, Lee SH, Shin DG, et al. Genetic Analysis of SCN5A in Korean Patients Associated with Atrioventricular Conduction Block. *Genomics Inform.* 2012 Jun;10(2):110-6.

[19] Huang H, Zhao J, Barrane FZ, Champagne J, Chahine M. Nav1.5/R1193Q polymorphism is associated with both long QT and Brugada syndromes. *Can. J. Cardiol.* 2006 Mar 15;22(4):309-13.

[20] Morita H, Wu J, Zipes DP. The QT syndromes: long and short. *Lancet.* 2008 Aug 30;372(9640):750-63.

[21] Wang Q, Chen S, Chen Q, Wan X, Shen J, Hoeltge GA, et al. The common SCN5A mutation R1193Q causes LQTS-type electrophysiological alterations of the cardiac sodium channel. *J. Med. Genet.* 2004 May;41(5):e66.

[22] Skinner JR, Chung SK, Montgomery D, McCulley CH, Crawford J, French J, et al. Near-miss SIDS due to Brugada syndrome. *Arch. Dis. Child.* 2005 May;90(5):528-9.

[23] Takahata T, Yasui-Furukori N, Sasaki S, Igarashi T, Okumura K, Munakata A, et al. Nucleotide changes in the translated region of SCN5A from Japanese patients with Brugada syndrome and control subjects. *Life Sciences.* 2003 Apr 11;72(21):2391-9.

[24] Hwang HW, Chen JJ, Lin YJ, Shieh RC, Lee MT, Hung SI, et al. R1193Q of SCN5A, a Brugada and long QT mutation, is a common polymorphism in Han Chinese. *J. Med. Genet.* 2005 Feb;42(2):e7; author reply e8.

[25] Winkel BG, Larsen MK, Berge KE, Leren TP, Nissen PH, Olesen MS, et al. The prevalence of mutations in KCNQ1, KCNH2, and SCN5A in an unselected national cohort of young sudden unexplained death cases. *J. Cardiovasc. Electrophysiol.* 2012 Oct;23(10):1092-8.

[26] Lahtinen AM, Noseworthy PA, Havulinna AS, Jula A, Karhunen PJ, Kettunen J, et al. Common genetic variants associated with sudden cardiac death: the FinSCDgen study. *Plos One*. 2012;7(7):e41675.

In: Sudden Death
Editors: Jiashin Wu and Jessica Wu

ISBN: 978-1-62618-825-9

Chapter IV

Predictors and Prevention of Sudden Cardiac Death

Yumei Hou, Jialu Hu, Indra Prasad Upadhyay, Zengyong Qiao, Ling Zhang and Sunny S. Po*

Heart Rhythm Institute, University of Oklahoma Health Sciences Center, Oklahoma City, OK, US

Abstract

Sudden cardiac death (SCD) indicates death following cardiac arrest with or without preexisting cardiovascular disease [1]. This mode of unexpected, natural death often occurs outside a hospital or emergency room and can be caused by any type of cardiovascular disease. The duration between the onset of symptoms and loss of consciousness (or death) is typically within one hour [1, 2]. SCD has the features of sudden onset, rapid progression and high mortality [1-3]. The incidence SCD is significantly higher in males. SCD is often caused by cardiac arrhythmias such as ventricular fibrillation (VF), ventricular tachycardia (VT), bradycardia/asystole or pulseless electrical activity as well as non-arrhythmic causes [3-10]. While ventricular arrhythmias were the leading cause of SCD, SCD is also strongly associated with coronary artery disease, left ventricular dysfunction, genetic disorders such as long QT syndrome and disturbances of the autonomic nervous system [3-10].

SCD is a common cause of death in industrialized countries. It was estimated that more than three million people die of SCD each year in the world [1-4, 6]. Using China as an example, the incidence of SCD was 41.84/10,000 persons/year [7]. Based on a population of 1.3 billion, the annual mortality of SCD in China was 544,000. Although the name SCD indicates that death occurs suddenly, warning signs or prodromes often existed prior to the fatal event but unfortunately were neglected by the victims and/or physicians. Identifying reliable predictors to prevent SCD has been a daunting challenge. Numerous techniques have been proposed to be valuable in preventing SCD, including electrophysiology study, T wave alternans, signal averaged ECG, autonomic nervous

* Correspondence: Sunny S. Po, MD, Ph.D. sunny-po@ouhsc.edu.

system activity, left ventricular ejection fraction, scars identified by cardiac MRI/echocardiography, genetic analysis, family history and exercise test [1-3,11-19]. Unfortunately, none of the aforementioned techniques can accurately predict SCD. More research is therefore needed to identify reliable predictors for SCD and provide more accurate risk stratification as well as appropriate preventive measures for patients at a significant risk of SCD.

Prevention of SCD

SCD prevention includes primary and secondary prevention. The former is to identify the population at a high risk before SCD occurs and provides specific therapy to prevent the 1st event of SCD. In theory, every individual carries a small risk of SCD but only a very small fraction of people in the general population eventually suffer from SCD. Moreover, the majority of SCD victims did not have the traditional risk factors for cardiovascular diseases or symptoms suggesting a high risk of SCD. The greatest challenge of primary prevention for SCD is to apply highly specific markers to identify a very small subgroup in the general population that is at a high risk of SCD and then provide preventive therapy only to this group of people. In sharp contrast, secondary prevention is less of a problem due to the wide-spread use of implantable cardioverter-defibrillator (ICD) in patients who survived SCD.

Multiple studies indicated that SCD is closely related to ventricular arrhythmias, depressed LV function, coronary artery disease (CAD) and cardiomyopathy [6-13]. It is simply not possible to provide every patient with these risk factors with an ICD. An extreme example is that in patients *appeared* to be at a very high risk of sudden death as a result of LV dysfunction from a recent (<40 days) myocardial infarction, the benefit of ICD to prevent SCD in this "apparent" very high risk group of patients has not been shown [9]. This "paradox" further underscores the necessity of developing highly specific, cost-effective risk stratification strategies to identify patients who are truly at a high risk of SCD.

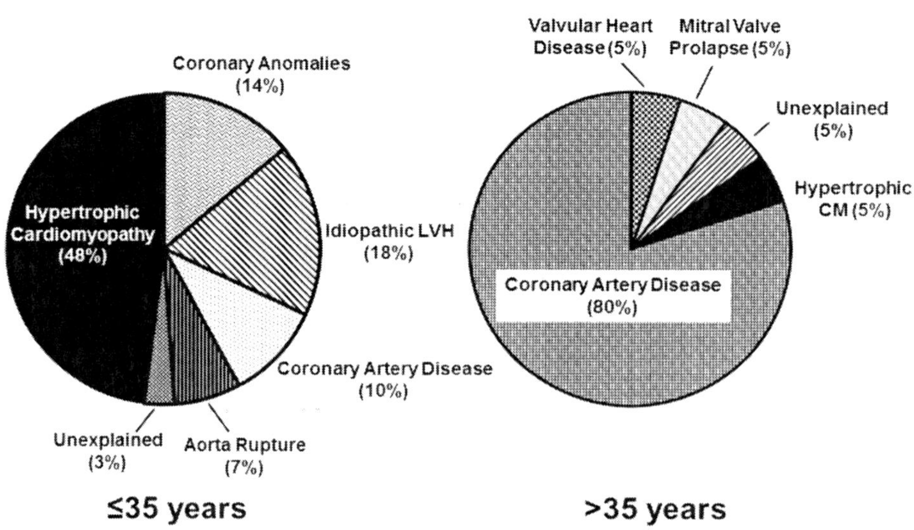

Figure 1. Causes of sudden cardiac death in competitive athletes.

SCD in Patients with Significant Cardiovascular Diseases

I. Coronary Artery Disease (CAD)

It was estimated that approximately 80% of all SCD in the US and Western Europe are related to CAD [1-3]. In SCD victims, the structural changes in the coronary arteries can be both acute and chronic. In an autopsy study of 171 SCD victims, Perper et al, reported that the majority of the victims had 3-4 major coronary arteries showing >75% luminal stenosis and similar changes were seen in 2 vessels in another 15% patients [20]. The risk of SCD is substantially higher in CAD patients in the presence of the following conditions: (a) multi-vessel diseases, diffuse coronary artery diseases and new thrombus in the coronary artery. In 100 patients with CAD who died suddenly (<6 hours), coronary artery thrombi were found in 74/100 patients [21]. No difference was found among the patients who died within 15 minutes, within 1 hour or after 1 hour. In the 26 patients without coronary artery thrombus, plaque fissuring was found in 21 patients. SCD in acute coronary syndrome is often caused by VF or VT as a result of ischemia and/or reperfusion arrhythmias. (b) CAD with prior history of SCD: Within a year following a successful resuscitation for SCD, the incidence of SCD caused by a recurrence of VF was as high as 30% [22-23] and (c) CAD associated with factors that lower the threshold for VF (e.g. excessive smoking, agitation or any conditions that markedly enhance the sympathetic tone). These factors tend to increase the release of catecholamines and increase myocardial oxygen demand, subsequent leading to VF and SCD.

While CAD is the most common cause of SCD in the general population, the causes of SCD in younger people are quite different (Figure 1). In competitive athletes, hypertrophic cardiomyopathy accounts for >50% SCD in younger athletes (≤35 y/o), followed by idiopathic LV hypertrophy (18%) and coronary anomalies (14%)(24). In contrast, CAD account for 80% of SCD in older competitive athletes (≥35 y/o). These differences provide important clues in terms of screening competitive athletes in different age groups to prevent SCD.

II. LV Systolic Dysfunction and Cardiomyopathy

LV ejection fraction (LVEF) <35% is the most widely accepted predictor for total mortality in heart failure patients but its value of predicting SCD varies with different etiologies of heart failure. In heart failure patients with NYHA class II, class III and class IV, SCD accounts for 64%, 59% and 33% of deaths, respectively (25). NYHA class IV patients are more likely to die of pump failure than SCD. The incidence of SCD in heart failure patients is known to be substantially higher in the presence of ventricular arrhythmias, particularly non-sustained ventricular tachycardia and frequent ventricular premature depolarizations (PVD) [13, 22]. Primary and secondary prevention of SCD in heart failure patients has been the focus of the ICD trials in the past two decades and the value of ICD for preventing SCD in these patients has been well established.

While CAD-related diseases cause >80% SCD, patients with dilated cardiomyopathy, hypertrophic cardiomyopathy (HCM) and arrhythmogenic RV cardiomyopathy (ARVC) account for nearly 10% of the SCD in adults [27, 28].

SCD among these patients with non-ischemic cardiomyopathy is more difficult to predict than that of the CAD patients. Electrolyte imbalance caused by diuretics, hyperactivity of the sympathetic nervous system, dispersion of refractoriness caused by antiarrhythmic drugs and other neurohormonal factors are known to predispose cardiomyopathy patients to SCD.

In a significant number of HCM patients, SCD occurred before 20 years of age [23-25]. The presence of the following findings indicate an increased risk of SCD in this group of patients: (a) survival of previous cardiac arrest such as VF, (b) frequent or long episodes of non-sustained VT recorded by Holter monitoring, (c) history of HCM-related premature sudden death in family, (d) unexplained syncope, particularly in young patients, (e) exercise-induced decrease in systolic blood pressure, (f) thickness of interventricular septum or LV wall larger than 30 mm and (g) pressure gradient across the LV outflow tract larger than 50 mm Hg. Early ICD implantation for primary prevention in these high risk patients had been proven to prevent arrhythmia death based on appropriate ICD shocks for VT/VF [28, 29]. The presence of more risk factors is associated with higher likelihood of appropriate ICD shocks too.

ARVC is a hereditary cardiomyopathy known to cause VT, VF and SCD. In addition, SCD is often related to exercise. Fibrous-fatty infiltration of the right ventricular myocardium is pathognomic of ARVC and is believed to cause ventricular tachyarrhythmia by providing reentrant substrates created by fatty tissue and fibrosis infiltrating the RV myocardium. Factors indicating a higher risk of SCD in ARVC patients include: (a) history of SCD, (b) unexplained syncope (c) sustained compromised VT, (d) severe right ventricular dilatation verified by cardiac MRI or echocardiolography, (e) left ventricular wall motion abnormality or impaired LV systolic function or (f) nonsustained VT. Although ARVC is known to be caused by mutations of the gene encoding desmosomes, the sensitivity and specificity of genetic testing for the use of risk stratification have not been established.

III. Cardiac Arrhythmias

Malignant ventricular arrhythmia is the leading risk factor of SCD. Malignant ventricular arrhythmias usually refer to arrhythmias with significant hemodynamic compromise and are likely progress to VF or SCD.

It is important to note that the incidence of out-of-hospital VF arrest in the Seattle area and probably the entire United States has been declining, presumably due to the nation-wide decline in the coronary artery disease mortality (Figure 2) [31]. However, the incidence of pulseless electrical activity and asystole did not show the same trend. While ventricular arrhythmias are often caused by structural heart diseases, SCD can be caused by conditions such as Wolff-Parkinson-White syndrome, long-QT syndrome or pharmacological agents in the absence of any detectable structural heart disease [32, 33].

Wolff-Parkinson-White syndrome, SCD is caused by rapid antegrade conduction to the ventricle over the accessory pathway that leads to VF and SCD. Inadvertent use of AV nodal blocking during preexcited AF may result in VF as well.

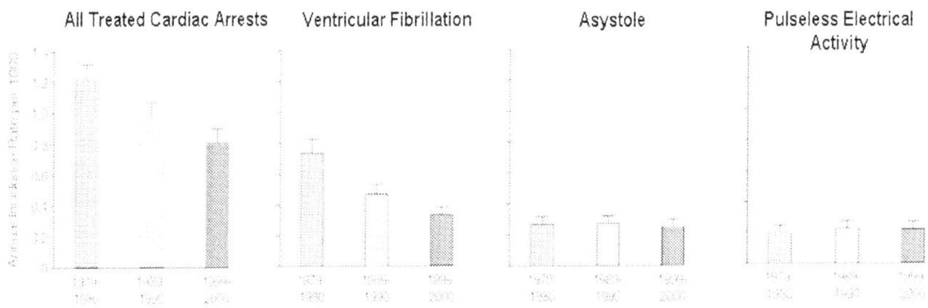

Figure 2. Age and Gender Adjusted Incidence Rate of Treated Out-of-Hospital Cardiac Arrest. The rates of the first recorded rhythms are represented as mean rates with 95% confidence intervals (error bars). Rates are adjusted in the Seattle, Washington population in 2000. The incidence of SCD decreased progressive in each decade, mainly due to a reduced incidence of VF as the first identified rhythm [31].

Wolff-Parkinson-White syndrome, SCD is caused by rapid antegrade conduction to the ventricle over the accessory pathway that leads to VF and SCD. Inadvertent use of AV nodal blocking during preexcited AF may result in VF as well.

IV. Valvular Heart Diseases and Congenital Heart Diseases

Among valvular heart diseases, severe aortic stenosis is most commonly associated with SCD. Although the incidence of SCD for severe symptomatic aortic stenosis is very high, patients with asymptomatic severe aortic stenosis is at a much lower risk of SCD, approximately 1% per year [34]. Mitral valve stenosis carries a high risk of strokes but SCD only accounts for a small number of deaths in these patients.

Other valvular disease as well as other untreated congenital heart diseases may lead to Eisenmenger syndrome (pulmonary hypertension and right-to-left shunt) and high incidence of SCD. Congenital heart diseases such as Tetralogy of Fallot, transposition of great arteries are also related to SCD because of a higher propensity to VT or VF. Importantly, late death can still occur after corrective surgery, indicating close follow-up is required in adults with corrected severe congenital heart diseases [1, 2, 35].

Predictors of SCD

Prevention of SCD remains exceedingly challenging despite the advances of medical technologies. Numerous minimally invasive or non-invasive methods to identify patients at a high risk of SCD have been developed. Although the benefit of electrophysiologic study in patients with ischemic cardiomyopathy and nonsustained VT had been widely accepted [13, 26], cost-effectiveness and risks of an invasive procedure preclude its use to risk stratify a large population of people.

In 2008, the Expert Consensus of AHA/ACC/HRS identified a number of non-invasive means for the purpose of risk stratification: LVEF, exercise capacity/functional status, conduction delay (QRS width, late potentials, fragmented QRS complex), repolarization abnormality (T wave alternans, QT dispersion, QT interval), imbalance of the cardiac autonomic nervous system (heart rate variability, heart rate turbulence, deceleration capacity, baroreceptor sensitivity) [5,36-40].

1. Left Ventricular Ejection Fraction (LVEF)

LVEF is a convenient and the most widely used means to predict the risk of SCD. The relationship between LV systolic dysfunction, malignant ventricular arrhythmias and SCD has been well established. The MUSTT trial found that LVEF less than 40% is a strong indicator of high risk for SCD. In addition, patients with LVEF less than 30% carrying a much higher risk of arrhythmia death total mortality [13,26,41].The MADIT-II trial randomized patients with history of prior myocardial infarction and depressed LV function to medical therapy and the ICD therapy [42]. The results showed that the mortality rate of the ICD group was reduced by 31%. The risk of ventricular arrhythmia in patients with LVEF between the 30 and 40% was 4.3% per year with a sensitivity of 59.1% and specificity of 77.8%.

Most of the large-scale randomized clinical trials to investigate the mortality benefits of ICD utilized EF less than 35-40% as the cut-off value for recruitment. Although LVEF is the most commonly used tools for risk stratification of SCD in heart failure patients, it is limited by its specificity and sensitivity, particularly primary prevention in non-ischemic dilated cardiomyopathy patients [3].

For instance, in heart failure patients received ICD for primary prevention, approximately 2/3 these patients never had an appropriate ICD discharge within 5 years, indicating that LVEF alone is not capable of identifying the real high risk patients who require primary prevention for SCD. It is therefore widely accepted that LVEF less than 35% is a good indicator for poor cardiovascular outcome but remains a poor indicator for ICD implantation. The false positive rate for predicting SCD remains high and inappropriate ICD shocks for atrial fibrillation or other supraventricular tachycardia continues to be a challenge.

2. New York Heart Association (NYHA) Functional Class

The NYHA class indication is a subjective evaluation for the severity of heart failure. It is helpful to predict the mode of death in heart failure patients. A significant number of the NYHA class II-III patients died of SCD but most of the class IV patients died of pump failure [1-3]. While ICD implantation significantly improved the survival rate of NYHA class II-III patients but the benefit for class IV patients remains debatable, mainly because the proportion of SCD decreases and death due to pump failure increases in class IV patients [1-3].

3. ECG Findings

Width of the QRS Complex

The width of the QRS wave of the 12 ECG is a non-invasive and highly reproducible means to assess ventricular depolarization as well as intraventricular and interventricular conduction delay. In patients with ischemic cardiomyopathy, QRS duration >120 ms is associated with higher incidence of SCD [3]. However, the association between QRS width and SCD in non-ischemic dilated cardiomyopathy patients is not well-established. Progressive increases in QRS width over time often suggest progression of the myocardial disease.

In patients with heart failure, increasing width of the QRS complex is an indicator of poor prognosis [43] because dysynchronization not only reduces the LV systolic function, it also increases the ventricular repolarization dispersion, leading to the development of ventricular tachyarrhythmias [44].

Factors such as bundle branch block, intraventricular conduction delay, coronary artery disease, cardiomyopathy, myocardial hypertrophy, electrolyte imbalance and ischemia all contribute to the widening of the QRS in CHF patients [43-46]. The value of using QRS width for risk stratification in heart failure patients is therefore limited.

QTc Interval

The QTc interval provides clues to both ventricular depolarization and repolarization. Prolonged QTc interval is associated with imbalance of the autonomic nervous system, hereditary channelopathy, pharmacological agents, cerebrovascular disease, brain injury and electrolyte imbalance. In the presence of prolonged QTc interval, either congenital or acquired, a ventricular pause followed by a premature ventricular beat (a long-short sequence) leads to great enhancement of the dispersion of ventricular refractoriness, setting the stage for torsade de pointe and subsequently SCD.

While prevention of SCD in acquired long QT syndrome is obviously removing the offending pharmacological agents or treating the underlying conditions such as electrolyte imbalance, preventing SCD in congenital long QT patients remains challenging due to a wide range of genetic mutations and triggering factors.

For instance, LQT2 and LQT3 patients are at low risk for SCD induced by exercise but LQT1 is known to be strongly related to exercise [47]. Using β-lockers to prevent SCD would work better for LQT1 patients than other forms of LQT syndrome patients.

Because of the dynamic nature of the QT interval and various factors that affect it, QTc interval and its derivatives (QT dispersion and QT variability) are yet to be proven to be effective in risk stratification for patients without congenital long QT syndrome.

Abnormal J-Wave

The J-point marks the end of the QRS complex, theoretically the moment when depolarization ends and repolarization starts. An abnormal J-point indicates the junctional point between the QRS complex and T wave is elevated by >0.1 mV [48, 49]. A problem of measuring the J-point is that the transition from depolarization (QRS complex) into repolarization (ST segment) may be delayed and subsequently obscures the J-point. While hypothermia and myocardial ischemia produce elevated J-point, two syndromes with elevated J-points have attracted enormous attention over the past decade: Brugada syndrome and early repolarization syndrome.

a. Brugada Syndrome

In 1992s, the Brugada brothers reported the association between right bundle branch block, ST elevation and nocturnal SCD among young male patients [50]. Based on findings of cellular electrophysiology, the ventricular tachyarrhythmia in Brugada syndrome patients was proposed to be caused by phase-II reentry [51]. The epicardium of the RV has significantly larger transient outward K^+ current (I_{TO}) than the RV endocardium. Mutations in the cardiac sodium channel (SCN5A) leads to unopposed epicardial repolarization by the I_{TO} current and subsequently marked shortening of the action potential duration. Phase II reentry is initiated by electrotonic current flowing from cells with longer action potentials to neighboring cells with shorter action potentials, leading to reentrant VT and consequently SCD. While Brugada syndrome was considered a repolarization disorder, a competing hypothesis ("depolarization hypothesis") was proposed in which ventricular tachyarrhythmia was thought to be caused by reentry as a result of the combination slow ventricular conduction due to sodium channel mutation and scars in the RV epicardium [48]. While syncope in Brugada syndrome patients heralds a high risk of SCD, primary prevention of SCD for Brugada syndrome patients remains a challenge as the risk of SCD in patients with Type-I Brugada ECG is only 0.5% per year [53].

b. Early Repolarization Syndrome

In 2008, Haissaguerre et al. reported a group of patients survived SCD caused by idiopathic VF whose baseline ECGs showed early repolarization pattern with J-point elevation >0.1 mV in the inferior and/or lateral leads (31% in SCD victims vs. 5% in control subjects, $p<0.001$). Moreover, the incidence of recurrence of VF was 14%, substantially higher than the control group [54]. Later studies confirmed these findings and also noted that patients with more diffuse pattern of early repolarization and ST segment with a horizontal-descending pattern carry a much higher risk of VF and SCD [55,56]. Although ECG pattern of early repolarization is far more common in patients suffered from idiopathic VF (SCD), early repolarization is a very common ECG finding, particularly in young adults. The vast majority subjects with early repolarization are not at a higher risk of SCD. Rosso et al. estimated that the incidence of idiopathic VF associated with early repolarization was 11:1,000,000. Such a high false positive rate precludes the use of early repolarization as a predictor for SCD [57, 58]. Whether diffuse early repolarization can be used as a predictor for SCD is to be determined.

Fragmented wide QRS Complex

Fragmented wide QRS (f-wQRS) is typically presented by relatively low amplitude associated with additional deflection or notch of the QRS complex in 12 lead ECG (59,60). f-wQRS is a hallmark of conduction delay and is often caused by myocardial scars as a result of structural heart disease such as myocardial infarction, congenital heart disease, arrhythmogenic RV cardiomyopathy and Brugada syndrome [59-63]. The presence of f-wQRS often indicates the presence of advanced diseases and it can be a useful tool for risk stratification of SCD. If f-wQRS is present in at least two adjacent ECG leads, it can be used to predict the presence of infarct scar(s) with the sensitivity, specificity, positive predictive value, and negative predictive value of 86.8%, 92.5%, 92.0%, and 87.5%, respectively (59,62). Das et al found that in patients of CAD, a significantly higher mortality exists in the f-wQRS group when compared with the group with wide QRS complex but without QRS fragmentation. Similar survival differences were also noted in patients with fragmented QRS in premature ventricular depolarizations.

Prior studies also indicate that f-wQRS may serve as a predictor for SCD in patients with prior myocardial infarction. In patients with prior MI, the death rate for patients with f-wQRS was 34% over 5.5 years, significantly higher than those without f-wQRS (26%), suggesting that f-wQRS may be a positive predictor for death in patients with prior MI [65]. Similar findings were reported in patients with non-ischemic cardiomyopathy in which 51% patients with f-wQRS received appropriate ICD therapy. f-wQRS is also associated with cardiomyopathy in the right ventricle. Peters et al. reported that f-wQRS was found in 85% patients with ARVC, indicating that f-wQRS may serve as an important criteria for the diagnosis of ARVC [61]. f-wQRS may have roles in early diagnosis of a ARVC and predicting the occurrence of VT or SCD. Morita et al. reported that f-wQRS was recorded in 43% of Brugada syndrome patients [62]. In Brugada syndrome patients, f-wQRS was found in 85%, 50%, 34% patients with ventricular tachyarrhythmia, syncope and without symptoms, respectively. In general, f-wQRS is a very helpful predictor with the advantages of an acceptable positive predictive value, reproducibility, non-invasiveness and low cost. At present, the value of fQRS for predicting SCD is limited only to patient with clinical evidence of myocardial scars or primary depolarization abnormality such as Brugada syndrome [60]. Its value in risk stratification for SCD is yet to be verified by large-scale clinical trials.

T-Wave Abnormality

Prior studies indicate that the changes in T wave in 12 lead ECG are very strong predictors for cardiovascular death, better than ST depression, left ventricular hypertrophy and QRS duration [64-66]. T wave alternans (TWA) manifest as beat-by-beat changes in the morphology, polarity or amplitude of the T waves, indicating the presence of substantial abnormality of ventricular repolarization and a high risk of developing ventricular tachyarrhythmia [64,65].

TWA may be difficult to observe clinically due to its small-scale changes in the micro volt range. Such micro-volt TWA has to be detected by special equipment.

If sustained alternans is detected at a heart rate <110 bpm, the result is considered positive. As "physiological" alternans may develop in normal subjects at a higher heart rate, a cut-off heart rate of 110 bpm provides better specificity [67]. The sensitivity of micro-volt TWA is enhanced by combining with exercise as micro-volt TWA would not be apparent until the heart rate is above a threshold heart rate.

Studies indicate that micro-volt TWA may provide prognostic information about VT/VF in patients suffered from MI [68,69] Importantly, micro-wave TWA offers a high negative predictive value for SCD in patients with both ischemic and non-ischemic cardiomyopathy [70-72]. If its high negative predictive value is proven by future large clinical trials, it may dramatically reduce the number of ICD implantation for primary prevention in heart failure patients.

Ventricular Late Potential

Ventricular late potential (VLP) manifests as high-frequency, low amplitude potentials at or after the end of the QRS complex [73-75]. Detection of VLP is often assisted by signal-averaged ECG to remove the noise in order to expose the low amplitude late potentials. VLP most commonly occurs in patients with prior MI or other cardiac diseases associated with myocardial scars in which surviving myocardial bundles traverse myocardial scars and form a large slow conduction zone.

A significant delay of the depolarization wavefront to exit this slow conduction zone therefore generates the late potentials. VLP indicates the presence of both marked heterogeneity of depolarization as well as repolarization, setting the stage for reentrant tachyarrhythmias. In patients with prior MI, the sensitivity and the specificity for VLP to prevent malignant tachyarrhythmias is 58-92% and 72-100% [77,78].

While VLP is a very useful tool for understanding the mechanism of ventricular tachyarrhythmia in patients with structural heart disease, its value is limited by the relatively low positive predictive value and the presence of bundle branch block or significant intraventricular conduction delay that seriously lower the sensitivity of detecting VLP.

4. Autonomic Nervous System

The normal cardiac rhythm is controlled by a coordinated and balanced action of the sympathetic and the parasympathetic nervous system. The sympathetic activity reduces the threshold for VT or VF but that parasympathetic activity exerts the opposite effect. There is no surprise that the incidence of SCD is increased in the presence of any imbalance toward sympathetic hyperactivity.

Heart Rate Variability (HRV)

HRV represents the minor change of the sinus cycle length during normal sinus rhythm. Power spectral analysis identifies several frequency bands in which high frequency (HF; 0.15-0.45 Hz), low frequency (LF; 0.05-0.15 Hz) and the ratio of LF/HF are commonly used to assess the autonomic function. The HF component is thought to represent the parasympathetic activity while the LF and particularly LF/HF reflect the sympathetic activity. HRV reflects the effects of the autonomic nervous system on regulating the sinus rhythm, particularly the balance between the sympathetic and parasympathetic nervous system [79, 80].

Since the cardiovascular system is often viewed as a system that is controlled by pressure, any factor that affects blood pressure can modulate the heart rate [80]. The best example is baroreflex which is triggered by changes in the blood pressure. The presence of mechanoreceptors in the atrium, ventricle, lungs as well as the aortic and carotid body function as sensors of the pressure at individual point.

The afferent inputs from these receptors were transmitted to the central nervous system by the autonomic nervous system. Through a series of reflexes occurring in the brain stem, the efferent autonomic nerve fibers maintain the homeostasis of the cardiovascular function. Low HRV is a good predictor for total mortality but not necessarily SCD in heart failure patients [79, 80]. The widespread use of beta blockers in heart failure patients also limits the role of HRV as a strong predictor for SCD in these patients.

Heart Rate Turbulence (HRT)

HRT presents the acceleration and then deceleration response of the sinus rate following a premature ventricular depolarization (PVD) (82). In other words, HRT reflects the sensitivity of the sinus node in response to a PVD and the sensitivity of the parasympathetic activity to modulate blood pressure. In comparison with HRV, HRT is less affected by the average heart rate, use of beta blocker and LVEF. In post-MI patients, patients with a low risk of SCD, HRT following a PVD was substantially more prominent than that of the patients with a higher risk of SCD in whom HRT was markedly reduced or even disappeared (82). The numerical quantification of HRT is represented by two values: turbulence onset (TO) and turbulence slope (TS). TO is defined as the difference between the mean of the first two sinus RR intervals after the PVD and the last two sinus RR intervals before the PVD, divided by the mean of the last two sinus RR interval before the PVD [82]. TS is defined as the maximum positive slope of a regression line assessed over any sequence of five consecutive sinus RR intervals within the first 20 sinus RR intervals following a PVD. TS ≤2.5 ms and TO≥0% may serve as a good predictor for SCD in patients with prior MI but its clinical utility will need further studies.

Deceleration Capacity of Rate (DC)

Bauer et al. proposed a new technique to examine the autonomic tone in order to risk stratify patients at lower risk of SCD (83). DC is determined by analyzing 24-hour Holter monitoring to determine the capacity of the heart rate to decelerate as an indicator of the parasympathetic tone and to predict the risk of SCD.

In patients with preserved DC (>4.5 ms), the risk of mortality is extremely low. In contrast, patients with lower DC (<2.5 ms) carry a high risk of mortality even with preserved LV. The results can be explained by a reduced parasympathetic tone that failed to protect the heart from malignant arrhythmias and the SCD.

Conclusion

Prevention of SCD continues to face ongoing challenges. First, most of the SCD occurred in the general population without the history of cardiac diseases.

To date, a measure that can reliably identify the high risk individuals in the general population is still lacking and the primary prevention of SCD in the general population is still out of reach. Second, the definition of SCD is not unified yet and the mechanisms underlying SCD are yet to be understood, leading to the discrepancies between the results of clinical trials and the epidemiology studies.

Third, most studies to prevent SCD were done in patients with cardiac diseases. The success of secondary prevention cannot be extrapolated to primary prevention of SCD. Fourth, the cost of ICD implantation is too high to serve as a means to prevent SCD in the general population.

In patients with significant risk factors for cardiovascular diseases or patients already suffering from mild to moderate cardiac diseases, aggressive lifestyle modification (e.g. smoking cession), aggressive treatment for hypertension, diabetes or hyperlipidemia, effective use of aspirin, beta blocker, ACE inhibitor/ARB may be the most effective means to prevent SCD in this population of patients.

References

[1] Myerburg R, Castellanos A. Sudden cardiac death. Zipes DP, Jalife J. Cardiac Electrophysiology: From Cell to Bedside. 5th ed.Philadelphia: *Saunders Elsevier*.2009:979-805.

[2] Myerburg RJ, Castellanos A.Cardiac arrest and sudden cardiac death [M].bIn:Libby P' Bonow RO.Mann DL.Zipes DP.eds.Braunwald'S heart disease,8th ed.Philadelphia: *Saunders Elsevier* .2012:845-884.

[3] Kong MH, Fonarow GC, Peterson ED, et al. Systematic review of the incidence of sudden cardiac death in the United States. *J. Am. Coll. Cardiol.*2011,57(7):794-801.

[4] Zheng ZJ, Croft JB, Giles W, Mensah GA. Sudden cardiac death in the United States, 1989 to 1998.*Circulation*,2001,104(18):2158-2163.

[5] Goldberger JJ, Cain ME, Hohnloser SH, Kadish AH, Knight BP, Lauer MS, Maron BJ, Page RL, Passman RS, Siscovick D, Siscovick D, Stevenson WG, Zipes DP; American Heart Association; American College of Cardiology Foundation; Heart Rhythm Society. American Heart Association/American College of Cardiology Foundation/Heart Rhythm Society scientific statement on noninvasive risk stratification techniques for identifying patients at risk for sudden cardiac death: a scientific statement from the American Heart Association Council on Clinical Cardiology Committee on Electrocardiography and Arrhythmias and Council on Epidemiology and Prevention. *Circulation*, 2008,118(14):1497-1518.

[6] Leslie LK, Cohen JT, Newburger JW, Alexander ME, Wong JB, Sherwin ED, Rodday AM, Parsons SK, Triedman JK. Costs and benefits of targeted screening for causes of sudden cardiac death in children and adolescents. *Circulation,* 2012,125(21):2621-2629.

[7] Hua W, Zhang LF, Wu YF, Liu XQ, Guo DS, Zhou HL, Gou ZP, Zhao LC, Niu HX, Chen KP, Mai JZ, Chu LN, Zhang S. Incidence of sudden cardiac death in China: analysis of 4 regional populations. *J. Am. Coll. Cardiol.*, 2009,54(12):1110-1118.

[8] Sweeney MO, Sherfesee L, DeGroot PJ, Wathen MS, Wilkoff BL. Differences in effects of electrical therapy type for ventricular arrhythmias on mortality in implantable cardioverter-defibrillator patients. *Heart Rhythm,* 2010,7(3):353-360.

[9] Hohnloser SH, Kuck KH, Dorian P, Roberts RS, Hampton JR, Hatala R, Fain E, Gent M, Connolly SJ; DINAMIT Investigators. Prophylactic use of an implantable cardioverter-defibrillator after acute myocardial infarction. *N. Engl. J. Med.* 2004,351(24):2481–2488.

[10] Moss AJ, Hall WJ, Cannom DS, Daubert JP, Higgins SL, Klein H, Levine JH, Saksena S, Waldo AL, Wilber D, Brown MW, Heo M. Improved survival with an implanted defibrillator in patients with coronary disease at high risk for ventricular arrhythmia. Multicenter Automatic Defibrillator Implantation Trial Investigators. *N. Engl. J. Med.* 1996,335(26):1933-1940.

[11] Myerburg RJ, Mitrani R, Interian A Jr, Castellanos A. Interpretation of outcomes of antiarrhythmic clinical trials: design features and population impact. *Circulation,* 1998,97(15):1514-1521.

[12] Huikuri HV, Tapanainen JM, Lindgren K, Raatikainen P, Mäkikallio TH, Juhani Airaksinen KE, Myerburg RJ. Prediction of sudden cardiac death after myocardial infarction in the beta-blocking era. *J. Am. Coll. Cardiol.,* 2003,42(4):652-658.

[13] Buxton AE, Lee KL, Fisher JD, Josephson ME, Prystowsky EN, Hafley GE. A randomized study of the prevention of sudden death in patients with coronary artery disease. Multicenter Unsustained Tachycardia Trial Investigators. N Engl J Med 2000, 342(17):1300-1305

[14] Walker ML, Rosenbaum DS. Repolarization alternans: implications for the mechanism and prevention of sudden cardiac death. *Cardiovasc. Res,* 2003, 57(3):599-614.

[15] Chow T, Kereiakes DJ, Bartone C, Booth T, Schloss EJ, Wal ler T, Chung ES, Menon S, Nallamothu BK, than PS. Prognostic utility of microvolt t-wave alternans in risk stratification of patients with ischemic cardiomyopathy. *J. Am. Coll. Cardiol.*,2006,47(9):1820-1827.

[16] Gerritsen J, Dekker JM, TenVoorde BJ, Kostense PJ, Heine RJ, BouterLM, Heethaar RM, Stehouwer CD. Impaired autonomic function is associated with increased mortality, especially in subjects with diabetes, hypertension, or a history of cardiovascular disease: *The hoorn study.Diabetes Care,*2001,24(10):1793-1798.

[17] Das MK, Khan B, Jacob S, Kumar A, Mahenthiran J. Significance of a fragmented QRS complex versus a Q wave in patients with coronary artery disease. *Circulation*, 2006,113(21):2495-501.

[18] Chopra NA, Knollmann BC. Genetics of sudden cardiac death syndromes. *Current Opinion in Cardiology*, 2011,26(3):196-203.

[19] Hookana E, Junttila MJ, Kaikkonen KS, Ukkola O, Kesäniemi YA, Kortelainen ML, Huikuri HV. Comparison of family history of sudden cardiac death in nonischemic and ischemic heart disease. Circ. Arrhythm. *Electrophysiol.*, 2012,5(4):757-761.

[20] Perper JA, Kuller LH, Cooper M. Arteriosclerosis of coronary arteries in sudden, unexpected deaths. *Circulation.* 1975,52(6 Suppl):III27-33.

[21] Davies MJ, Thomas A. Thrombosis and acute coronary-artery lesions in sudden cardiac ischemic death. *N. Engl. J. Med.*, 1984,310(18):1137-1140.

[22] Poole JE, Johnson GW, Hellkamp AS, Anderson J, Callans DJ, Raitt MH, Reddy RK, Marchlinski FE, Yee R, Guarnieri T, Talajic M, Wilber DJ, Fishbein DP, Packer DL, Mark DB, Lee KL, Bardy GH. Prognostic importance of defibrillator shocks in patients with heart failure. *N. Engl. J. Med.*, 2008,359(10):1009-1017.

[23] Moss AJ, Greenberg H, Case RB, Zareba W, Hall WJ, Brown MW, Daubert JP, McNitt S, Andrews ML, Elkin AD; Multicenter Automatic Defibrillator Implantation Trial-II (MADIT-II) Research Group. Long-term clinical course of patients after termination of ventricular tachyarrhythmia by an implanted defibrillator. *Circulation,* 2004,110(25):3760-3765.

[24] Zipes DP, Wellens HJ. Sudden cardiac death. *Circulation,*1998 ,98(21):2334-2351.

[25] MERIT-HF Study Group. Effect of metoprolol CR/XL in chronic heart failure: Metoprolol CR/XL Randomised Intervention Trial in-Congestive Heart Failure (MERIT-HF). *Lancet.* 1999 Jun 12;353(9169):2001-2007.

[26] Buxton AE, Lee KL, Hafley GE, Wyse DG, Fisher JD, Lehmann MH, Pires LA, Gold MR, Packer DL, Josephson ME, Prystowsky EN, Talajic MR; MUSTT Investigators. Relation of ejection fraction and inducible ventricular tachycardia to mode of death in patients with coronary artery disease: an analysis of patients enrolled in the multicenter unsustained tachycardia trial. *Circulation,* 2002,106(19):2466-2472.

[27] Zipes DP, Camm AJ, Borggrefe M, Buxton AE, Chaitman B, Fromer M, Gregoratos G, Klein G, Moss AJ, Myerburg RJ, Priori SG, Quinones MA, Roden DM, Silka MJ, Tracy C, Priori SG, Blanc JJ, Budaj A, Camm AJ, Dean V, Deckers JW, Despres C, Dickstein K, Lekakis J, McGregor K, Metra M, Morais J, Osterspey A, Tamargo JL, Zamorano JL, Smith SC Jr, Jacobs AK, Adams CD, Antman EM, Anderson JL, Hunt SA, Halperin JL, Nishimura R, Ornato JP, Page RL, Riegel B; American College of Cardiology; American Heart Association Task Force; European Society of Cardiology

Committee for Practice Guidelines; European Heart Rhythm Association; Heart Rhythm Society. ACC/AHA/ESC 2006 guidelines for management of patients with ventricular arrhythmias and the prevention of sudden cardiac death: a report of the American College of Cardiology/American Heart Association Task Force and the European Society of Cardiology Committee for Practice Guidelines (Writing Committee to Develop guidelines for management of patients with ventricular arrhythmias and the prevention of sudden cardiac death) developed in collaboration with the European Heart Rhythm Association and the Heart Rhythm Society. *Europace,* 2006,8(9):746-837.

[28] Frenneaux MP. Heart. Assessing the risk of sudden cardiac death in a patient with hypertrophic cardiomyopathy, 2004,90(5):570-575.

[29] Maron BJ, Spirito P, Shen WK, Haas TS, Formisano F, Link MS, Epstein AE, Almquist AK, Daubert JP, Lawrenz T, Boriani G, Estes NA 3rd, Favale S, Piccininno M, Winters SL, Santini M, Betocchi S, Arribas F, Sherrid MV, Buja G, Semsarian C, Bruzzi P. Implantable cardioverter-defibrillators and prevention of sudden cardiac death in hypertrophic cardiomyopathy. *JAMA*, 2007, 298(4):405-412.

[30] Basso C, Corrado D, Bauce B, Thiene G. Arrhythmogenic right ventricular cardiomyopathy. *Circ. Arrhythm. Electrophysiol.,* 2012, 5(6):1233-1246.

[31] Cobb LA, Fahrenbruch CE, Olsufka M, Copass MK. Changing incidence of out-of-hospital ventricular fibrillation, 1980-2000. *JAMA*, 2002, 288(23):3008-3013.

[32] Bennett MT, Sanatani S, Chakrabarti S, Deyell MW, Krahn AD. Assessment of genetic causes of cardiac arrest. *Can. J. Cardiol.*, 2013,29(1):100-110.

[33] Obeyesekere MN, Leong-Sit P, Massel D, Manlucu J, Modi S, Krahn AD, Skanes AC, Yee R, Gula LJ, Klein GJ. Risk of arrhythmia and sudden death in patients with asymptomatic preexcitation: a meta-analysis. *Circulation,* 2012,125(19):2308-2315.

[34] Rosenhek R, Binder T, Porenta G, Lang I, Christ G, Schemper M, Maurer G, Baumgartner H. Predictors of outcome in severe, asymptomatic aortic stenosis. *N. Engl. J. Med.*, 2000,343(9):611-617.

[35] Koyak Z, Harris L, de Groot JR, Silversides CK, Oechslin EN, Bouma BJ, Budts W, Zwinderman AH, Van Gelder IC, Mulder BJ. Sudden cardiac death in adult congenital heart disease. *Circulation*, 2012,126(16):1944-1954.

[36] Tikkanen JT, Wichmann V, Junttila MJ, Rainio M, Hookana E, Lappi OP, Kortelainen ML, Anttonen O, Huikuri HV. Association of early repolarization and sudden cardiac death during an acute coronary event. *Circ. Arrhythm. Electrophysiol.,* 2012,5(4):714-718.

[37] Carey MG.Electrocardiographic Predictors of Sudden Cardiac Death. *J. Cardiovasc. Nurs.*, 2008,23(2):175-182.

[38] El-Menyar A, Asaad N. T-wave alternans and sudden cardiac death. *Crit. Pathw. Cardiol.*, 2008,7(1):21-28.

[39] Narayanaswamy S. High resolution electrocardiography. *Indian Pacing Electrophysiol. J.* 2002,2(2):50-56.

[40] Okin PM, Devereux RB, Fabsitz RR, Lee ET, Galloway JM, Howard BV. Principal component analysis of the T wave and prediction of cardiovascular mortality in American Indians: the Strong Heart Study. *Circulation*,2002,105(6):714-719.

[41] Daoud EG, Hummel JD, Rhodes TE.Management of sudden cardiac death risk in the very early postmyocardial infarction period. *Curr. Opin. Cardiol.,* 2010, 25(3):253-261.

[42] Moss AJ, Zareba W, Hall WJ, Klein H, Wilber DJ, Cannom DS, Daubert JP, Higgins SL, Brown MW, Andrews ML; Multicenter Automatic Defibrillator Implantation Trial II Investigators. Prophylactic implantation of a defibrillator in patients with myocardial infarction and reduced ejection fraction. *N. Engl. J. Med*, 2002,346(12):877-883.

[43] Kurl S, Mäkikallio TH, Rautaharju P, Kiviniemi V, Laukkanen JA. Duration of QRS complex in resting electrocardiogram is a predictor of sudden cardiac death in men. *Circulation*, 2012,125(21):2588-2594.

[44] Zareba W, Klein H, Cygankiewicz I, Hall WJ, McNitt S, Brown M, Cannom D, Daubert JP, Eldar M, Gold MR, Goldberger JJ, Goldenberg I, Lichstein E, Pitschner H, Rashtian M, Solomon S, Viskin S, Wang P, Moss AJ; MADIT-CRT Investigators.Effectiveness of Cardiac Resynchronization Therapy by QRS Morphology in the Multicenter Automatic Defibrillator Implantation Trial-Cardiac Resynchronization Therapy (MADIT-CRT). *Circulation*,2011,123(10):1061-1072.

[45] Rautaharju PM, Prineas RJ, Zhang ZM. A simple procedure for estimation of the spatial QRS/T angle from the standard 12-lead electrocardiogram. *J. Electrocardiol.*, 2007,40(3):300-304.

[46] Pietrasik G, Goldenberg I, Zdzienicka J, Moss AJ, Zareba W. Prognostic significance of fragmented QRS complex for predicting the risk of recurrent cardiac events in patients with Q-wave myocardial infarction. *Am. J. Cardiol.*, 2007,100(4):583-586.

[47] Schwartz PJ, Priori SG, Spazzolini C, Moss AJ, Vincent GM, Napolitano C, Denjoy I, Guicheney P, Breithardt G, Keating MT, Towbin JA, Beggs AH, Brink P, Wilde AA, Toivonen L, Zareba W, Robinson JL, Timothy KW, Corfield V, Wattanasirichaigoon D, Corbett C, Haverkamp W, Schulze-Bahr E, Lehmann MH, Schwartz K, Coumel P, Bloise R. Genotype-phenotype correlation in the long-QT syndrome: gene-specific triggers for life-threatening arrhythmias. *Circulation*, 2001,103(1):89-95.

[48] Antzelevitch C, Yan GX. J wave syndromes. *Heart Rhythm*, 2010,7(4):549-558.

[49] Surawicz B, Macfarlane PW. Inappropriate and confusing electrocardiographic terms: J-wave syndromes and early repolarization. *J. Am. Coll. Cardiol.*, 2011,57(15):1584-1586.

[50] Brugada P, Brugada J. Right bundle branch block, persistent ST segment elevation and sudden cardiac death: a distinct clinical and electrocardiographic syndrome. A multicenter report. *J. Am. Coll. Cardiol.*,1992, 20(6):1391-1396.

[51] Antzelevitch C. Genetic, molecular and cellular mechanisms underlying the J wave syndromes. *Circ. J.*, 2012,76(5):1054-1065.

[52] Meregalli PG, Wilde AA, Tan HL. Pathophysiological mechanisms of Brugada syndrome: depolarization disorder, repolarization disorder, or more? *Cardiovasc. Res.*, 2005,67(3):367-378.

[53] Probst V, Veltmann C, Eckardt L, Meregalli PG, Gaita F, Tan HL, Babuty D, Sacher F, Giustetto C, Schulze-Bahr E, Borggrefe M, Haissaguerre M, Mabo P, Le Marec H, Wolpert C, Wilde AA. Long-term prognosis of patients diagnosed with Brugada syndrome: Results from the FINGER Brugada Syndrome Registry. *Circulation*, 2010,121(5):635-643

[54] Haïssaguerre M, Derval N, Sacher F, Jesel L, Deisenhofer I, de Roy L, Pasquié JL, Nogami A, Babuty D, Yli-Mayry S, De Chillou C, Scanu P, Mabo P, Matsuo S, Probst V, Le Scouarnec S, Defaye P, Schlaepfer J, Rostock T, Lacroix D, Lamaison D, Lavergne T, Aizawa Y, Englund A, Anselme F, O'Neill M, Hocini M, Lim KT, Knecht

S, Veenhuyzen GD, Bordachar P, Chauvin M, Jais P, Coureau G, Chene G, Klein GJ, Clémenty J. Sudden cardiac arrest associated with early repolarization. *N. Engl. J. Med.,* 2008,358(19):2016-2023.

[55] Tikkanen JT, Junttila MJ, Anttonen O, Aro AL, Luttinen S, Kerola T, Sager SJ, Rissanen HA, Myerburg RJ, Reunanen A, Huikuri HV. Early repolarization: electrocardiographic phenotypes associated with favorable long-term outcome. *Circulation,* 2011,123(23):2666-2673.

[56] Tikkanen JT, Anttonen O, Junttila MJ, Aro AL, Kerola T, Rissanen HA, Reunanen A, Huikuri HV. Long-term outcome associated with early repolarization on electrocardiography. *N. Engl. J. Med.*, 2009,361(26):2529-2537.

[57] Rollin A, Maury P, Bongard V, Sacher F, Delay M, Duparc A, Mondoly P, Carrié D, Ferrières J, Ruidavets JB. Prevalence, prognosis, and identification of the malignant form of early repolarization pattern in a population-based study. *Am. J. Cardiol.* 2012 Nov 1;110(9):1302-1308.

[58] Rosso R, Kogan E, Belhassen B, Rozovski U, Scheinman MM, Zeltser D, Halkin A, Steinvil A, Heller K, Glikson M, Katz A, Viskin S. J-point elevation in survivors of primary ventricular fibrillation and matched control subjects: incidence and clinical significance. *J. Am. Coll. Cardiol.,* 2008,52(15):1231-1238.

[59] Das MK, Suradi H, Maskoun W, Michael MA, Shen C, Peng J, Dandamudi G, Mahenthiran J. Fragmented wide QRS on a 12-lead ECG: a sign of myocardial scar and poor prognosis. *Circ. Arrhythm. Electrophysiol.,* 2008,1(4):258-268.

[60] Das MK, Saha C, El Masry H, Peng J, Dandamudi G, Mahenthiran J, McHenry P, Zipes DP. Fragmented QRS on a 12-lead ECG: a predictor of mortality and cardiac events in patients with coronary artery disease. *Heart Rhythm,* 2007,4(11):1385-1392.

[61] Peters S, Trümmel M, Koehler B. QRS fragmentation in standard ECG as a diagnostic marker of arrhythmogenic right ventricular dysplasia-cardiomyopathy. *Heart Rhythm,* 2008,5(10):1417-1421.

[62] Morita H, Kusano KF, Miura D, Nagase S, Nakamura K, Morita ST, Ohe T, Zipes DP, Wu J. Fragmented QRS as a marker of conduction abnormality and a predictor of prognosis of Brugada syndrome. *Circulation,* 2008, 118(17):1697-1704.

[63] Korhonen P, Husa T, Konttila T, Tierala I, Mäkijärvi M, Väänänen H, Ojanen J, Vehtari A, Toivonen L. Fragmented QRS in prediction of cardiac deaths and heart failure hospitalizations after myocardial infarction. *Ann. Noninvasive Electrocardiol.,* 2010,15(2):130-137.

[64] Papadakis M, Basavarajaiah S, Rawlins J, Edwards C, Makan J, Firoozi S, Carby L, Sharma S. Prevalence and significance of T-wave inversions in predominantly Caucasian adolescent athletes. *Eur. Heart J.,* 2009,30(14):1728-1735.

[65] Marcus FI. Prevalence of T-wave inversion beyond V1 in young normal individuals and usefulness for the diagnosis of arrhythmogenic right ventricular cardiomyopathy /dysplasia. *Am. J. Cardiol.*, 2005,95(9):1070-1071.

[66] Zabel M, Acar B, Klingenheben T, Franz MR, Hohnloser SH, Malik M. Analysis of 12-lead T-wave morphology for risk stratification after myocardial infarction. *Circulation,* 2000,102(11):1252-1257.

[67] Hohnloser S; Zipes DP, Jalife J. Cardiac Electrophysiology: From Cell to Bedside. 5th ed.Philadelphia: *Saunders Elsevier*. 2009:p887.

[68] Ikeda T, Saito H, Tanno K, Shimizu H, Watanabe J, Ohnishi Y, Kasamaki Y, Ozawa Y. T-wave alternans as a predictor for sudden cardiac death after myocardial infarction. *Am. J. Cardiol.*, 2002,89(1):79-82.

[69] Ikeda T, Yoshino H, Sugi K, Tanno K, Shimizu H, Watanabe J, Kasamaki Y, Yoshida A, Kato T. Predictive value of microvolt T-wave alternans for sudden cardiac death in patients with preserved cardiac function after acute myocardial infarction: results of a collaborative cohort study. *J. Am. Coll. Cardiol.*, 2006,48(11):2268-2274.

[70] [68] Hohnloser SH, Klingenheben T, Bloomfield D, Dabbous O, Cohen RJ. Usefulness of microvolt T-wave alternans for prediction of ventricular tachyarrhythmic events in patients with dilated cardiomyopathy: results from a prospective observational study. *J. Am. Coll. Cardiol*, 2003 ,41(12):2220-2224.

[71] [69] Bloomfield DM, Bigger JT, Steinman RC, Namerow PB, Parides MK, Curtis AB, Kaufman ES, Davidenko JM, Shinn TS, Fontaine JM.Microvolt T-wave alternans and the risk of death or sustained ventricular arrhythmias in patients with left ventricular dysfunction. *J. Am. Coll. Cardiol.*, 2006,47(2):456-463.

[72] Chow T, Kereiakes DJ, Bartone C, Booth T, Schloss EJ, Waller T, Chung ES, Menon S, Nallamothu BK, Chan PS. Prognostic utility of microvolt T-wave alternans in risk stratification of patients with ischemic cardiomyopathy. *J. Am. Coll. Cardiol.*, 2006,47(9):1820-1827.

[73] Simson MB. Use of signals in the terminal QRS complexted identify patients with recurrent ventricular tachycardia after myocardial infarction. *Circulation*, 1981, 64:(2):235-242.

[74] Yamada T, Fukunami M, Shimonagata T, Kumagai K, Kim J, Sanada S, Ogita H, Hori M, Hoki N. Prediction of the effectiveness of long-term beta blocker treatment for dilated cardiomyopathy by signal averaged electrocardiography. *Heart*,1998,79(3):256-261.

[75] Kuchar DL, Thorburn CW, Sammel NL.Signal-averaged electrocardiogram for evaluation of recurrent syncope. *Am. J. Cardiol.*, 1986,58(10):949-953.

[76] Simson MB. Use of signals in the terminal QRS complex to identify patients with ventricular tachycardia after myocardial infarction. *Circulation*, 1981,64(2):235-242.

[77] Rozanski JJ, Mortara D, Myerburg RJ, Castellanos A. Body surface detection of delayed depolarizations in patients with recurrent ventricular tachycardia and left ventricular aneurysm. *Circulation*, 1981,63(5):1172-1178.

[78] Denes P, Santarelli P, Hauser RG, Uretz EF. Quantitative analysis of the high-frequency components of the terminal portion of the body surface QRS in normal subjects and in patients with ventricular tachycardia. *Circulation*, 1983,67(5):1129-1138.

[79] Singer DH, Martin GJ, Magid N, Weiss JS, Schaad JW, Kehoe R, Zheutlin T, Fintel DJ, Hsieh AM, Lesch M. Low heart rate variability and sudden cardiac death. *J. Electrocardiol.*, 1988,21 Suppl:S46-55.

[80] Malik M, Camm AJ. Heart rate variability. *Clin. Cardiol*, 1990,13(8):570-576.

[81] Goldberger JJ, Jacobson JT. Relationship of blood pressure to heart rate in isolated systolic hypertension. *J. Investig. Med.*, 2011,59(8):1228-1232.

[82] Schmidt G, Malik M, Barthel P, Schneider R, Ulm K, Rolnitzky L, Camm AJ, Bigger JT Jr, Schömig A.Heart-rate turbulence after ventricular premature beats as a predictor of mortality after acute myocardial infarction. *Lancet,* 1999,353(9162):1390-1396.

[83] Bauer A, Kantelhardt JW, Barthel P, Schneider R, Mäkikallio T, Ulm K, Hnatkova K, Schömig A, Huikuri H, Bunde A, Malik M, Schmidt G.Deceleration capacity of heart rate as a predictor of mortality after.myocardial infarction: cohort study. *Lancet*, 2006, 367(9523):1674-1681.

In: Sudden Death
Editors: Jiashin Wu and Jessica Wu

ISBN: 978-1-62618-825-9

Chapter V

Pathophysiology, Risks, Preventive and Therapeutic Strategies in Sudden Cardiac Death

Shyam Gelot[1], Catherine Law[2] and Srinivas M. Tipparaju[3]*
[1]Department of Pharmacotherapeutics and Clinical Research,
USF College of Pharmacy, Tampa, FL, US
[2]Department of Cardiovascular Sciences,
USF Morsani College of Medicine, Tampa, FL, US
[3]Department of Pharmaceutical Sciences,
USF College of Pharmacy, Tampa, FL, US

Abstract

Sudden cardiac death (SCD) is a clinical problem worldwide and the majority of patients with coronary artery disease are at risk of sudden cardiac death. Predisposition to high blood pressure, diabetes, environment, obesity, age, genes, and other factors further increase the risk of death in patients with heart disease. The exact etiology for the disease remains elusive; nonetheless, clinical assessment and preemptive strategies have improved the outcomes in recent years. Therapeutic options for clinicians and health care providers are very limited; therefore, research focusing on translational aspects of sudden cardiac death would help in further understanding the basis of the disease and may provide novel therapeutic options.

This chapter discusses the standard of care given and identifies the specific advantages and disadvantages ofto each step in patient care. Present understanding of the disease and pathophysiological basis shows "how" the disease progresses in patients.The cross talk between treatment options and disease basis offers new insights in the area of sudden cardiac death that will be useful for researchers and clinicians in this area.

* Corresponding Author: Srinivas M. Tipparaju, MPharm, PhD, 12901 Bruce B Downs Blvd, MDC030, USF Health College of Pharmacy, Tampa, FL 33612; Phone# 813-974-7195, Fax# 813-974-9885, Email: stippara@health.usf.edu.

Introduction

Sudden cardiac death (SCD) is a clinical problem worldwide and the majority of patients with coronary artery disease carry the risk of sudden cardiac death. SCD is often referred to as an unexpected death due to a cardiovascular cause within one hour of change in clinical status [1-3].

These events are most likely due to structural heart disease that is undiagnosed, especially coronary heart disease. [4] Because the time of when the person experiences loss of consciousness and hemodynamic instability is not always witnessed, the definition of SCD often encompasses an unexpected death that occurred within a 24-hour time frame.[2][2]SCD has also been described as the resulting death following sudden cardiac arrest (SCA). [1,5] SCA refers to the cessation of cardiac activity such that there is no blood circulation and a loss of normal breathing. [5]

Despite advances in cardiopulmonary recitation training and public use of automated external defibrillators, patients who experience SCA out of the hospital have less than a 5 five percent chance of survival. [4] The specific causes of sudden cardiac arrest will be described later in the chapter; however, for unknown reasons, there has been an increase in last two decades inof pulseless electrical activity (PEA) and asystole in last two decades. [4]

Epidemiology

The true incidence of SCD is uncertain; however, it is estimated that there are between 180,000 to 450,000 cases in the United States each year. [2] The large range in the annual incidence is most likely due to a lack of consistent definition to use as inclusion criteria in the epidemiologic studies as described in the introduction.

Additionally, these estimates are predominately based on retrospective studies evaluating death certificates. [6] The reported incidences may be a poor reflection of the true number of people who suffer SCD if solely based on evaluation of death certificates. [7]

A more ideal and accurate method for estimating the true incidence would be through prospective analysis. In one recent study, Chugh and colleagues evaluated, prospectively, the number of patients who suffered SCD. The study concluded that the incidence of SCD in 2003, in one Oregon County, was 5.6%. When the authors compared the prospective analysis with the death certificate based method of evaluating SCD, only 19% of these diagnoses were shown to be true positives with the death certificate method. [7]

Age

Despite not knowing the true incidence of SCD, it is well accepted that the risk of SCD increases with age (Figure 1). The annual incidence in of persons less than age 35 appears to be 1 per 100,000, while in adults greater than 50 years of age, the incidence increases to 1 per 1000 events per year. [2, 8]

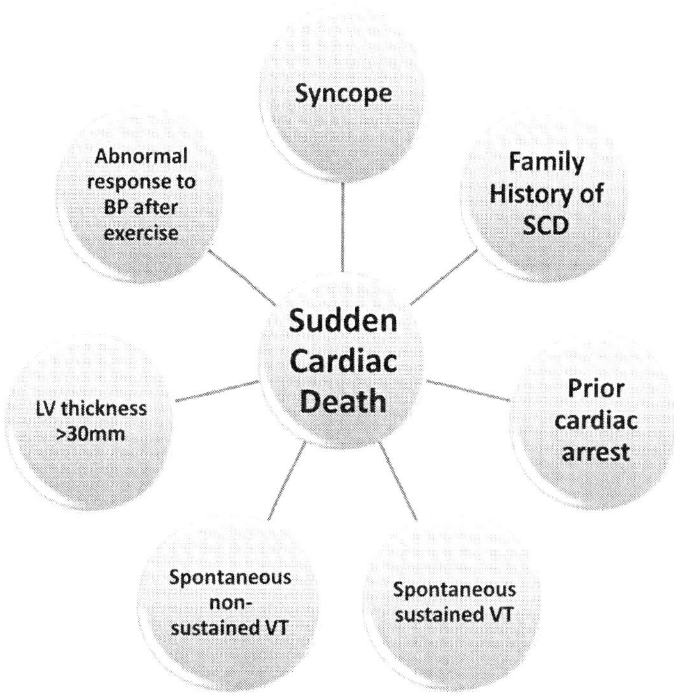

Figure 1. Major risk factors for sudden cardiac death.

Gender

In addition to age, it appears that women seem to have less risk of developing SCD. The annual incidence is 3 to 4 times higher in men. Even after menopause, the incidence in women who participated in the World Health Initiative was still low (2.4 for every 10,000 events) [8].

Race

Race appears to have some influence on the risk of SCD. Epidemiologic studies show that African- Americans have higher rates of SCD while Hispanic populations have fewer incidences. In addition, African-Americans have less chance of survival than Caucasians after a SCA event. [8, 9]

Etiology

The causes of SCD are vast, including both structural and non-structural heart disease. Examples of structural heart disease include conditions such as coronary heart disease (CHD), hypertrophic and dilated cardiomyopathy. Medications, electrolyte imbalance, Brugada syndrome, Wolff-Parkinson-White syndrome are examples of non-structural heart disease.

Structural Heart Disorders

Coronary Artery Disease

Approximately 80% of patients who suffer from SCD have coronary artery disease (CAD). As described in the previous section, the rate of SCD increases with age. With increased age, there is a greater risk of atherosclerotic coronary artery disease leading to SCD. [2] Ischemic heart diseases and its subsequent effects, such as myocardial infarction (MI) and arrhythmic events comprises the majority of SCD. [1]

Sadly, inIn most of the cases, coronary artery disease is undiagnosed prior to death. If the patient survives a MI, the risk of mortality is four times higher in the 30-day window post-MI. [10] This is largely due to the increased risk of developing subsequent malignant arrhythmias, such as ventricular tachycardia and ventricular fibrillation.

Non-atherosclerotic coronary artery disorders leading to SCD are not as common, nevertheless, a very important consideration. Examples of this include emboli resulting from endocarditis, coronary artery vasospasm, and mechanical obstruction from coronary artery dissection.

Dilated Cardiomyopathy and Heart Failure

Dilated cardiomyopathy (DCM) along with hypertrophic cardiomyopathy (described in next section) represent the second largest cardiac cause of SCD. [13] Approximately 10% of SCD can be attributed to DCM. [14]

DCM is a common cause of heart failure. Approximately 30% of patients with heart failure will experience SCD, but it appears the risk of SCD increases in patients with worsening left ventricular function. The etiology is not fully understood, but may be related to arrhythmias induced by stretching of the His-Purkinje fibers producing reentrant ventricular tachycardia [1, 15] It is well established that SCD occurs in patients with heart failure with reduced ejection fraction; however, there is little information on HF in patients with preserved ejection fraction (>45%). [12]

Hypertrophic Cardiomyopathy (HCM)

It is estimated that the incidence of SCD in these patients with HCM is 2-4% per year in adults and up to 6% in children and adolescents. [11] Obstructive HCM (versus non-obstructive HCM) appears to be more fatal, in which, 70% of these patients suffer from ventricular arrhythmias and ultimately SCD. [1]

Specific mechanisms that cause sudden cardiac death are multifactorial and need further investigation. There is a strong family history of patients with HCM who die from SCD. It is believed that there is a genetic component responsible, which mutations in beta-myosin heavy chain and alpha-tropomyosin gene have been identified. [11]

Other

Other structural heart diseases that are linked with SCD include congenital heart disease, arrhythmogenic right ventricular dysplastic cardiomyopathy (ARVD), and valvular disease such as mitral valve prolapse and aortic stenosis.

Non-Structural Heart Disorders

Electrophysiological (EP) Conditions

Brugada syndrome is a disease caused by alterations in ion channels in cardiac myocytes that alter membrane potential. It is a genetic disorder and in roughly 50% of the time it is autosomal dominant, generally in young males.

This disease is characterized by ECG changes, specifically right bundle branch block and ST elevations in the anterior precordial leads. A mutation in the SCNA5 gene, which expresses for voltage gated sodium channels are thought to be the cause in a small percentage of patient with SCD.

Wolff-Parkinson-White Syndrome, is another example of EP abnormality that places patients at risk for SCD, due to rapid ventricular conduction in the accessory pathway. [17] Although SCD is thought to be less common in these patients (1 in 1000 patients), there have been very few prospective studies, with long-term outcomes [17].

Electrolyte Imbalance

Electrolyte imbalance, specifically hypokalemia, hypophosphatemia, and hypomagnesaemia can increase the risk of sudden death.

Hypokalemia, defined as potassium levels less than 3.5 mEq/L, can reduce the electrical action potential across myocardium.

If severe hypokalemia occurs (less than 2.5 mEq/L), this can cause decreased myocardial contraction, ECG changes, and induce arrythmias. [16]

Additionally, low serum phosphate levels (less than 2.7 mg/dL) can decrease myocardial contractility and lead to death. [17]

Severely low magnesium levels (less than 1mg/dL) can lead to ECG changes, induce malignant arrhythmias such as *Torsades de pointes*, and subsequently death. [17] It is always prudent to check laboratory values and correct by replacing the deficient electrolyte.

Medication

Antiarrhythmic drugs, specifically class IA agents (e.g, quinidine, procainamide, and disopyramide), are known to cause prolongation of the QTc interval. These agents increase the risk of *Ttorsades de pointes*.Other commonly used non-cardiac QTc prolonging drugs have a three-fold increased risk of SCD. [18] Examples include psychotropic agents (e.g.

haloperidol, lithium, risperidone and tricyclic antidepressants) and antibiotics (e.g.clarithromycin, azithromycin, and trimethoprim-sulfamethoxazole) [14, 18, 19].

Assessment and Diagnostic Workup

Taking a thorough history is imperative for identifying those at risk of sudden cardiac death. Because the incidence of SCD is highest amongst patients with CAD, it is logical that the risk factors for SCD are similar to that for CAD. The risk factors that should be screened for are smoking, diabetes, hypertension, dyslipidemia, obesity/physical inactivity, and a family history of CHD.

In addition, the onset of prodromal symptoms such as palpitations, presyncope and syncope may raise suspicion for high risk of SCD. Palpitations are usually sudden in its onset and may result in syncope. Other times, abrupt collapse and loss of consciousness without any warning that usually last for seconds may raise suspicion for conduction defects and structural heart disease. As mentioned above, risk factors for sudden cardiac death include structural heart disease. Thus, symptoms relating to structural heart disease such as chest discomfort and dyspnea should be noted. In addition, as mentioned above, a thorough drug history should be taken as some drugs can worsen QT prolongation, making the patient more susceptible to ventricular arrhythmias. Physical examination can lead to diagnosis of structural heart problems.

Risk Factors

Smoking

Cigarette smoking is an independent risk factor for sudden cardiac death. In a recent study, 101,018 female participants were followed for 30 years. This study found that there was a 2.4 fold higher increased risk for SCD in those patients that smoked. [20] Even a low consumption of 1-14 cigarettes still carried a 1.84 fold higher risk of SCD and 8% increased risk of SCD every five years. [20] Another smaller study, with a mean follow-up time of 8 years, showed a higher incidence of SCD (8.1%) in current smokers. Additionally, this study showed that persons who never smoked and those that quit smoking experienced the same incidence of SCD of 4.6%. [21]

Exercise

It is recommended for individuals to get at least 30 minutes of moderate intensity exercise everyday. However, sometimes it is reported that physically fit persons and trained athletes die from SCD. The most likely cause of SCD in young athletes is HCM. SCD appears to be very rare in 1 event per every 36.5 million hours of moderate exercise. [22]

Family History

In some cases there may be a genetic predisposition in developing certain cardiac disorders, which may place an individual at a higher risk of sudden cardiac death. A family history of premature death before the age of 50 is a strong independent marker of susceptibility to ventricular arrhythmias and SCD. Future research is needed in the genetics area to determine specific mutations encoding for membrane potential ions and linking this to fatal ventricular arrhythmias. Examples include KCNH2, KCNQ1, SCN5A, KCNE1, and KCNE2 for Long-QT syndrome, SCN5A for Brugada syndrome, and Pkp2 and Dsp for ARVC. [23]

Noninvasive Evaluation

Physical examination can lead to suspicion of heart problems and often in the cardiology office, the patient will undergo a 12 lead ECG to detect both evidence of arrhythmias or evidence of structural abnormalities such as left ventricular hypertrophy. However, the change of detecting the arrhythmias on a single ECG is rare and thus continued monitoring with a Holter, event monitor or loop recorder may be necessary.

Echocardiogram is also performed as it allows evaluation of systolic and diastolic dysfunction, regional wall abnormalities, myocardial thickness and valvular disorders. In the American Society of Echocardiography, it is highly recommended for those patients at increased risk for developing SCD or ventricular arrhythmias such as those with HCM, ARVD, dilated cardiomyopathy, those who have survived an acute myocardial infarction, or relatives of patients with inherited disorders associated with SCD.

Ischemic workup is especially important in both those who have suffered a cardiac arrest and those who are at high risk of developing SCD since most events occur in the setting of coronary artery disease. Ischemic workup can involve a stress test or coronary angiography.

Other cardiac imaging modalities such as MRI have visualization in detecting infiltration cardiomyopathies as well as ARVD. Cardiac positron emission tomography (PET) can be used in detecting cardiac sarcoid.

Pathophysiology

The basis for sudden cardiac death is not entirely known; however, recent evidence suggests that patients with a family history of sudden cardiac death are at higher risk for SCD. This area of investigation has been a major focus for researchers, particularly as it relates to Brugada Syndrome [24] , Long-QT (LQT1, 2 and 3) syndromes have revealed that the mutations associated with ion channels that regulate the functioning in the heart are abnormal and may be causing thecause sudden cardiac death. [25] Single nucleotide polymorphisms (SNP) in sodium channels (Nav) that have been identified are directly related to action potential changes leading to ECG abnormalities in patients. Given the few pharmacological options supported by compelling evidence, the use of ICD's in patients with risk of SCD is the standard of care.

The etiology of SCD is not entirely known, but studies indicate that,,at a fundamental level, hypertension may lead to cardiomyopathy and if left untreated can lead to decompensated hypertrophy and increase the propensity for sudden cardiac death. The role of ion channels in cardiac hypertrophy has been studied in detail using animal models to identify trans-aortic coarctation (TAC), LAD occlusion, and mutations to specific gene of interest. Investigators have demonstrated that ion channels (Ca, K, Na) are modulated both at functional and expressional level and affect the performance of the heart. [26, 27] Among the potassium channels (Kv1-12), the Kv4.x, which regulates the transient outward current fast (Ito_{fast}) is significantly down regulated and causes action potential prolongation. Therefore, the major problem at the repolarization level is depletion of its reserve. The mechanisms relating to depletion of repolarization in sudden cardiac death remains relatively unknown. In recent years, investigations have been focused on identifying the molecular mechanisms in β-adrenergic (β-AR) system stimulated hypertrophy models using isoproterenol induced hypertrophy with a focus to decipher the biochemical mechanism. [28]

In addition, research has been attempting to elucidate the role of Kv4.2 and key mediators that regulate the Kv channel activity in hypertrophy and sudden death. Investigators have utilized the β-AR stimulated model of hypertrophy to test the role of Kv channels in physiological and pathological hypertrophy [29].

It has been shown that isoproterenol causes hypertrophy in wild type mice; therefore, one can utilize this tool to evaluate the role of Kv4.2 using transgenic mice along with mediators such as KChIP2 (potassium channel interacting protein 2), Irx5 (Iroquois protein), and NfkB (nuclear factor k) in the heart. The role of Kvβ subunits has not been evaluated in cardiac hypertrophy and myocardial ischemia.

The shaker potassium channel subunits (Kvβ1-3) that co-assemble with Kv channels bind pyridine nucleotides with high affinity; however, the physiological significance of this binding has not been evaluated. Previously, studies have evaluated the role of Kvβ subunits and its property to modulate Kv1.5 currents upon binding to pyridine nucleotides. It has been demonstrated that pyridine nucleotides modulate the gating and kinetics of the Kv1.5 channel [30, 31]. Based on these studies Kvβ1 and Kvβ3 restore or accelerate the Kvβ induced inactivation of Kv1.5 current whereas Kvβ2 causes a hyperpolarization shift in the Kv1.5 midpoint of activation [32, 33]. The current understanding is lacking as to how physiological ratios or bulk changes in pyridine nucleotides (NAD(P)H and NAD(P)) in the cells may be modulating Kv currents in the heart and altering action potential. Therefore, understanding the role of voltage gated potassium channels (Kv) along with its subunits will provide additional new tools for developing the biochemical and physiological basis of this disease and potentially develop new therapeutics.

Patients in intensive care units are often put on oxygen treatment with the idea to deliver more oxygen systemically; however, recent studies indicate that oxygen treatment may cause hypertrophy and cardiac complication. [34] Based on these investigations,; it is plausible that Kv channel may be playing a major role in sudden cardiac death.

Prevention of Sudden Cardiac Death

Prevention of SCD can be divided into primary and secondary prevention. Primary prevention of sudden cardiac death refers to the avoidance of the first malignant arrhythmia, usually ventricular fibrillation or ventricular tachycardia. Secondary prevention refers to the deterrence of another life-threatening arrhythmia. The management of both primary and secondary prevention is implantable cardioverter-defibrillators (ICDs)

Primary Prevention

Implantable Cardioverter-Defibrillators

Using ICDs as a form of primary prevention is largely based on patients with a prior MI and are at risk for arrhythmias and heart failure due to ischemic or nonischemic cardiomyopathy. There have been three large randomized controlled trials that support the use of ICDs For in patients who have ischemic cardiomyopathy there have beenthreelarge randomized controlled trials that support its use: MUSTT, MADIT-I, and MADIT-II. [35-37] ICD implantation is largely based on inclusion criteria in these studies. The MUSTT Trial included patients with a left ventricular ejection fraction (LVEF) of ≤ 40%, MADIT-I study included patients with LVEF of ≤35%, and MADIT-II included patients with LVEF of ≤30%. Other inclusion criteria in the studiesy were non-sustained ventricular tachycardia, a previous MI, and inducible ventricular arrhythmias on EP studies. For the trials, MUSTT, MADIT-I, and MADIT-II all showed benefit of ICD placement with a relative risk for SCD of 0.29, 0.25, and 0.39, respectively. [35-37] The SCD-HeFT trial included 2,521 patients with HF (NYHA class II and III) due to either ischemic or non-ischemic cardiomyopathy who had a LVEF ≤ 35%. [38] Patients were divided into conventional therapy plus either placebo, amiodarone, or ICD placement. This study showed that amiodarone had no benefit on survival; however, ICD therapy showed a decrease in mortality by 23% at the five year mark. Another trial, the DEFINITE study, evaluated patients with nonischemic cardiomyopathy. [39].

Indication	Classification	Level of Evidence
Hemodynamically unstable sustained VT without any reversible cause	Class I	A
LVEF <35% because of MI, 40 days post MI, NYHA class II or III	Class I	A
LVEF < 30 because of MI, at least 40 days post MI, and NYHA class I	Class I	A
Nonischemic DCM with LVEF ≤ 35% and NYHA class II or III	Class I	B
Non-sustained VT and LVEF < 40% because of MI, and VT/VF on EP study	Class I	B
Sustained VT and Structural heart disease	Class I	B
Idiopathic syncope and VT/VF on EP study	Class I	B

Figure 2. ICD placement Class I recommendations[42].Class I represents situations when the benefit for implantation of an ICD clearly outweighs the risk involved. Level of evidence of "A" means that there were several randomized control trials or meta-analyses evaluating ICD use.

Indication	Classification	Level of Evidence
Idiopathic syncope, nonischemic cardiomyopathy, and LV dysfunction	Class IIa	C
Sustained VT and normal or near normal ventricular function	Class IIa	C
HCM with ≥ 1 risk factor for SCD	Class IIa	C
ARVD with ≥ 1 risk factor for SCD	Class IIa	C
Brugada syndrome and documented VT that did not lead to SCA	Class IIa	C
Brugada syndrome with syncope	Class IIa	C
Long-QT syndrome experiencing syncope and/or VT while on beta adrenergic blockers	Class IIa	C
Non hospitalized patients awaiting transplantation	Class IIa	C
Cardiac sarcoidosis, giant cell myocarditis, Chagas disease	Class IIa	C
Catecholaminergic polymorphic VT with syncope and/or sustained VT while receiving beta adrenergic blockers	Class IIa	C

Figure 3. ICD placement Class IIa recommendations[42]. Class IIa represents clinical situations when it is beneficial for implantation of an ICD, however there is still risk involved. Level of evidence "C" means that only a consensus opinion or case reports exist for that particular situation.

Indication	Classification	Level of Evidence
Long-QT syndrome and risk factors for SCD	Class IIb	B
Non-ischemic heart disease with LVEF ≤35% and NYHA class I	Class IIb	C
Syncope and advanced structural heart disease, in which there is no known cause	Class IIb	C
Familial cardiomyopathy associated with SCD	Class IIb	C
LV noncompaction	Class IIb	C

Figure 4. ICD placement Class IIb recommendations[42].Class IIb represents situations in which implantation may be appropriate; however, there is a very strong potential for risk with the procedure.

This study included patients with LVEF less than 36%, NYHA class I, II or III, and a history of non-sustained ventricular tachycardia. The patients were then randomized to conventional therapy of beta-adrenergic receptor blockers and angiotensin converting enzyme inhibitors (ACE) or implantation of an ICD. At two years time the mortality rate was 14.1% with the conventional medication group and 7.9% with the ICD group. [39] This study was important because it emphasized the benefit for ICD placement in patients with non-ischemic cardiomyopathy and not just in patients with CAD. While there is a clear benefit to using ICDs, the timing of placement is also an important consideration. The DINAMIT trial (332 patients) and the IRIS trial (898 patients) failed to show an improvement in annual mortality when ICD was placed within the first month after an MI. [40, 41] The DINAMIT trial included patients who had an MI in the last 6 to 40 days, LVEF ≤35 and a heart rate ≥ 80 bpm. The IRIS trial, on the otherhand, enrolled patients who had an MI within the last 5-31 days, had LVEF ≤ 40 and HR ≥ 90 bpm. Based on these trials, the 2008 American College of Cardiology/American Heart Association/Heart Rhythm Society guidelines recommend ICD placement for patients who have suffered an MI with persistent decrease in ejection fraction for 40 days since the last MI despite optimal medical treatment, and if giving the patient an ICD that the patienty would have a survival of more than one year. [42] (See figures 2-4 for specific recommendations). There is contention as to what the specific LVEF should be in clinical practice; however, based on the trials most institutions use a cutoff of ≤ 35%.

Pharmacotherapy

Because the incidence of SCD is greatest amongst individuals with CAD, pharmacological primary prevention should be optimized for agents that increase oxygen supply, decrease myocardial demand, and help to reduce ventricular remodeling. Examples include agents such as beta-adrenergic receptor blockers, ACE inhibitors or angiotensin receptor blockers (ARBs).

Amiodarone is an antiarrhythmic agent that has been investigated for primary prevention of SCD, but has had conflicting results in studies. Studies Data from these studies, such as the CHF-STAT, showed no benefit in SCD or all-cause mortality with amiodarone and SCD-HeFT, as mentioned earlier, found no improvement in all-cause mortality when amiodarone was compared to ICD and placebo. [38,43] The GESICA study was one of the few major studies that showed a benefit to using amiodarone versus no treatment in reducing SCD. [44] In this trial, however, the investigators were not blinded to the treatment groups. Studies, such as EMIAT and CAMIAT, did not show benefit in cardiac mortality;, both trials did show a reduction in arrhythmic deaths. [45, 46] Additionally, a post-hoc analysis of both of these studies showed a synergistic benefit for using beta blockers with amiodarone in prevention of SCD [47].

Secondary Prevention

As with primary prevention, ICDs are the main treatment modality for secondary prevention. Other options for consideration in secondary prevention are ablation and antiarrhythmic medications; however, these options have not been as effective as ICDs in precluding SCD.

Implantable Cardioverter-Defibrillators

Three major trial (CASH, CIDS, and AVID) investigated the use of ICD in patients who survived SCA due to ventricular arrhythmias. [48-50] The CASH and CIDS studies lacked enough power to be statistically significant but showed positive results favoring patients in the ICD groups. 288 patients participated in the CASH study and were randomized to an ICD placement group, amiodarone, metoprolol, or propafenone. There was a 61% higher mortality rate of participants in the propafenone group and investigators prematurely stopped this arm of the study. [48] For the other groups the primary outcome was all cause mortality with a minimum follow-up time of two years. The ICD group had a 23% reduction in all cause mortality compared to the metoprolol and amiodarone arm. This reduction, however, was not statistically significant. The CIDS trial studied 659 patients, who had a SCA secondary to ventricular tachycardia or fibrillation, and randomly assigned them to either an amiodarone group or an ICD placement group. The results from this trial like the CASH study were not powered enough and thus there was no statistically significant difference in either group in all cause mortality or arrhythmic death. The AVID trial was the first of these trials and had significant power compared to the previously described two trials. This study investigated 1,016 patients who survived a SCA due to ventricular tachycardia/ventricular fibrillation, or had LVEF $\leq$ 40%. Patients were randomized to either sotalol, amiodarone or an ICD group. This study was terminated early due to a clear benefit in the ICD group in overall survival compared to the antiarrhythmic drugs (a 27% relative risk reduction in all cause mortality at two years' time). [50]

Conclusion/Future

Sudden cardiac death is a condition which investigators have ascertained a great deal of knowledge in the last few decades; however, there is much more to be discovered. While true incidence of SCD remains unknown, risk factors such as family history and CAD places patients at a much higher risk. The focus of research is drawn to identifying specific genes, in cases of family history that may place patients at a higher risk.; Tthese genes often encode for specific voltage gated ion channels. Further genetic and translational research is needed to help understand the basis of SCD. With our current understanding and results from major clinical trials, ICDs remain the one of the best options for both primary and secondary prevention of SCD.

Acknowledgments

The authors acknowledge the funding received from NIH (HL102171), USF COP seed grant and startup funding to SMT.

References

[1] Bonow R, Mann D, Zipes D. (2012). Braunwald's Heart Disease 9th edition. Philidelphia, PA. Elsevier.

[2] Deo, R and Albert, C. Epidemiology and Genetics of Sudden cardiac Death. *Circulation*. 2012; 125:620-637.

[3] Lloyd-Jones D, Adams RJ, Brown TM et al. Heart Discase and stroke statistics-2010 update: a report from the American Heart Association. *Circulation*. 2010:121:e46-e215.

[4] John, R, Tedrow U, Koplan B et al. Ventricular arrhythmias and sudden cardiac death. *Lancet.* 2012 Oct 27;380(9852):1520-9.

[5] ACC/AHA Task Force on Clinical Data Standards (ACC/AHA/HRS Writing Committee to Develop Data Standards on Electrophysiology), Buxton AE, Calkins H, Callans DJ, et al. *Circulation.* 2006;114(23):2534.

[6] Zheng, ZJ, Croft, JB, Giles, WH. et al. Sudden cardiac death in the United States, 1989 to 1998. *Circulation.* 2001:104:2158.

[7] Chugh SS, Jui J, Gunson K. Current burden of sudden cardiac death: Multiple source surveillance versus retrospective death certificate-based review in a large U.S. community. *J. Am. Coll. Cardiol.* 2004; 44:1268.

[8] Bertoia M, Allison M, Manson J. Risk factors for sudden cardiac death in post-menopausal women. *J. Am. Coll. Cardiol.* 2012; 60:2674.

[9] Becker L, Han B, Meyer P. et al. Racial differences in the incidence of cardiac arrest and subsequent survival. The CPR Project. *N. Engl. J. Med.* 1993; 329:600-606.

[10] Adabag A, Therneau T, Gersh B et al. Sudden death after myocardial infarction. *JAMA.* 2008; 300:2022-2029.

[11] Spirito P, Seidman C, McKenna W et al. The management of hypertrophic cardiomyopathy. *N. Engl. J. Med.* 1997;336:775-785.

[12] Adabag S, Smith, L, Anand I et al. Sudden cardiac death in heart failure patients with preserved ejection fraction. *Journal of Cardiac Failure.* 2012; 18 (10):749-754.

[13] Huikuri, H, Castellanos A, Myerburg R. Sudden Death Due to Cardiac Arrhythmias. *N. Engl. J. Med.* 2001; 345(20): 1473-1482.

[14] Zipes, D, Wellens H. Clinical Cardiology: New Frontiers Sudden Cardiac Death. *Circulation.* 1998:2334-2351.

[15] Tomaselli G, Beuckelmann D, Calkins H et al. Sudden cardiac death in heart failure: The role of abnormal repolarization. Circulation. 1994; 90:2534-39.Kraft M, Btaiche I, Sacks G.

[16] Fitzsimmons P, McWhirter P, Peterson D, Kruyer W. The natural history of Wolff-Parkinson-White syndrome in 228 military aviators: A long-term follow-up of 22 years. *Electrophysiology.* 2001; 143(3): 503-536.

[17] Treatment of electrolyte disorders in adult patients in the intesive care unit. *Am. J. Health-Sys. Pharm.* 2005; 62:1663-82.

[18] Straus S, Sturkenboom M, Bleumink G et al. Non-cardiac QTc-prolonging drugs and the risk of sudden cardiac death. *Eur. Heart J.* 2005; 26(19): 2007-2012.

[19] Straus S, Bleumink G, Dieleman J, et al. Antipsychotics and the risk of sudden cardiac death. *Arch. Intern. Med.* 2004;164:1293-97.

[20] Sandhu R, Jimenez M, Chiuve S. Smoking, smoking cessation, and risk of sudden cardiac death in women. *Circ. Arrhythm. Electrophysiol.* 2012; 5(6): 1091-7.

[21] Goldenberg I, Jonas M, Tenenbaum A et al. Current smoking cessation, and the risk of sudden cardiac death in patients with coronary artery disease. *Arch. Inter. Med.* 2003; 163(19): 2301-5.

[22] Whang W, Manson J, Hu F, et al. Physical exertion, exercise and sudden cardiac death in women. *JAMA.* 2006;295:1399-1403.

[23] Krahn A, Healey J, Chauhan V. Systematic Assessment of Patients with Unexplained Cardiac Arrest: Cardiac Arrest Survivors with Preserved Ejection Fraction Registry (CASPER). *Circulation.* 2009; 120:278-285.

[24] John R, Tedrow U, Koplan B, et al. Ventricular arrhythmias and sudden cardiac death.*Lancet.* 2012;380(9852):1520-9.

[25] Saenen J, Vrints C. Molecular aspects of the congenital and acquired Long QT Syndrome: clinical implications. *J. Mol. Cell. Cardiol.* 2008; 44(4):633-46.

[26] Marionneau C, Brunet S, Flagg TP, Distinct cellular and molecular mechanisms underlie functional remodeling of repolarizing K+ currents with left ventricular hypertrophy. Circ. Res. 2008 Jun 6;102(11):1406-15.

[27] Sugiyama S, Ozawa T. Biochemical basis for reperfusion arrhythmias. *J. Mol. Cell. Cardiol.* 1987 Oct;19Suppl 5:67-75.

[28] Oudit GY, Crackower MA, Eriksson U, et al. Phosphoinositide 3-kinase gamma-deficient mice are protected from isoproterenol-induced heart failure.Circulation.2003 Oct 28;108(17):2147-52.

[29] Tur J, Chapalamadugu KC, Panguluri SK and Tipparaju SM. Role of voltage gated potassium channel subunit Kvβ1.1 in cardiac hypertrophy.USF Health Research Day, Feb 2013, Abstract).

[30] Tipparaju SM, Saxena N, Liu SQ, Kumar R, Bhatnagar A. Differential regulation of voltage-gated K+ channels by oxidized and reduced pyridine nucleotide coenzymes. *Am. J. Physiol. Cell. Physiol.* 2005 Feb;288(2):C366-76.

[31] Tipparaju SM, Liu SQ, Barski OA, Bhatnagar A. NADPH binding to beta-subunit regulates inactivation of voltage-gated K(+) channels. *Biochem. Biophys. Res. Commun.* 2007, 27;359(2):269-76.

[32] Tipparaju SM, Li XP, Kilfoil PJ, Xue B, Uversky VN, Bhatnagar A, Barski OA. Interactions between the C-terminus of Kv1.5 and Kvβ regulate pyridine nucleotide-dependent changes in channel gating. *Pflugers Arch.* 2012;463(6):799-818.

[33] Kilfoil PJ, Tipparaju SM, Barski OA, Bhatnagar A. Regulation of ion channels by pyridine nucleotides. *Circ. Res.* 2013;112(4):721-41.

[34] Moradkhan R, Sinoway LI. Revisiting the role of oxygen therapy in cardiac patients. J. Am. Coll. Cardiol.2010 Sep 21;56(13):1013-6.

[35] Moss A, Hall W, Cannom D, et al. Improved survival with an implanted defibrillator in patients with coronary disease at high risk for ventricular arrhythmia. Multicenter Automatic Defibrillator Implantation Trial Investigators. *N. Engl. J. Med.* 1996; 335:1933.(MADIT).

[36] Moss A, Zareba W, Hall W. Prophylactic implantation of a defibrillator in patients with myocardial infarction and reduced ejection fraction. *N. Engl. J. Med.* 2002;346:877-83. (MADIT II).

[37] Buxton AE, Lee K, Fisher et al. A randomized study of the prevention of sudden death in patients with coronary artery disease. Multicenter Unsustained Tachycardia Trial Investigators. *N. Engl. J. Med.* 1999; 341:1882.(MUSTT).

[38] Bardy G, Lee K, Mark D, et al. Amiodarone or an implantable cardioverter-defibrillator for congestive heart failure. *N. Engl. J. Med.* 2005;352 (3): 225 (SCD-HeFT).

[39] Kadish A, Dyer A, Daubert JP. Prophylactic defibrillator implantation in patients with nonischemic dilated cardiomyopathy. *N. Engl. J. Med.* 2004 20;350(21):2151-8. (DEFINITE).

[40] Hohnloser S, Kuck K, Dorian P. Prophylactic use of an implantable cardiovert-defibrillator after acute myocardial infarction. *N. Engl. J. Med.* 2004; 351(24):2481.(DINAMIT).

[41] Steinbeck G, Andresen D, Seidl K et al. Defibrillator implantation early after myocardial infarction. *N. Engl. J. Med.* 2009; 361 (15):1427. (IRIS).

[42] Epstein A, DiMarco J, Ellenbogen K, et al. ACC/AHA/HRS 2008 Guidelines for device-based therapy of cardiac rhythm abnormalities. *Circulation*. 2008; 117(21):e350.

[43] Singh S, Fletcher R, Fisher S. Amiodarone in patients with congestive heart failure and asymptomatic ventricular arrhythmia. Survival Trial of Antiarrhythmic Therapy in Congestive Heart Failure. *N. Engl. J. Med.* 1995; 333:77. (CHF-STAT).

[44] Doval H, Nul D, Grancelli H, et al. Randomised trial of low-dose amiodarone in severe congestive heart failure. Grupo de estudio de la sobrevida en la insuficienciacardiaca en Argentina (GESICA). *Lancet* 1994; 344: 493.

[45] Camm AJ, Julian D, Janse G. The European Myocardial Infarct Amiodarone Trial. *Am. J. Cardiol.* 1993;72(16):95F-98F. (EMIAT).

[46] Cairns JA, Connolly SJ, Roberts R.Randomised trial of outcome after myocardial infarction in patients with frequent or repetitive ventricular premature depolarisations. *Lancet.* 1997;349(9053):675-82. (CAMIAT).

[47] Boutitie F, Boissel JP, Connolly SJ.Amiodarone interaction with beta-blockers: analysis of the merged EMIAT (European Myocardial Infarct Amiodarone Trial) and CAMIAT (Canadian Amiodarone Myocardial Infarction Trial) databases. *Circulation* 1999 May 4 99 2268-2275.

[48] Kuck K, Cappato R, Siebels J, et al. Randomized comparison of antiarrhythmic drug therapy with implantable defibrillators in patients resuscitated from cardiac arrest : the Cardiac Arrest Study Hamburg (CASH). *Circulation*. 2000; 102(7): 748-54.

[49] Connolly S, Gent M, Roberts R, et al. Canadian implantable defibrillator study (CIDS): a randomized trial of the implantable cardioverter defibrillator against amiodarone. *Circulation.* 2000; 101(11): 1297-302.

[50] The Antiarrhythmics versus Implantable Defibrillators (AVID) Investigators. A comparison of antiarrhythmic-drug therapy with implantable defibrillators in patients resuscitated from near-fetal ventricular arrhythmias. *N. Engl. J. Med.* 1997; 337(22): 1576.

In: Sudden Death
Editors: Jiashin Wu and Jessica Wu

ISBN: 978-1-62618-825-9

Chapter VI

Sudden Cardiac Death in Athletics: Scope of the Problem and Emergency Response

Eric E. Coris[1], Frances Sahebzamani[2], Steve Walz[3], Anne Curtis[4], Eduardo Gonzalez[5], Leon Anijar[5] and Kira Zwygart[5]

[1]The University of South Florida, Morsani College of Medicine, Department of Family Medicine,Department of Orthopaedics and Sports Medicine, Tampa, FL, US
[2]The University of South Florida, College of Nursing, Tampa, FL, US
[3]USF Department of Athletics, Tampa, FL, US
[4]Department of Internal Medicine, University of Buffalo, Buffalo, NY, US
[5,6,7]The University of South Florida, Morsani College of Medicine, Tampa, FL, US

Abstract

Sudden cardiac death (SCD) is the leading cause of exertional death in athletes. An understanding of the most common causes of SCD in athletes can in some cases, equip the team physician to optimize detection and treatment prior to an emergency event. Assessing and carefully planning an emergency SCD response, customized to the sport and venue can improve response time and maximize the chances of a successful resuscitation. AED utilization as early in the process as possible is critical in the emergency action plan in SCD cases.

Our knowledge of the utility of non-invasive cardiovascular screening methodologies continues to expand. Many sports medicine programs in Europe and in the United States are employing routine non-invasive cardiovascular screening in the pre participation evaluation of high level competitive athletes to attempt to screen for occult congenital cardiac disease. Further study in the area of cardiac screening in high level athletes is critical in elucidating the role of non-invasive cardiovascular screening, and its role in the prevention of SCD.

Incidence

Introduction

Exceeding 300,000 cases annually, sudden cardiac death (SCD) is the leading cause of death in the United States. [1,2] SCD is also the leading cause of death in athletes. [3] Defined as occurring within one hour of participation in sports, [4] exercise-related SCD occurs in 1-5 cases per one million athletes per year. Of the approximately 25 million competitive athletes in the United States, there are 25-125 documented cases of SCD per year, which likely represents a significant underestimation. [5] The National Federation of High School Coaches estimates 10-25 cases of SCD per year in individuals younger than 30 years. [6] The overall occurrence rate of SCD in high school athletics is estimated to be 1:100,000 to 1: 300,000 athletes/ year. [7] Despite concerted national efforts to identify the ideal mechanism for detecting and preventing these events, cardiovascular collapse as the cause of athletic fatalities in high school and collegiate athletics outnumbers death from trauma by 2:1. [8]

SCD in older athletes (>35 years of age) is most often related to atherosclerotic coronary artery disease resulting in myocardial infarction. However, in young athletes (<35 years of age), the majority of cases are caused by defined and hereditary cardiovascular disorders. Cardiac electrical instability, due to these underlying pathologies, deteriorating into fatal ventricular tachycardia or ventricular fibrillation, appears to be the most common immediate cause of death. [1,5,9,10]

To better elucidate the clinical, pathological and demographic profile of sudden deaths in young (< age 35) athletes, Maron and colleagues conducted a systematic retrospective analysis of 158 sudden deaths in athletes reported during the years 1985 – 1995 and found that 85% of these sudden deaths in competitive athletes represented a spectrum of structural cardiovascular abnormalities. [11] The majority of these athletes were involved in high school sports (62%), with collegiate athletes a distant second (22%), and professional athletes ranking third (7%). Of the athletes that experienced sudden death, 90% were male, 44% were African American and only 18% reported experiencing any prodromal symptoms prior to the event. From a sport-specific standpoint, 68% of these deaths occurred during football and basketball participation, likely a participation based statistic, but also potentially an intensity-related phenomenon. 90% of these athletes collapsed during, or immediately after, a training session or competition.

Unfortunately, while symptoms or family history of SCD may precede the event,the majority of reported episodes of arrest are the first manifestation of disease in an “apparently healthy” individual. Many athletes are capable of exceptionally high levels of performance for long periods of time, despite harboring occult and potentially lethal cardiovascular malformations. [11] As SCD events are highly traumatic to the family, the involved sports team and the surrounding community, such events tend to prompt public outcry for increased efforts by sports medicine professionals to detect, prevent and respond aggressively to these rare but catastrophic events.

To address this complex issue, significant resources have been targeted on strategies to improve detection of at-risk athletes through the pre-participation examination. Although extensive non-invasive cardiovascular testing has yielded modest benefits, [12] the ability of the pre-participation examination to optimally identify all athletes with underlying cardiovascular predispositions to sudden cardiac arrest has been limited and attempts at broad-based implementation of various non-invasive cardiovascular screening techniques have been ineffective. [7,13-16] Given the relative rarity of cardiovascular events in otherwise healthy athletes, an extremely sensitive and specific screening test, clearer, indications and guidelines for implementation are needed to improve outcomes and the cost-effectiveness of screening programs. [17]

Another major approach to this complex issue has been to support aggressive implementation of emergency response protocols and automatic defibrillators to optimally respond to a sudden cardiac arrest event. [18] While there has been significant progress in the development of nationally standardized recommendations in emergency action planning, [19] particularly from the National Athletic Trainer's Association, [20] the successfuluse of defibrillation devices in the young athlete has been less than the use of defibrillation devices in the general population. [21] We will further discuss these studies later in the chapter.

Ultimately, successful efforts to identify at risk athletes and improve intervention outcomes will require further research to develop optimal pre-participation evaluation examination strategies and to identify best practice methods for the detection and management of the spectrum of underlying cardiac pathologies commonly associated with arrest in active youth,as well as the continued pursuit of optimal response to arrest episodes.

Causes

Greater than 20 structural or functional cardiac pathologies have been identified as causes of sudden cardiac death in athletes. [22] One of the early champions for systematically analyzing the underlying pathology and clinical characteristics of SCD in order to prevent and protect young athletes is Dr. Barry Maron. In 1996, Dr. Maron published his landmark study which systematically collected and evaluated data on sudden death in a large sample of reported sudden deaths of athletes. [11] His data sources for this analysis included news media accounts, the National Center for Catastrophic Sports Injury Research registry, the cardiovascular pathology registry of Baylor University Medical Center, interviews with family members and the institutions involved with the event as well as autopsy and toxicology findings. His reported findings of the pathology found at autopsy revealed a predominance of hypertrophic cardiomyopathy (26%) and aberrant coronary arteries (13%) as the major underlying causes of sudden death among these athletes. Of cases studied, only 18% of the athletes reported symptoms associated with the cardiovascular system in the preceding 36 months prior to death (i.e. chest pain, exertional dyspnea, syncope, or dizziness). Further, 115 of the athletes had standard pre-participation examinations performed. Of these, only 3% were suspected of having cardiovascular disease and only 1 athlete (0.9%) had the correct cardiovascular abnormality identified. [11]

The lack of standardization in the quality and type of pre-participation physical examination performed on these athletes, as well as the high rate of unrecognized cardiovascular disease, illustrates the need for health care professionals, particularly in the sports medicine community, to explore adjunctive means for preventing and/or treating SCD. [23]. SCD in older athletes (>35 years old) is most often related to coronary artery disease, [4] with the incidence of SCD increasing with age. [24] Incidence rates of SCD increases when older populations of vigorous exercisers are included resulting in estimates of SCD incidence approaching 1:15,000 to 1:18,000. [25] Most of these deaths, young and old, are thought to be related to electrical instability leading to ventricular tachycardia and, eventually, ventricular fibrillation. [4, 26]

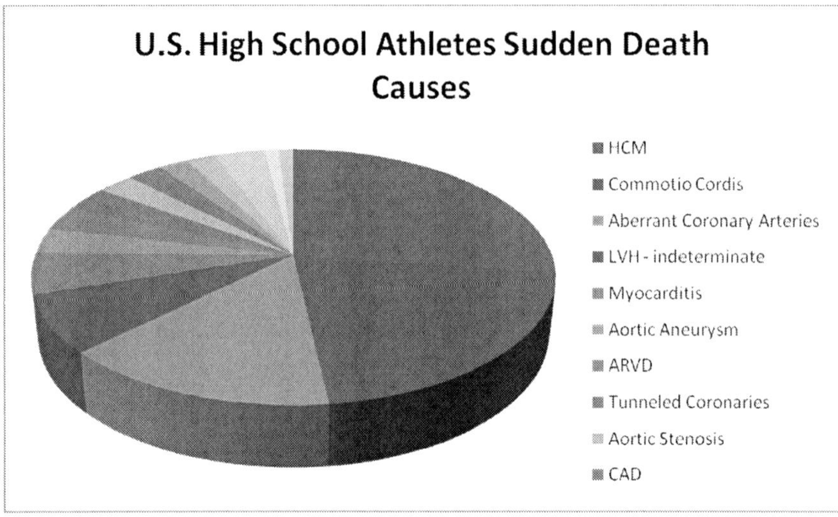

Data from Maron, JACC, 2005.

Specific Causes

Hypertrophic Cardiomyopathy

The single most common cardiac abnormality leading to SCD in the United States is hypertrophic cardiomyopathy. [11] Responsible for approximately 26% of all SCD events in U.S. athletes, it is the most significant cardiac pathology with which the sports medicine community struggles. Affecting approximately 1 in every 500 adults in the U.S., it appears to have a fairly equal male: female genetic distribution ratio.

In Maron's study, hypertrophic cardiomyopathy was more prevalent in African-American athletes compared with Caucasian athletes (48% vs. 26%; $p = .01$). Less prevalent in the athletic population, likely due to selection and some screening practices, the mortality rate is 6% per year in children and adolescents with HCM, and 1-3% per year in adults. [12]

Eleven mutant genes with over 200 specific mutations in these genes have been identified and implicated in the development of clinical hypertrophic cardiomyopathy. [27] Mutations involving the Beta-myosin heavy chain, the myosin-binding protein C, and the cardiac troponin T are responsible for approximately 50% of the population's HCM. Of these mutations, the Beta-myosin heavy chain mutations and the troponin T mutations tend to create the highest risk, while the cardiac myosin-binding protein C and alpha-tropomyosinmutations tend to be of lower risk. HCM is generally inherited via an autosomal dominant pattern.Pathologic disease of the myocardium typically develops in adolescence in conjunction with rapid growth of the body. [27] Only 60% of all individuals with HCM have an affected first degree relative, due in large part to the occurrence of spontaneous mutations. [28].

SCD Cause	Percentage
Hypertrophic Cardiomyopathy	26
CommotioCordis	20
Aberrant Coronary Arteries	14
LVH-indeterminate	7
Myocarditis	5
Ruptured Aortic Aneurysm	3
ARVD	3
Tunneled Coronary Arteries	3
Aortic Stenosis	2.5
CAD	2.5
Dilated CM	2
Myxomatous MV	2
Asthma	2
Heat stroke	1.5
Drug Abuse	1
Long QT syndrome	1

Data from Maron, JACC, 2005.

Evaluation of the pathology and morphology of the heart with HCM demonstrates a larger than normal heart with a particularly enlarged left ventricle. [27] Total left ventricular mass is increased without compensatory dilation of the chamber; thus, ventricular filling is decreased in diastole. Thickness of the ventricular septum is typically markedly increased from 15 to 50 mm, with less than 13 mm considered to be the upper limit of the normalseptum thickness. [5, 27] The marked septal hypertrophy is particularly asymmetric when compared to the left ventricular free wall, causing the characteristic left ventricular outflow tract obstruction. [22] Also commonly seen in the setting of HCM is significant anterior motion of the mitral valve during systole. [29] Microscopic pathology reveals abnormally small arteries, with "myocardial disarray" and a complex, disorganized arrangement of the myocytes with interstitial fibrosis. [30]

On clinical evaluation, HCM is typically asymptomatic. [31] Patients may present, however, with exertional chest pain, shortness of breath, dizziness, or syncope with exertion. Findings on physical examination may include a laterally displaced, enlarged point of maximal impulse. A systolic murmur may be heard, typically at the left lateral sternal border, which is characteristically increased by maneuvers that decrease preload. The Valsalva maneuver or a squatting-to-standing position change should induce the murmur on auscultation. This murmur is in contrast to more flow-dependent benign murmurs which will often become quiet or disappear with these maneuvers.

Electrocardiographic (ECG) testing is fairly sensitive for HCM; with a sensitivity greater than 90%. [31,32] Characteristic findings include left ventricular hypertrophy, abnormal axis, q waves, and ST-T wave changes. [22, 31, 32] The ECG, however, can be normal, particularly in cases of non-obstructive, or less obstructive, disease. In cases of non-obstructive HCM, the sensitivity of ECG drops to approximately 75%. Asymmetric septal hypertrophy, systolic anterior motion of the mitral valve, abnormal diastolic filling, and often, diminished left ventricular cavity size can all be seen on echocardiogram. [16, 33, 34] Cardiac MRI, particularly with contrast, can often identify the abnormal myocardium if the diagnosis is in doubt. Genetic testing is available but can approach or exceed $4500. [31, 35]

For more info, please see: http://genetics.med.harvard.edu/seidman/cg3

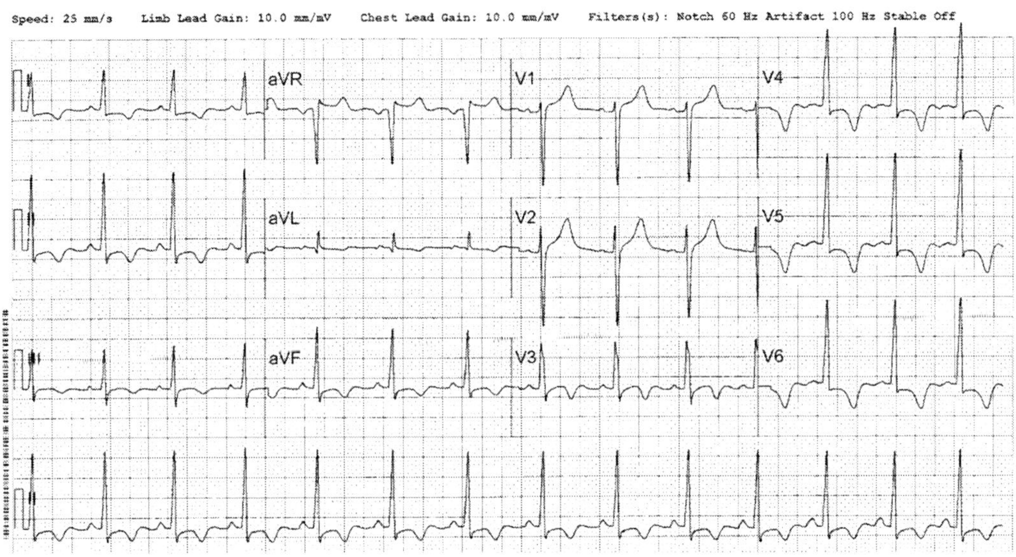

12 Lead EKG with typical findings of Hypertrophic Cardiomyopathy in an 18 year old female.

Commotio Cordis

Responsible for 20% of all SCD in U.S. athletes, commotiocordis is of particular risk for athletes participating in high velocity ball sports and represents a traumatic cause of SCD. [36, 37] A sudden forceful impact to the chest wall during ventricular repolarization can induce electrical instability leading to asystole or ventricular fibrillation which is the hallmark for the condition. [37] The mean age of fatalities from commotion cordisis 13 years of age. Symptoms of the dysrhythmia are usually absent prior to the event [37] and there are typically nounderlying cardiac abnormalities found at autopsy. Although rapid defibrillation is the treatment of choice, defibrillation attempts are often unsuccessfulas many athletes deteriorate immediately into asystole [21, 22]. Thus the resuscitation rate is usually low and approximately 15%, even with appropriate rapid response. Currently, anational commotiocordis registry is tracking injuries and response which is expected to provide important information in furthering our understanding of this deadly condition.

Coronary Arterial Abnormalities

The second leading cause of non-traumatic SCD is represented by a group of disorders of the coronary arteries. [1, 4, 18, 22, 34, 38, 39] Anomalous origin of the left anterior descending arteryfrom the right aortic sinus is the most common of a variety of congenital anomalies of the coronary vessels. [12] Tunneled coronaries, myocardial bridging, single coronary arteries, and others anomalies have been found to contribute to transient myocardial ischemia during intense activity that then induces malignant arrhythmia, often ventricular tachycardia/ventricular fibrillation. [10, 40]. Although these anomalies are most often asymptomatic, approximately 1/3 of athletes will experience angina, syncope, or exertional dyspnea prior to an SCD event. [41] In one study conducted in the United States and Italy, 10 out of the12 athletes found to have underlying coronary abnormalities also reported cardiac symptoms prior to death. [42] Symptoms may play an important role in the identification of at risk athletes as the physical examination for arterial abnormalities is typically unremarkable. [26] Equally challenging is the fact that the resting echocardiogram, andthe exercise treadmill stress testing are often also normal. [7, 12, 40, 43, 23, 44, 4, 23]

In the study cited above, nine athletes with arterial abnormalities had normal resting ECGs; six of these athletes also had normal exercise stress testing in addition to the routine ECG. [42] Although segmental wall motion abnormalities may be seen on stress echocardiography, a definitive diagnosis is often made by coronary angiography, computed tomography of the coronary arteries, or magnetic resonance imaging. [31, 34, 42]

Myocarditis

Inflammation or infection in the myocardial tissue can lead to electrical instability and SCD in athletes. Involvement of the conduction system can also lead to fatal complete heart block. [10, 26, 34] While cardiac inflammation is typically related to a Coxsackie B viral infection (approximately 50%), cardiac inflammation can be cause by a large number of organisms. [45, 46] Affected individuals may present with chest pain, dyspnea, syncope, and/or dizziness, but they mayalso present with more systemic symptoms related to the infectious process. [45]. Fever, chills, nausea, vomiting, upper respiratory symptoms, diarrhea, and/or sore throat may be present. However, an athletes' presenting symptom is often the SCD event. [5, 18, 21, 46].

Clinically, athletes at risk may be identified by symptoms of infection as mentioned above or of by symptoms associated with cardiac involvement including chest pain, dyspnea, syncope or dizziness. [46] On physical examination, they may present with signs associated with congestive heart failure such as distended neck veins, a laterally displaced and enlarged PMI, an audible S3 gallop, rales, or peripheral edema, and/or hepatojugular reflux. [34, 45, 46]. The chest x-ray may be normal, but may also demonstrate cardiomegaly or pulmonary edema. [45] The ECG may indicate myocarditis through characteristic ST segment elevation, but sensitivity for the ECG is relatively low and often highly variable (10-50%). [34, 45, 46] Echocardiographic examination may demonstrate myocardial hypokinesis, a depressed ejection fraction, or may be normal. Cardiac MRI with contrast may be helpful in demonstrating myocardial inflammation [46]. Definitive diagnosis for myocarditis depends on a myocardial biopsy. [46] Histologic analysis may demonstrate myocardial inflammation and/ idiopathic myocardial scarring. [46, 47] It has been postulated that myocardial scarring generates the arrhythmogenic focus in some asymptomatic athletes with SCD events. [5, 10, 45]. Treatment for myocarditis is targeted towards the clinical cardiac disease, treatment of any underlying heart failure, and to protecting the heart from excessive stress during the active phase of the disease. Echocardiography, electrophysiology and stress testing may be utilized to document resolution of the condition and the absence of arrhythmogenic potential. [1, 5, 26, 45].

Marfan's Syndrome

Accounting for only 2% of SCD in U.S. athletes, Marfan's syndrome represents a cluster of clinical characteristics which the sports physician and cardiologist must recognize. Marfan's syndrome is a clinical diagnosis which is associated with an autosomal dominant inherited connective tissue disorder occurring in approximately 1 in 10,000 individuals. [46]

An athlete with this condition will often have a family history significant for Marfan's syndrome. The physician's ability to diagnose and subsequently monitor Marfanoid athletes to reduce their risk of SCD is unique among the major causes of SCD and warrants additional attention. Marfan's is one of a family of connective tissue disorders that leads to an increased risk of progressive dilatation of the aortic root, potentially leading to dissection and/or rupture of the aorta resulting in massive hemorrhage, pericardial tamponade, coronary artery dissection, acute aortic valve insufficiency, and congestive heart failure. [46, 48]. Marfan's syndrome is frequently asymptomatic but does have characteristic morphologic/clinical findings related to the connective tissue pathology. [48] Marfanoid athletes are characteristically tall and thin with an accompanying long thin facies. They often have disproportionately long limbs, with an arm span greater than their height and an upper body to lower body ratio of more than one standard deviation below the mean [46] Hyperextension of joints and significant overlap of the thumb and fifth digit when circumferentially wrapped around the thin wrist is another common finding. [46, 48, 49] Kyphoscoliosis and anterior thoracic deformities such as pectusexcavatum and carinatum are often present [49]. Once an athlete with Marfan's syndrome has been identifiedby the clinical characteristics of the syndrome, an echocardiagram is recommended to evaluate for evidence of aortic root dilation. These athletes are then subsequently screened by serial echocardiograms on a 6 month, or yearly, basis to monitor for aortic root dilation. [46, 48]An ophthalmic exam is also required to evaluate for the presence of ectopialentis. Depending on the results of these evaluations and the sport, the athlete must be limited from participating in inappropriate activity. [49].

Marfan's Syndrome Major Diagnostic Criteria

Major criteria

Skeletal – must have at least four

1. Pectuscarinatum
2. Pectusexcavatum
3. Arm span greater than height
4. Reduced upper trunk to lower segment ratio
5. Positive wrist sign (thumb overlaps little finger wrapped around opposite wrist)

6. Positive thumb sign
7. Scoliosis, greater than 20 degrees
8. Spondylolisthesis
9. PesPlanus
10. Protrusion Acetabulae

Cardiovascular

1. Ascending aortic dilation or aneurysm
2. Ascending aortic dissection

Spinal Dura

1. Dural ectasia

Long QT Syndromeand Ion Channel Disorders

Long QT Syndrome

Long QT syndrome is a rare (1% of all SCD episodes in U.S.) but dramatic result of a group of congenital ion channel defects that may lead to SCD in an athlete. [3] By current estimations, approximately 1 in 10,000 Americans have prolonged QT syndrome. [3, 50] In this syndrome, the period of the cardiac cycle between ventricular firing and repolarizationknown as the QT interval is longer than normal. In men this period of the cardiac cycle is considered prolonged if the interval, after correction for rate, is greater than, or equal to, 440 ms. In women, the corrected QT interval is considered prolonged if it is greater than, or equal to, 460 ms.

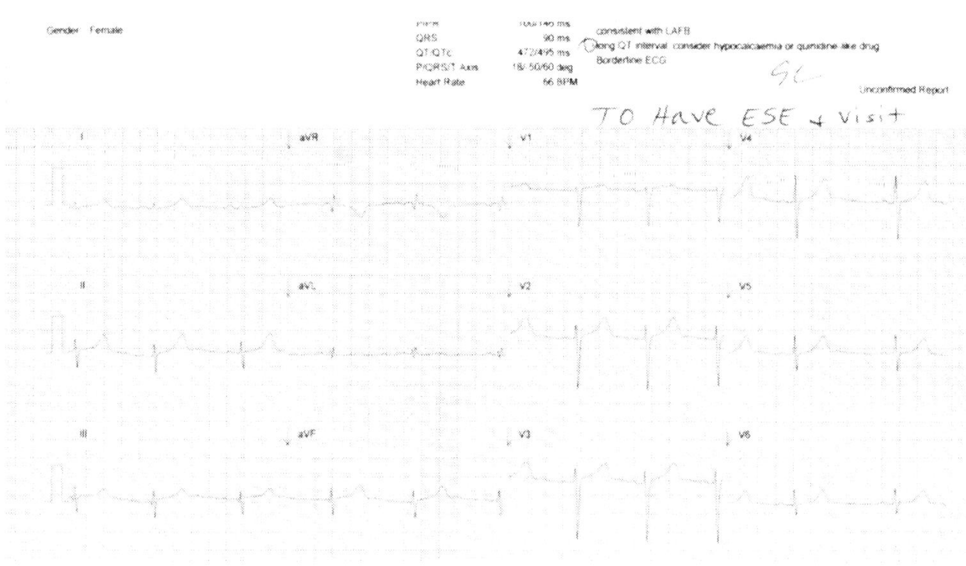

12 Lead EKG with typical findings of Long QT syndrome.

Of those individuals with long QT syndrome, 60% are likely to have a positive family history of long QT or SCD. [3, 50] One third of all patients present with symptoms referable to the disorder; with palpitations, seizures, and syncope being most common. [23, 51] The heart is structurally normal in most patients, with the primary abnormality being a tendency toward life-threatening ventricular arrhythmias resulting from an ion channel defect.While these syndromes tend to be asymptomatic, a catecholamine surge or extreme stress may induce a SCD. [3, 9, 48] Statistically, these syndromes are likely underreported due to inconclusive autopsy findings that are common in deaths resulting from these disorders. [50]

Long QT syndrome can be identified on ECG by a prolonged QT interval.. [1, 3, 31, 32] Occasionally, only an atypical U wave may be seen. In the related Brugada syndrome, the ECG will demonstrate evidence of an incomplete right bundle branch block and ST segment elevations in the right precordial leads, with a structurally normal heart. Genetic testing may allow identification of the disease and the underlying subtype. Genetic testing may detect up to 75% of the most common genetic mutations leading to prolonged QT syndrome (QT1, QT2, QT3, QT5, QT6). The three major types of testing for this condition target slightly different genetic tendencies. The Comprehensive Cardiac Ion Channel Analysis provides analysis for variants in all five suspected genes, and is the most comprehensive test. In contrast, the Sodium Channel Analysis only targets the SCN5A gene and is most appropriate in cases of suspected Brugada Syndrome. There is also a family-specific analysis to identify the specific subtype of prolonged QT syndrome that is carried in the family genome. [3, 31, 48] Genetic testing, however, can be expensive and often requires repeated negotiations with the patient's insurance company for reimbursement. Resources for additional information on these genetic tests can be found on www.familion.com.

Interestingly, of the four major subtypes of long QT syndrome that account for the majority of mutations, each has a different predictable trigger that precedes a SCD episode. [3, 27, 31, 50] In QT1, the common trigger is swimming. Although these athletes may tolerate an extreme level of exertion associated with most types of activities, the unique cardiovascular demands of swimming typically produce a sudden death event by triggering a malignant tachyarrhythmia, often ventricular tachycardia decompensating into ventricular fibrillation. In QT2, the most common trigger is extreme emotion. Often a frightening surprise will send athletes with prolonged QT2 into an aberrant tachyarrhythmia and SCD. In contrast, the most common trigger for QT3is not activity, but inactivity. The malignant tachyarrhythmia seems to erupt almost spontaneously during low levels of activity. In QT4, the most common trigger of a SCD episode is a sudden malignant tachyarrhythmia precipitated by a loud noise, such as an alarm clock.

Treatment often involves therapy with B-blockers, a pacemaker and/or an implantable cardiac defibrillator (ICD),as well as refraining from activity likely to provoke the dysrhythmia.However, a growing number of athletes, after extensive consultation and assessment, are returning to competitive sport even with an ICD in place. [31, 52] Please refer to the chapter on the athlete with an implanted device.

Wolff-Parkinson-White Syndrome (WPW)

Unlike the channelopathies, WPW is a result of an accessory pathway connecting the atrium to the ventricle that can promote the development of "re-entrant tachycardias". Typically manifesting as a relatively benign intermittent supraventricular tachycardia (SVT), patients will often present with symptoms of palpitations, dizziness, or lightheadedness. [26,

34, 53] The ECG during an episode may demonstrate a narrow complex tachycardia. Once the episode resolves and the patient returns to normal sinus rhythm, a characteristic "delta wave" can be seen.

The typical appearance of a delta wave is a slurred, early upstroke in the QRS complex. [26, 31] The acute episode of SVT can often be terminated with stimulation of the vagal system. Maneuvers such as unilateral carotid sinus massage, the Valsalva maneuver, or even facial immersion in ice water, will often break the tachycardia and return the patient to normal sinus rhythm. [53] If not, often a calcium channel blocker or adenosine can break the abnormal rhythm.SCD is rare in WPW syndrome, but it can occur, particularly with rapid ventricular rates during atrial fibrillation that may degenerate into ventricular fibrillation. In cases of aborted SCD in WPW, or for patients with recurrent or severe symptoms, an electrophysiology study with radiofrequency catheter ablation of the abnormal accessory pathway should be performed. [53]

Arrhythmogenic Right Ventricular Dysplasia

Arrhythmogenic right ventricular dysplasia (ARVD), also known as arrhythmogenic right ventricular cardiomyopathy, is a genetic disorder characterized by right ventricular enlargement and dysfunction associated with potentially life-threatening ventricular arrhythmias. The incidence of SCD in athletes with ARVD is estimated to be 0.5/100,000 persons/year. [54] Typically, the disease becomes manifest during adolescence and early adulthood, with a male predominance. ARVD is the most common pathological finding in athletes who have died suddenly in the Veneto region of Italy, accounting for approximately one-fourth of fatal events. The identification of ARVD as the cause of SCD in the United States is much less frequent, with an estimated incidence of 3%. [46].

ARVD is a genetic disorder with autosomal dominant transmission in about one-third of cases. In many cases it is recognized to be a desmosomal disease caused by defective cell adhesion proteins such as desmoplakin, plakoglobin, and others. [55] There is also a mutation in the cardiac ryanodine receptor that has been identified as the cause of ARVD in other patients. Progressive myocyte death occurs with fibro-fatty infiltration. Thinning of the right ventricle walloccurs, along with localized aneurysmal dilatationThe disease primarily affects the right ventricle, with a much lower incidence of left ventricular dysfunction.

Athletes with ARVD have a 5.4-fold increased risk of dying during competitive sports than when they are sedentary. [54] The reasons for this observation are not known, but may relate to increases in right ventricular afterload during exertion along with denervation hypersensitivity to catecholamines that may lead to an increase in ventricular arrhythmiasduring exercise. Athletes with ARVD may present with palpitations or syncope, but others may be asymptomatic when first evaluated. Physical examination is usually normal unless extensive disease and right ventricular failure is present. The typical ECG abnormality in an individual with ARVD manifests as T wave inversions in the right precordial leads beyond V1.

Ventricular arrhythmias, including premature ventricular beats and ventricular tachycardia, are frequent and usually have a left bundle branch block morphology. Signal-averaged electrocardiography is typically abnormal as well. The diagnosis may be confirmed by noninvasive imaging studies such as echocardiography, angiography, or magnetic resonance imaging. In some cases, endomyocardial biopsy is used to demonstrate fibro-fatty infiltration of the right ventricle.

The diagnosis of ARVD in an athlete would lead to disqualification from sports participation, given the high risk of SCD during competition. ICDs are often implanted in symptomatic individuals.

Immediate Treatment

Following a thorough pre-participation exam, the next step in prevention of SCD is the implementation of a well-consideredemergency action plan (EAP). Careful planning and consideration must be taken into account when developing the EAP. Several factors must be considered including, but not limited to, the physical facilities, emergency equipment requirements, designated personnel, communication strategies, and the local hospital settings. Due to its high participation levels and variety of venues, athletics has become a key EAP target, not only for athletes, but for coaches, staff, and spectators as well. [21, 56] The National Athletic Trainers' Association (NATA) and the National Collegiate Athletic Association (NCAA) have developed statements and positions regarding the EAP and its utilization for sporting events [20, 56].

The following components have been identified as fundamental to the organization and development of a comprehensive EAP: [20]

Personnel -mandating personnel trained in cardiopulmonary resuscitation (CPR), AED, and First Aid. It is imperative to have all key personnel who are directly involved with the athletes trained in emergency care. Key personnel may include coaches, athletes, administrators, equipment managers, and officials. The implementation of the EAP is not limited onlyto those who are certified in emergency care. Personnel not trained in emergency care can be instrumental in coordinating communication, directing emergency medical response teams to the correct location, and in helping to maintain the area around the emergency situation. These individuals need to be accounted for in the EAP.

Equipment- having the appropriate equipment on-site, or nearby, assists in the smooth implementation of the EAP. [18] One of the most essential pieces of emergency equipment is the Automated External Defibrillator (AED).[57] Access to an AED is critical in many SCD cases and can mean the difference between saving, or losing, a life. [18, 20, 21] Other equipment needed for CPR would include masks and oxygen supplies. Personnel participating in the EAP must befamiliar with and trained to use the necessary equipment. [18]

Communication- a communication device could easily be listed in the equipment section as the most essential piece of emergency rescue equipment. Access to communications in the event of an emergency including SCD's, should be the first step in initiating an EAP. The EAP should clearly identify where the closest landline is located, who should have cell phones on site, and/or who is in charge of radio communication. In the event radio communication is utilized, protocol should be developed which clearly designates the duties of the person receiving the emergency message and how they should proceed to relay or coordinate messages. It is critical that the designated person authorized to make the emergency call to 911 be knowledgeable accurate about the correct information needed to be provided to the dispatcher and trained to remain calm while listening to the dispatcher and accurate in relaying any action to be initiated. Key elements of a 911 call include: 1) the nature of emergency; 2) the patient's symptoms; 3) current care being given to the patient; 4) approximate age of patient, and 5) any medical history that can be ascertained from the patient, or those involved in his/her care. Specifically, concern regarding a cardiac event must be relayed to the dispatcher as, often; it is possible to expedite AED arrival to the scene, even prior to full EMS response.

Venue - the EAP should be specific to the venue in which a given sporting event takes place. For example, intercollegiate athletics programs will need to have an EAP for each sport and for each practice site.

Even practice sites used for only a short period of time will require a plan in anticipation of an emergency. Recommended items for each venue include: 1) means of communication (eg., landlines for phone access, radio devices, cell phones); 2) access to the field or court; 3) the location of and keys for gated access that may facilitate or hinder emergency access, and 4) the location of the nearest AED. Hospital access from the site is another consideration and should be included in the plan.

Emergency Care Facilities - access to the hospital based emergency department and personnel is a key strategic component of any comprehensive EAP. It is important to communicate beforehand with the emergency facility closest to your venue and to establish how information can best be relayed to these emergency providers during an emergency event. Making prevenient contact with the hospital and local EMT's/Paramedics can help establish a more efficacious implementation of the EAP when applied in an emotionally charged setting.

Practice and Review - the EAP should not only be reviewed but should also be practiced at each site. The importance of practicing the EAP prior to an event cannot be overstated. A verbal review of the EAP procedures with personnel involved in the emergency plan is important, but implementing a practice run with selected simulation scenarios for the EAP at specific venues will enhance the ultimate performance of the plan. The results of these practice runs should be well documented and indicate any changes in the plan.

The NATA consensus statement on Emergency Planning in Athletics is a thorough, detailed document that forms a comprehensive blueprint for customizing an EAP for anyathletic venue. The NCAA guidelines for Emergency Care and Coverage (NCAA Sports Medicine Handbook) is another source for universities and colleges to help design, construct, and implement an emergency action plan. While the statistics show that the survival rate of a SCD is low, especially in cases of young, otherwise healthy athletes, the numbers also show that there have been successful outcomes with revival attempts. Well planned EAP procedures play an integral part in those successful cases of survival.

AED Utilization - NCAA Collegiate experience

In 2002, Coris et. al., examined current AED access, ownership, and utilization among National Collegiate Athletic Association (NCAA) Division 1 athletic departments. [18] Of the 186 (61%) of 303 institutions responding to the survey, 72% (133) reported having access to AED units for their athletic programs, either through departmental ownership of the units or through the university system or local emergency medical services, while slightly more than half, 54% (101), reported departmental ownershipof AED units for their programs.The mean number of total students attending the responding departments' institutions was 16,360 (SD = 11,026.00) with a reported 498 (SD = 222) mean number of varsity athletes per institution. [18]. At the time of the survey, 8.6% (16) of the 133 programs with either access to, or ownership, of AED units reported having had to use the AED in an SCD event since purchase.

Victims of Sudden Cardiac Death

Reported recipients of the AED interventions included: 62.5% (10) officials, fans, and athletic department staff; 18.7% (3) athletes; and 6.25% (1) event involving a department's coach. Twelve and one-half percent (2) reported having had to use their AED units multiple times since purchase. [21]

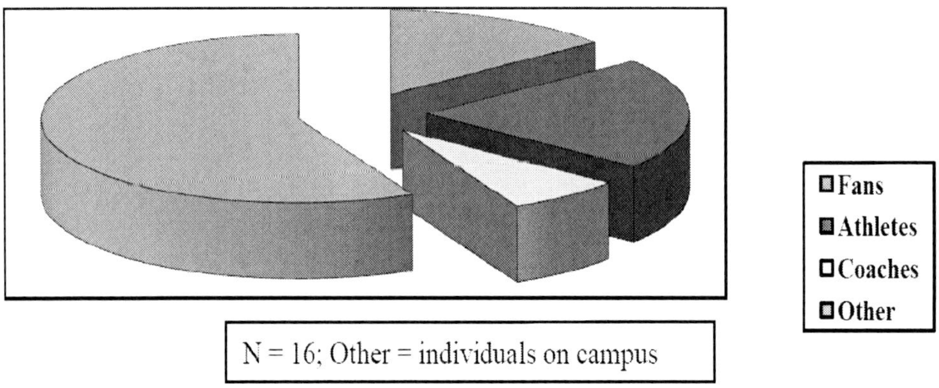

NCAA Experience with Sudden Cardiac Death

Cases of AED utilization reported by athletic departments are outlined in the table above. Twenty percent of AED uses were attributed to student athletes, with 33% of utilizations for athletic department staff, and 47% for fans. Defibrillation was actually administered in 53% of AED unit applications. Time to shock was an average of 3.4 minutes, with average EMS response time of 8.2 minutes for those events without EMS on site. Reported survival in this university athletic department setting for SCD was 0% for students, 75% for staff, 57 % for fans, and 61% overall. [21] Eighty-eight percent of the reported AED interventions occurred during athletic events or training venues, with the exception of two events which occurred on campus locations unrelated to the athletic department.

Of departments directly involved with the AED unit intervention (67%), 56% reported the AED units as easy to use, with all 16 respondents denying problems specifically with the units during the SCD event.

Case #	Patient	Outcome	Time to Shock	Location	EMS response time
1	Student-athlete	Head athletic trainer notified 5-10 minutes after event, defibrillator applied within 9 minutes, non-shockable, deceased	No shock	Student weight room	11 min
2	Student-athlete	Pt with cardiac history, reported chest pain, monitored within 30 seconds, survived, diagnosis: non-cardiac chest pain	No shock	Practice field	8-10 min
Case #	Patient	Outcome	Time to Shock	Location	EMS response time
3	Student-athlete	Defibrillator applied within 90 seconds, non-shockable rhythm (PEA), deceased, diagnosis: hypertrophic cardiomyopathy	No shock	Campus rec ctr	8 min
4	Coach	Defibrillator applied within 2 minutes, non-shockable rhythm, deceased, diagnosis: myocardial infarction	No shock	Bleachers	Unknown
5	Graduation attendee	Suspected MI, Defibrillator applied in 5-7 min, no shock advised, survived to hospital discharge	No shock	Gymnasium	10 minutes
6	Lecture attendee	Defibrillator x 3, once more by EMS, survived to discharge, diagnosis: MI	2 min	Lecture hall	5-10 min
7	Staff	Monitored, survived to discharge	No shock	Training room	7 min
8	Football official	Defibrillator applied within one minute, ventricular fibrillation noted, defibrillated x1, survived to hospital discharge, diagnosis: myocardial infarction	55 sec	Football stadium	Immediate, on site
9	Fan	Defibrillated x1, survived to discharge	< 5 min	Arena	Immediate, on site
10	Fan	Defibrillated x2, resumed normal sinus rhythm, survived to hospital discharge	< 2.5 min	Basketball arena	Within 5 min
11	Fan	CPR provided until EMS arrival, no defibrillation prior, patient did not survive, diagnosis: MI	5-10 min	Basketball arena	5-10 min
12	Fan	VF/VT, Defibrillated x3, resumed normal sinus rhythm, survived to hospital discharge	4 min	Parking area	Within 5 min
13	Fan	VF/VT, Defibrillated x1, resumed normal sinus rhythm, survived to hospital discharge	2 min	Unknown	15 min
14	Fan	Notified within minutes, Defibrillated x 1, presumed VF/VT, precipitated non-shockable rhythm, did not survive	3 min	Stadium	5 min
15	Fan	Hockey trainer notified, EMS on site, CPR immediately, Defibrillator applied in 7-8 min due to crowd related delay, non shockable rhythm, did not survive, diagnosis: massive MI	No shock	Hockey arena	On site

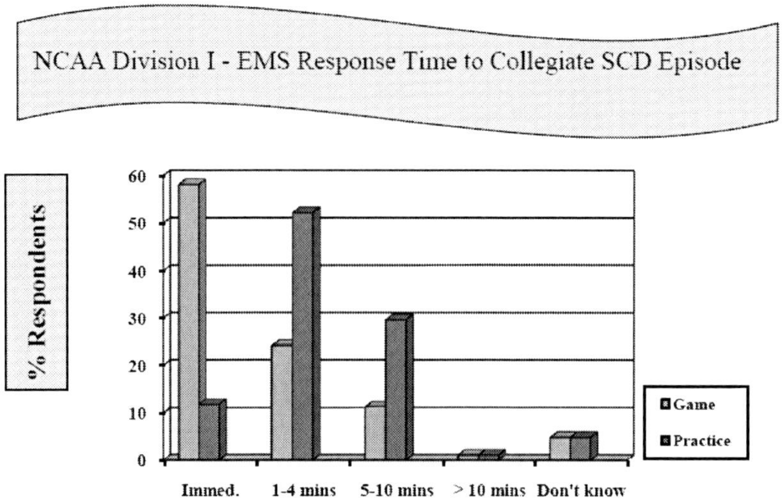

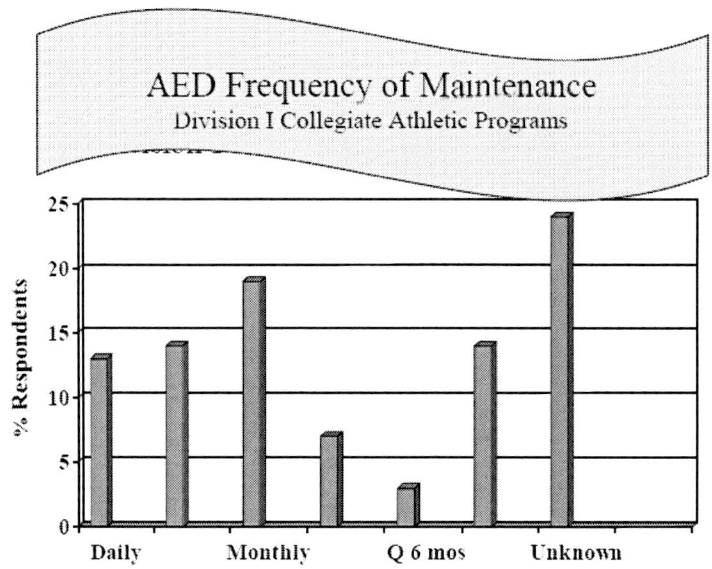

N=133

The previous tables illustrate AED unit program utilization and maintenance policies for the sub-sample, which were not significantly different from the total sample of NCAA respondents. When compared with the total sample of Division I Athletic departments reporting access to or ownership of AED units (n = 133), departments reporting having experienced an SCD event were significantly more likely to report a greater number of units per department (4.5 *SD* = 2.7 vs. 2.84 *SD* = 2.4; t = -2.32, p = .03) at a greater per unit cost ($2568.00 *SD* = $1115.00 vs. $1872.00 *SD* = $1597.00, T= -2,21, p < .03) than departments without an SCD event. Five (31%) of departments reported purchasing additional AED units to expand their program since their initial implementation of their AED programs, three (18.5%) reported that they were actively attempting to fund additional units, while 50% reported no changes in their current AED programs.

Case 1

As a 20 year old softball pitcher is making her way back to the mound during routine pitching drills, she reaches up to her head as she states she “doesn’t feel good” and then suddenly collapses face first to the turf. Her athletic trainer, witnessing her fall, rushed to her aid. There did not appear to be any trauma involved in the incident. After a log rolling maneuver, assessment of her airway revealed that she had some dirt in her mouth, but that her airway was otherwise unobstructed. There was no evidence of respiration and she was beginning to appear cyanotic peripherally, and then centrally. The emergency action plan was activated.

AED Tracing of Case 1. SCD

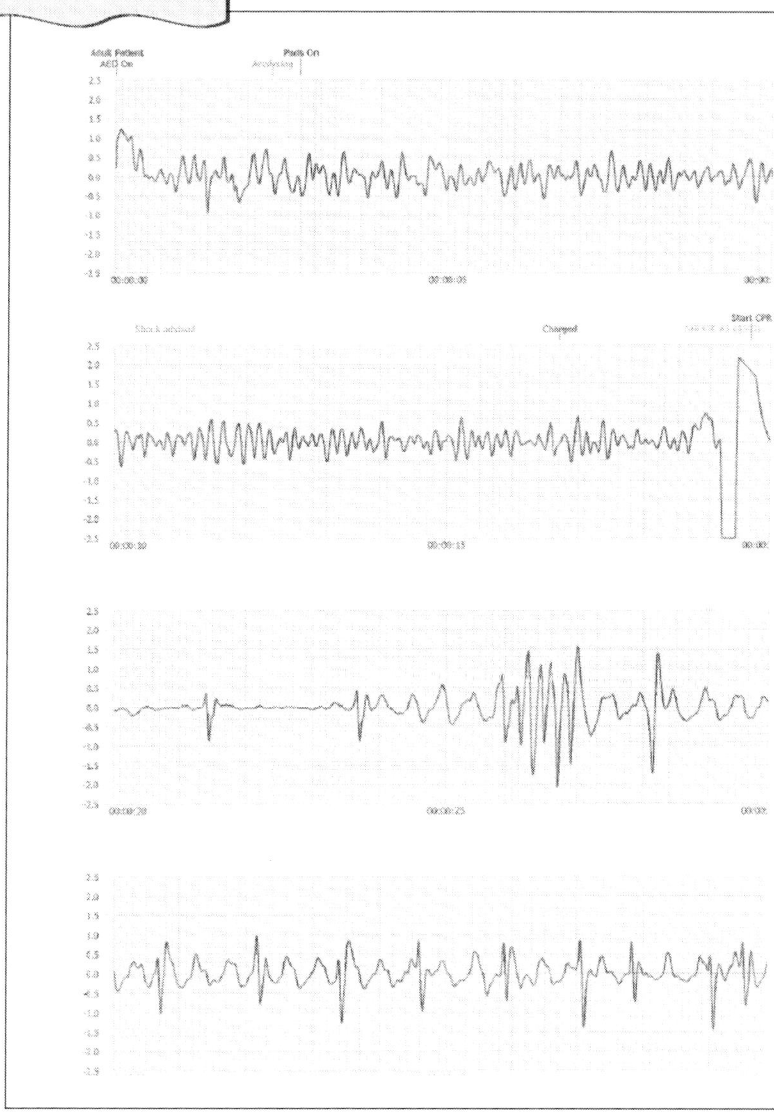

Following the look, listen, and feel protocol, no respiration or pulse could be found and CPR was immediately initiated. The AED was called for and chest compressions and rescue breaths were begun by one person CPR while awaiting the AED. Upon arrival of the AED, approximately one and a half minutes later, chest pads were applied and a shock was advised. All were cleared and one shock was delivered. Return of color was witnessed in the athlete and gasping respirations were observed. A pulse was palpated and the patient was placed on her side in the recovery position. Two minutes later, the AED advised another shock, but the patient was alert and responsive at the time, and the AED pads were removed. After the initial shock event, she converted to a sinus tachycardia with a right bundle branch block. EMS arrived approximately 5 minutes after the initial shock event. At this time, she was still responsive and found to be in a normal sinus tachycardia rhythm with a right bundle branch block.

The patient was placed on oxygen, an IV was started, and she was placed on a transport gurney and subsequently taken to the nearest ER. In the emergency room, her ECG showed a mild U wave and a right bundle branch block, but was otherwise normal.The chest x-ray was normal and her labs revealed mild hypokalemia.The rest of her labs were normal, and the patient was admitted to a cardiac care unit for observation.

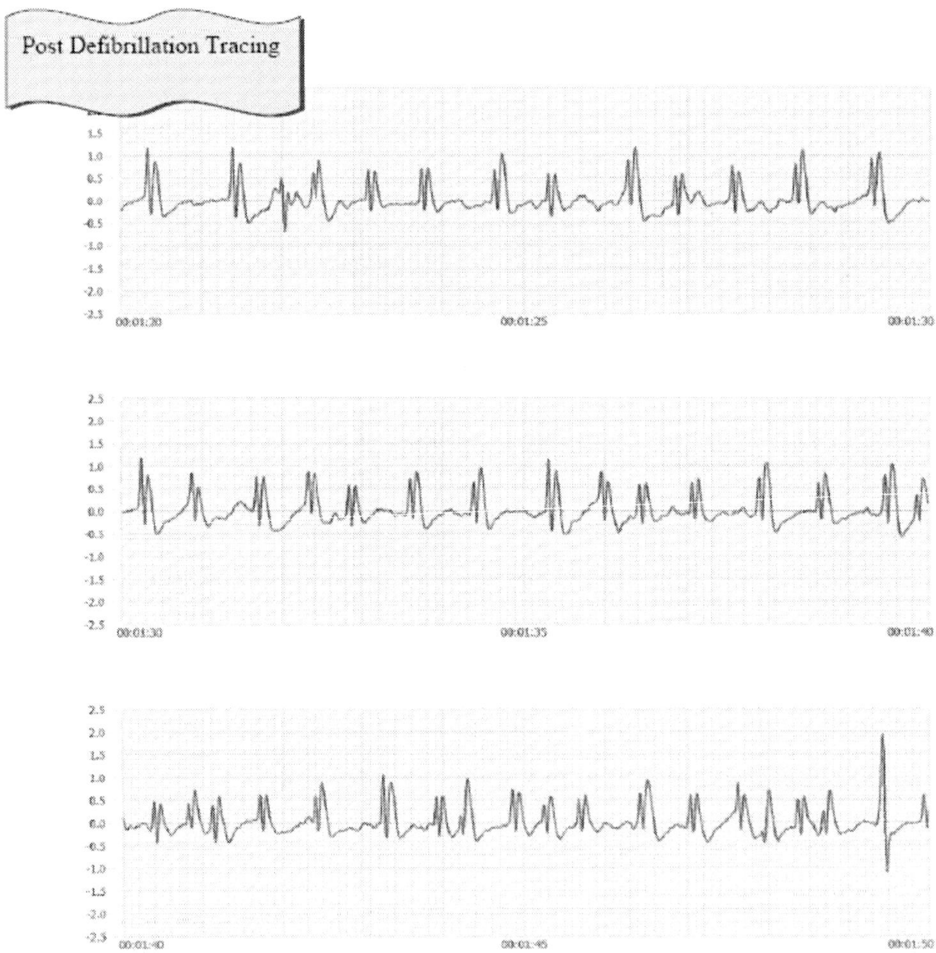

No further ectopy or ventricular arrhythmia was noted. Echocardiogram andcardiac MRI were normal, with normal muscle signal and normal take off of the coronary arteries.

Given the patient's SCD event, extensive discussion with the patient and her parents was completed and an implantable cardiac defibrillator was placed in her left axilla. The patient tolerated the procedure well and was discharged home after hospital day 3.

Conclusion

There are a variety of cardiac conditions, many asymptomatic that can lead to sudden death. Pre-participation examinations can identify some athletes at risk and should be done in accordance with the AHA guidelines [7] for pre-participation examination, and by the recommendations for the Preparticipation Physical Evaluation endorsed by the American Academy of Family Physicians, the American Academy of Pediatrics, The American College of Sports Medicine, the American Medical Society for Sports Medicine, the American Orthopaedic Society for Sports Medicine, and the American Osteopathic Academy of Sports Medicine. [17] Many cardiovascular abnormalities will not be identified by even the most thorough pre-participation evaluation. As more data becomes available in the U.S., the role of non-invasive cardiovascular screening in the large-scale pre-participation examinations, particularly relating to the screening ECG, may become clearer. Currently almost half of U.S. Division I intercollegiate athletic programs utilize non-invasive cardiac testing in their pre-participation screening programs. [58] Further research into the underlying causes of SCD in athletes is also ongoing and should provide invaluable insights into and recommendations for the detection and treatment of underlying cardiac disease in athletes.

Finally, a robust emergency action plan is imperative to optimally respond to the inevitable emergencies that will infrequently, but emergently, present themselves to the sports medicine team. Establishing, teaching, and practicing this plan may save lives that otherwise would be lost to this diverse collection of hidden disorders.

References

[1] Huikuri HV CA, Myerburg RJ. Sudden Death Due to Cardiac Arrhythmias. *New England Journal of Medicine* 2001;345(20):1473-1482.

[2] Gillum RF. Sudden Coronary Death in The United States. *Circulation* 1989;79:756-765.

[3] Ackerman MJ. The Long QT Syndrome: Ion Channel Diseases of the Heart. *Mayo Clinic Proceedings* 1998;73:250-269.

[4] Basilico F. Current Concepts: Cardiovascular Disease in Athletes. *American Journal of Sports Medicine* 1999;27(1):108-121.

[5] Futterman LG MR. Sudden Death in Athletes: An Update. *Sports Medicine* 1998;26(5):335-350.

[6] Van Camp SP. Sudden Death. *Clinics in Sports Medicine* 1992;11:273-289.

[7] Maron BJ TP, Puffer JC, et al. Cardiovascular Pre-Participation Screening of Competitive Athletes. *Circulation* 1996;94(4):850-856.

[8] Cantu RC. Congenital Cardiovascular Disease: The Major Cause of Athletic Death in High School and College. *Medicine and Science in Sports and Exercise* 1992;24:279-280.

[9] Myerburg RJ KK, Castellanos A. Sudden Cardiac Death: Structure, Function, and Time-Dependance of Risk. *Circulation* 1992;85(supplement I):I2-I10.

[10] Maron BJ. Triggers for Sudden Cardiac Death in the Athlete. *Cardiology Clinics* 1996;14(2):195-210.

[11] Maron BJ SJ, Poliac LC, et al. Sudden Death in Young Competitive Athletes. *JAMA* 1996;276(3):199-204.

[12] Maron BJ, Thompson PD, Ackerman MJ, Balady G, et.al. Recommendations and Considerations Related to Preparticipation Screening for Cardiovascular Abnormalities in Competitive Athletes: 2007 Update. *Circulation* 2007;115:1643-1655.

[13] Fuller CM MC, Spring DA. Prospective Screening of 5,615 High School Athletes for Risk of Sudden Cardiac Death. *Medicine and Science in Sports and Exercise* 1997;29:1131-1138.

[14] Maron BJ BS, Wesley YE, et al. Results of Screening a Large Group of Intercollegiate Competitive Athletes for Cardiovascular Disease. *Journal of the American College of Cardiology* 1987;10:1214-1221.

[15] Murray PM CJ, Heath DL, et al. The Role of Limited Echocardiography in Screening Athletes. *American Journal of Cardiology* 1995;76:849-850.

[16] Lewis JF MB, Diggs JA, et al. Preparticipation Echocardiographic Screening for Cardiovascular Disease in a Large Predominantly Black Population of Collegiate Athletes. *American Journal of Cardiology* 1989;64:1029-1033.

[17] Matheson GO, Boyajian-O'Neill LA, D C, Dexter W, et.al. Preparticipation Physical Evaluation: Third Edition. 3 ed. Minneapolis, New York City: McGraw-Hill Companies, 2005.

[18] Coris EE SF, Walz SJ, Ramirez AM. Automated External Defibrillators in Division I Athletics. *American Journal of Sports Medicine* 2004;32(3):744-754.

[19] White RD HD, Bugliosi TF. Seven Years' Experience With Early Defibrillation By Police and Paramedics in an Emergency Medical Services System. *Resuscitation* 1998;39:145-151.

[20] Drezner JA, Courson RW, Roberts WO, Mosesso VN, et.al. Interassociation Task Force Recommendations on Emergency Preparedness and Management of Sudden Cardiac Arrest in High School and College Athletic Programs: A Consensus Statement. *Journal of Athletic Training* 2007;41(1):143-158.

[21] Coris EE, Miller E, Sahebzamani F. Sudden Cardiac Death in Division I Collegiate Athletics. *Clinical Journal of Sports Medicine* 2005;15(2):89-91.

[22] Bille K, Figueiras D, Schamasch P, Kappenberger L, et.al. Sudden Cardiac Death in Athletes: the Lausanne Recommendations. *European Journal of Cardiovascular Prevention and Rehabilitation* 2006;13:859-875.

[23] Wingfield K, Matheson GO, Meeuwisse WH. Preparticipation Evaluation: An Evidence-Based Review. *Clinical Journal of Sports Medicine* 2004;14(3):109-122.

[24] Maron BJ PL, Roberts WO. Risk of Sudden Cardiac Death Associated With Marathon Running. *Journal of the American College of Cardiology* 1996;28:428-431.

[25] Siscovick DS WN, Fletcher RH, et al. The Incidence of Primary Cardiac Arrest During Vigorous Exercise. *New England Journal of Medicine* 1984;311:874-877.

[26] Link MS, Homoud MK, Wang PJ, Estes NAM. Cardiac Arrhythmias in the Athlete. *Cardiology in Review* 2001;9(1):21-30.

[27] Maron BJ, Towbin JA, Thiene G, Antzelevitch, et.al., . Contemporary definitions and classification of the cardiomyopathies: an American Heart Association Scientific Statement from the Council on Clinical Cardiology, Heart Failure and Transplantation Committee; Quality of Care and Outcomes Research and Functional Genomics and Translational Biology Interdisciplinary Working Groups; and Council on Epidemiology and Prevention. *Circulation* 2006;113(14):1807-1816.

[28] Maron BJ, Roberts WC, Epstein SE. Sudden Death in Hypertrophic Cardiomyopathy: a profile of 78 patients. *Circulation* 1982;65:1388-1394.

[29] Shah JS, Tome Esteban MT, Thaman R, Sharma R, et.al. Prevalence of Exercise Induced Left Ventricular Outflow Tract Obstruction in Symptomatic Patients with Non-obstructive Hypertrophic Cardiomyopathy.Heart. *Heart* 2007.

[30] Maron BJ, Gohman TE, Aeppli D. Prevalence of Sudden Cardiac Death During Competitive Sports Activities In Minnesota High School Athletes. *Journal of the American College of Cardiology* 1998;32:1881-1884.

[31] Lawless CE, Best TM, . Electrocardiograms in athletes: interpretation and diagnostic accuracy. *Med Sci Sports Exerc* 2008;40(5):787-798.

[32] Corrado D, Basso C, Pavei A, Michieli P, Schiavon M, G T. Trends in sudden cardiovascular death in young competitive athletes after implementation of a preparticipation screening program. *JAMA* 2006;296(13):1593-1601.

[33] Feinstein RA CE, Oh MK. Echocardiographic Screening As Part of a Preparticipation Examination. *Clinical Journal of Sports Medicine* 1993;3:149-152.

[34] Koester MC. A Review of Sudden Cardiac Death in Young Athletes and Strategies for Preparticipation Cardiovascular Screening. *Journal of Athletic Training* 2001;36(2):197-204.

[35] Cardiology ACo. ACC/ESC Clinical Expert Consensus Document on HCM. *Journal of the American College of Cardiology* 2003;42(9).

[36] Orliaguet G FM, Riou B. The Heart in Blunt Trauma. *Anesthesiology* 2001;95(2).

[37] Perron AD BW, Erling BF. Commotio Cordis: An Underappreciated Cause of Sudden Cardiac Death in Young Patients: Assessment and Management in the ED. *American Journal of Emergency Medicine* 2001;19(5):406-409.

[38] Kyle JM LJ, Elkins G. Planning for Scholastic Cardiac Emergencies: The Ripley Project. *The West Virginia Medical Journal* 1999;95(September/October):258-260.

[39] Berger S DA, Friedberg DZ. Sudden Cardiac Death in Infants, Children, and Adolescents. *Pediatric Clinics of North America* 1999;46(2):221-227.

[40] Thiene G, Basso C, Corrado D. Is Prevention of Sudden Death in Young Athletes Feasible:. *Cardiologia* 1999;44:497-505.

[41] Liberthson RR, Dinsmore RE, Fallon JT. Aberrant coronary artery origin from the aorta: report of 18 patients, review of the literature and delineation of natural history and management. *Circulation* 1979;59:748-754.

[42] Basso C, Maron BJ, Corrado D, Thiene G. Clinical profile of congenital coronary artery anomalies with origin from the wrong aortic sinus leading to sudden death in young competitive athletes. *Journal of the American College of Cardiology* 2000;35:1493-1501.

[43] Moss AJ. Sudden Cardiac Death and National Health. *Pacing and Clinical Electrophysiology* 1993;16:2190-2191.

[44] Weidenbener EJ KM, Waller BF, et al. Incorporation of Screening Echocardiography in the Preparticipation Examination. *Clinical Journal of Sports Medicine* 1995;5:86-89.

[45] Bresler MJ. Acute Pericarditis and Myocarditis. *Emergency Medicine* 1992;24:35-51.

[46] Maron BJ, Ackerman MJ, Nishimura RA, Pyeritz RE, Towbin JA, Udelson JE. Task Force 4: HCM and other cardiomyopathies, mitral valve prolapse, myocarditis, and Marfan syndrome. *Journal of the American College of Cardiology* 2005;45(8):1340-1345.

[47] Lecomte D, Fornes P, Fouret P, Nicholas G. Isolated myocardial fibrosis as a cause of sudden cardiac death and its possible relation to myocarditis. *Journal of Forensic Science* 1993;38:617-621.

[48] Maron BJ, Chaitman BR, Ackerman MJ, Bayés de Luna A, et.al. Working Groups of the American Heart Association Committee on Exercise, Cardiac Rehabilitation, and Prevention; Councils on Clinical Cardiology and Cardiovascular Disease in the Young.Recommendations for physical activity and recreational sports participation for young patients with genetic cardiovascular diseases. *Circulation* 2004;109(22):2807-2816.

[49] McKeag DB. Preparticipation screening of the potential athlete. *Clinics in Sports Medicine* 1989;8:373-397.

[50] Kapetanopoulos A, Kluger J, Maron BJ, Thompson PD. The congenital long QT syndrome and implications for young athletes. *Med Sci Sports Exerc* 2006;35(5):816-825.

[51] Reiserdorff EJ, Prodinger RJ. Sudden Cardiac Death in the Athlete. *Emergency Medical Clinics of North America* 1998;16:281-294.

[52] Lawless CE. Implantable Cardiac Defibrillators in Athletes. *Clinical Journal of Sports Medicine* 2008.

[53] Sarubbi B. The Wolff-Parkinson-White electrocardiogram pattern in athletes: how and when to evaluate the risk for dangerous arrhythmias.. The opinion of the paediatric cardiologist. *J Cardiovasc Med* 2006;7(4):271-8.

[54] Basso C, Corrado D, Thiene G. Arrhythmogenic right ventricular cardiomyopathy in athletes: diagnosis, management, and recommendations for sport activity. *Cardiology Clinics* 2007;25:415-422.

[55] Rampazzo A, Nava A, Malacrida S, et al. Mutation in human desmoplakin domain binding to plakoglobin causes a dominant form of arrhythmogenic right ventricular cardiomyopathy. *American Journal of Human Genetics* 2002;71:1200-6.

[56] Anderson, Courson, Kleiner. *Journal of Athletic Training* 2002; 37(1):99-104.

[57] Cummins RO OJ, Thies WH, et al. Improving Survival From Sudden Cardiac Arrest: The Chain of Survival Concept. *Circulation* 1991;83:1832-1847.

[58] Coris EE, Sahebzamani F, Curtis A, et al., Preparticipation cardiovascular screening among National Collegiate Athletic Association Division I Institutions, BJSM, September 2012.

In: Sudden Death
Editors: Jiashin Wu and Jessica Wu
ISBN: 978-1-62618-825-9

Chapter VII

The Roles of Electrical Cardiac Systole in Sudden Death

Francisco R. Breijo Márquez[1,*] ***and Manuel Pardo Rios***[2]
[1]School of Medicine, Commemorative Hospital, Boston, MA, US
[2]School of Medicine and Dentistry, University Research Institute on Aging, University of Murcia, Spain

Abstract

The definition for sudden death had to be explained in many other chapters of this book. So I will not go in more details regarding it. The sudden death in the absence of structural heart disease is uncommon, but when it appears, has a very significant clinical impact because many of the victims are young. In relatively recent form it has given special attention to particular conditions expressed in repolarization electrocardiographic on QT interval, whose relationship with the functionality of some ion channels in the membrane cell has prompted its designation as "channelopathies". But the QT-interval alteration is not unique.

Keywords: Electrical cardiac systole disturbances, long and short QT-syndromes, the short PR-interval disturbances, sudden cardiac death

The Electrical Cardiac Systole

Disorders in the electrical cardiac systole can be very dangerous for sudden death, as some cardiac entities previously cited on this book. Its role in sudden death is very important. Before anything else, it is essential to know what is considered as "electrical cardiac systole". For some authors it would be from the beginning of the Q-wave until the ending of T-wave.

* E-mail: frbm@gmx.us. frbreijo@aol.com.

In contrast for other authors, including us, it would be from the beginning of the P-wave until the ending of T-wave, including the P- wave and the PR- interval.

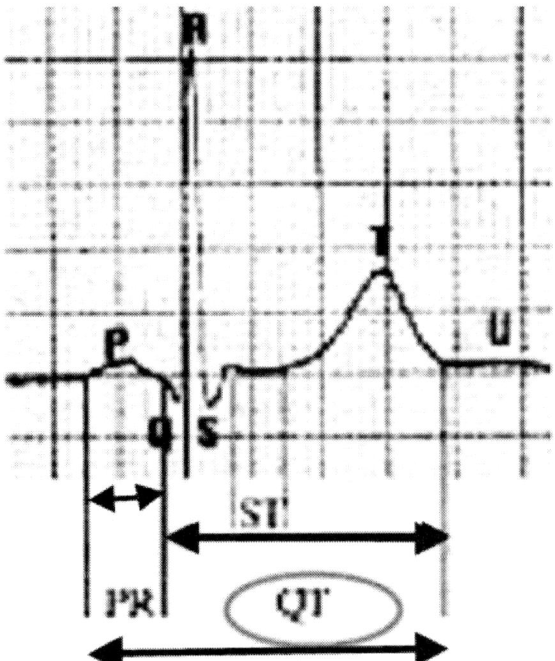

ELECTRICAL CARDIAC SYSTOLE AND ITS COMPONENTS

The P- wave, representing atrial activation, the PR- interval is the time from the beginning of atrial activation until the beginning of ventricular activation. The QRS complex represents the ventricular activation. The ST segment and the T- wave represent ventricular repolarization. The QT-interval is the duration of ventricular activation and its recovery. The U-wave probably represents post-depolarization in the ventricles.

In ELECTROGRAM study its normal image would be the below:

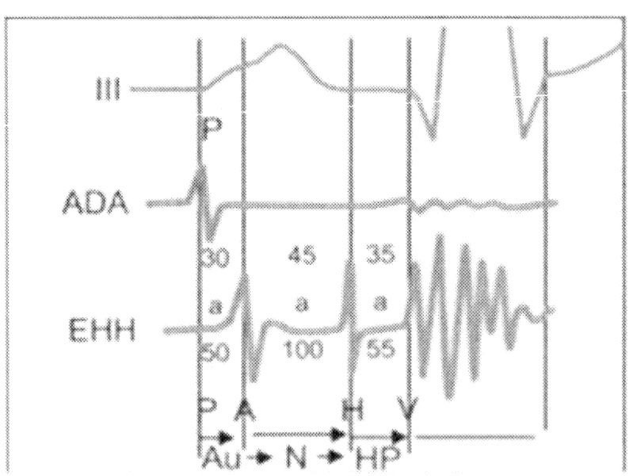

Different areas of the PR- interval. ADA = high right atrium. EHH = His bundle interval electrogram. PA = From the high right atrium to the beginning of the P wave in the ECG to the first fast deflection of the lower right atrium; this represents the right intra-atrial conduction, its normal value ranges are between 30 and 50 ms. AH = From the first fast ECG atrial deflection under (A) to the His bundle deflection (H), this represents the intranodal conduction and its normal value ranges are between 45 and 100 ms. The HV-interval value, distance between the His bundle and ventricular muscle its normal length is between 35 and 55 ms.

Standard values in length for waves and intervals in an ECG tracing.

P-WAVE. LESS THAN 0.12 SEC. IN LENGTH.
PR-INTERVAL. 0.12 SEC. TO 0.20 SEC. IN LENGTH.
QRS COMPLEX. 0.08 SEC. TO 0.12 SEC. IN LENGTH.
QT-INTERVAL. * 0.40 SEC. TO 0.44 SEC. IN LENGTH. *(ACCORDING THE FORMULAS OF BAZETT AND FRIDERICIA)

It comprises from the beginning of the ventricular complex (Q wave) to the end of the T wave. It measures approximately 0.36 s on average in normal people with a normal heart rate. While overall the QT-interval should be less than half of the interval between two successive R- waves, this rule applies only when the heart rate is normal. Ashmann have established a table that relates the heart rate with the length of the QT interval (QTc corrected).

Duration of QT interval related to the frequency heart rate (QTc)

50 0,414- 0,425 SEC.
60 0,386- 0,396 SEC
70 0,361- 0,371 SEC
80 0,342- 0,352 SEC
90 0,321- 0,330 SEC
100 0,297- 0,305 SEC
120 0,283- 0,291 SEC
150 0,252 -0,258 SEC

(According with Ashmann)

The upper limits of these measures should not exceed 10% or more. If so, it would be pathological. However, there are tables for us that are much more useful.

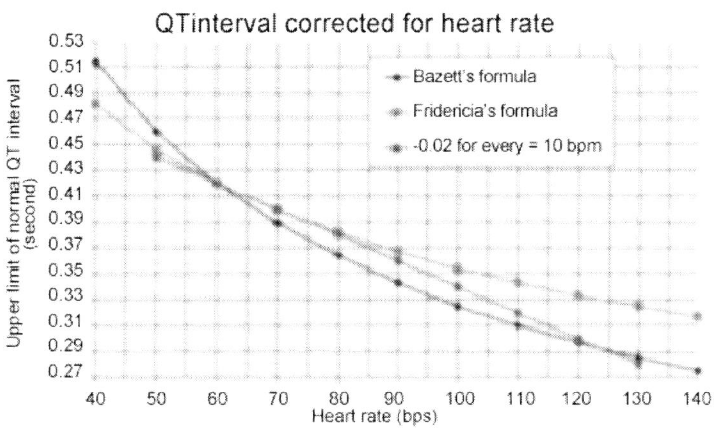

These table types are very useful when we trying to find out if a QT-interval is normal, short or long (prolonged) in relation to the heart rate.

The More Acquaintances Alterations in the Cardiac Electrical Systole

1°. SHORT PR-INTERVAL DISEASES.
2° CARDIAC BLOCKADES.
3° QRS-COMPLEX ALTERATIONS.
4° LONG QT SYNDROME.
5° SHORT QT SYNDROME.

1. Short Pr-Interval

Any ECG analysis with a PR- interval value less than 0.12 sec differentiates clinical entities with an early ventricular activation, also called 'ventricular pre-excitation', which means that the ventricular activation is produced much earlier than it should be expected when the stimulus is from sinus node, and conduction system is normal. This is so because there are fibers or anomalous conduction pathways that are independent of the normal A-V electrical conduction, connecting the auricles to the ventricles. Since these entities are often associated with paroxysmal tachycardia, is very useful known personal antecedent of episodes of tachycardia and syncope, and also to know if there have fast palpitations with beginning and ending suddenly, which may be a likeness for these pathologies. Currently, we are recognizing four forms of ventricular preexcitation with different electrophysiological substrates. One is quite unknown yet: the clinical entity with a short PR and short QT together on the same ECG tracing (Breijo's Pattern).

These are:

WOLF-PARKINSON-WHITE.
LOWN-GANONG-LEVINE.
MAHAIM SYNDROME.
BREIJO'S PATTERN.

A. Wolff-Parkinson-White

Between 1929 -1930, Wolff, Parkinson, and White described a cardiological entity in a series of patients who had a bundle branch block pattern on electrocardiography (ECG); they found, a short PR interval, and paroxysmal tachycardia [1,2]. Most of patients were young teenagers.

Preexcitation was defined by Durrer et al.[2] in 1970 with the following statement, Preexcitation exists, if in relation to atrial events, the whole or some part of the ventricular muscle is activated earlier by the impulse originating from the atrium than would be expected if the impulse reached the ventricles by way of the normal specific conduction system only.

While the vast majority of persons with Wolff-Parkinson-White (WPW) syndrome remain asymptomatic throughout their lives, there is a risk of sudden death associated with the syndrome, and is due to very fast tachyarrhythmias (more than 200-250 bpm) that trigger off in the person and that are produced by presence of this accessory pathway [3,4].

During episodes of supraventricular tachycardia, the individual may experience palpitations dizziness, difficulty breathing, and sometimes fainting. An ECG displays the typical "delta wave". The individuals with WPW syndrome have an accessory pathway atrioventricular conduction known as the bundle of Kent. In honour to Kent, who in 1893, found muscle lateral connections in the ring of atrioventricular node, and he thought they were normal atrioventricular connections and however corresponds to an abnormal electrical communication between the atria and ventricles [5]. This accessory pathway does not share the properties of AV node, so that electrical activity can lead to a significantly higher rate than the AV node. A rapid heartbeat is potentially dangerous because it can cause hemodynamic instability.

In some cases, the combination of an accessory pathway can trigger a ventricular fibrillation, the leading cause of sudden cardiac death. The bundle of Kent is present in a small percentage of the overall population. This pathway is a conduction bundle of tissue that can be found either between the left atrium and left ventricle, in this case as type A preexcitation or between the right atrium and right ventricle, in this case as type B preexcitation. The problems arise when this pathway creates electrical circuits that avoid the AV node. The AV node has the property of decreasing the speed of electrical impulses. When performing an abnormal electrical connection through this pathway, tachyarrhythmia is produced [6].

In an individual asymptomatic for WPW syndrome this is usually diagnosed by a surface electrocardiogram. It is a typical feature of this syndrome, the delta wave, which is manifested in the slope of the principle of the ascending branch of the R wave, being less pronounced than usual. After a few hundredths of a second, the slope returns to normal. This delta wave, which is verified before and during the initial phase of the R wave carries to a shortening of PR interval and lengthening of the duration of the QRS complex as well as ventricular repolarization disorders. Atrial fibrillation is extremely frequent in symptomatic patients for WPW [6, 7]. If the patient experiences episodes of atrial fibrillation, the ECG will show a wide QRS complex and a polymorphic tachycardia. This combination of atrial fibrillation and WPW is considered very dangerous. In individuals with WPW syndrome, the electrical activity that starts in the sinus node travels through the accessory pathway as well as across the atrioventricular node to activate the ventricles through both paths. Since no accessory pathway slows down the electrical impulse (which does make the AV node), this first activates the ventricles through the accessory pathway, and immediately through the AV node. This causes a short PR interval and the presence of delta waves. It is usual that patients with a manifest WPW have often more of an accessory pathway. The treatment depends on the individual risk stratification [8,9]. This is performed to determine if individuals with WPW syndrome are at risk for sudden cardiac death (SCD), which in these individuals is due to the propagation of an atrial arrhythmia to the ventricles at a very high rate. The individuals with WPW syndrome in which delta waves disappear with the increased heart rate are those who have the lowest risk of sudden death [8-9]. This is because the loss of the delta wave proves that the accessory pathway can not conduct the electrical impulses to a high rate (in the antegrade direction). Generally, these individuals have no fast conduction the accessory pathway during episodes of atrial fibrillation. Classic ECG findings that are associated with Wolff-Parkinson-White syndrome include the following:

PRESENCE OF A SHORT PR INTERVAL (< 120 MS)
A WIDE QRS COMPLEX LONGER THAN 120 MS WITH A SLURRED ONSET OF THE QRS WAWE FORM PRODUCING A DELTA WAVE IN THE EARLY PART OF QRS
SECONDARY ST-T WAVE CHANGES.

The location of the accessory pathway, in descending order of frequency, is 53%, the left free wall, 36%, posteroseptal, 8%, right free wall, and 3%, anteroseptal. The presence of concealed accessory pathway accounts for approximately 30% of patients with apparent Supra Ventricular Tachycardia referred for EPS. These patients do not have true Wolff-Parkinson-White syndrome because no delta wave is present, but they do have the potential for orthodromic tachycardia. Patients with mitral valve prolapse can have an association with WPW, but the mechanism is unclear. Wolff-Parkinson-White syndrome is found in persons of all ages but most patients with Wolff-Parkinson-White syndrome present during childhood. However, a second peak of presentation is noted in school-aged children and in teenagers. This interesting bimodal age-distribution is due to permanent or transitory loss of preexcitation during childhood in some patients and during youth. In asymptomatic patients, antegrade conduction across the accessory pathway may spontaneously disappear with advancing age. Once identified and appropriately treated, WPW syndrome is associated with an excellent prognosis, including the potential for permanent cure through catheter ablation. Asymptomatic patients with only preexcitation on ECG generally have a very good prognosis. Patients with a family history of Sudden Cardiac Death or significant symptoms of tachyarrhythmias have worse prognoses. However, even in patients with asymptomatic WPW, the risk of Sudden Cardiac Death is increased above that of the general population.

Some studies hypothesized that 2 mechanisms are involved in the pathogenesis of AF in patients with Wolff-Parkinson-White syndrome: one is related to the abnormal pathway that predisposes the atria to fibrillation, and the other is independent from the abnormal pathway and is related to increased atrial vulnerability present in these individuals [4,5]. According to the literature, risk factors for the development of AF in the setting of WPW syndrome include advancing age (2 peak ages for AF occurrence are recognized, one at 30 years and the other at 50 years), male gender, and prior history of syncope.

Wolff-Parkinson-White (ECG 12 Leads)

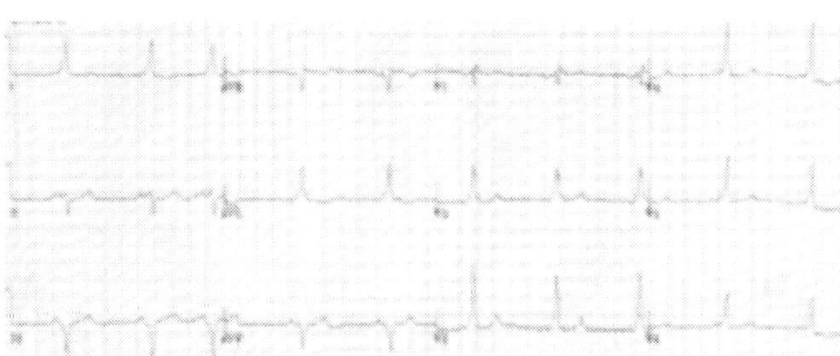

Detail on V3

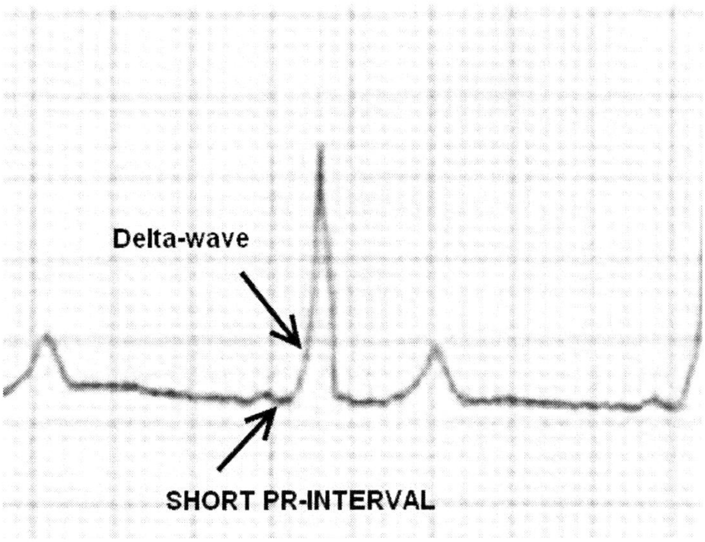

Electrophysiological Image

A Wolff-Parkinson-White during sinus rhythm. Negative delta wave in V1 and positive in V5, with a short PR -interval. On the right, an episode of atrial fibrillation with high preexcitation in the same leads, symptomatic for syncope and need immediate electrical cardioversion. The first three rows correspond to the DII electrocardiographic leads V1 and V5, and the following four intracavitary proximal AV junction, AV junction distal ablation catheter and right ventricle.

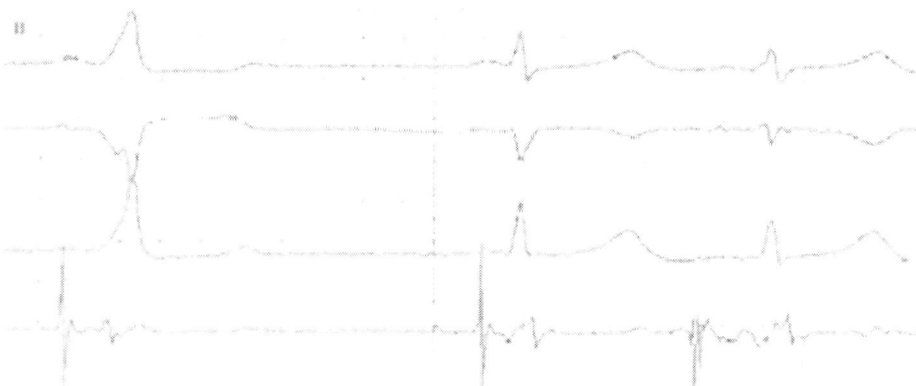

In many more occasions that we can think, Wolff-Parkinson-White can go together to other cardiac electrical disease [10]. The cryptogenic Wolff-Parkinson -White is not uncommon. We will put two graphic examples.

- Wolff-Parkinson-White alongside a Long QT interval.
- Cryptogenic Wolff-Parkinson-White, with sudden cardiac death as a final result.

Wolff-Parkinson-White alongside a Long Qt Interval [10]

(Breijo-Marquez FR, Pardo Ríos M (2011) Wolff-Parkinson-White and Prolonged "Q-T" Patterns in the Same Electrocardiographic Record. J Clinic Experiment Cardiol 2:118. doi:10.4172/2155-9880.1000118.)

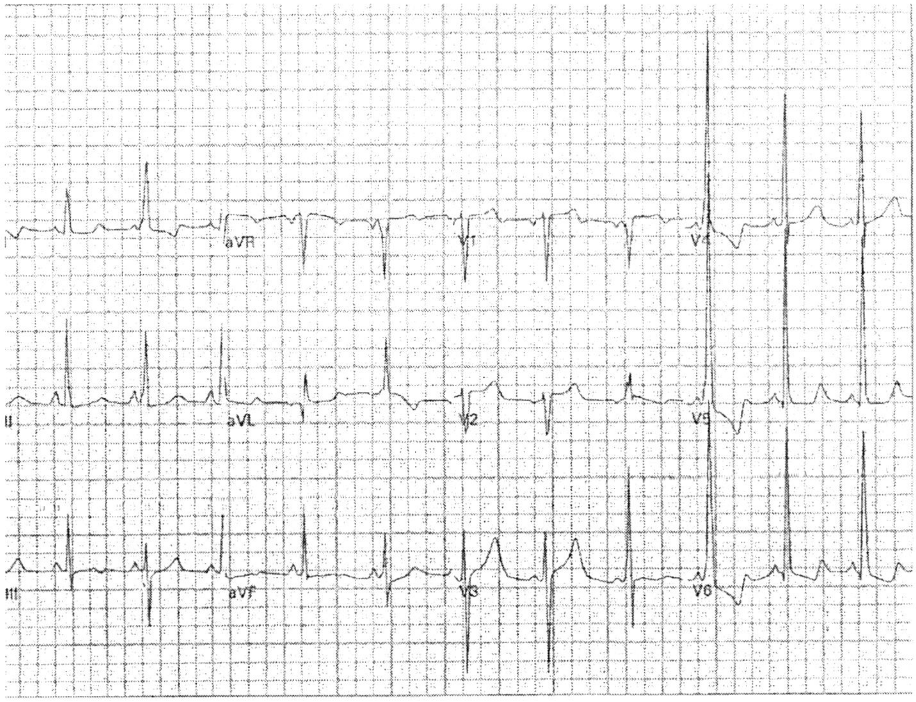

Electro-physiology Study. In the EPS graphic can be seen (arrow) typical signs of a WPW: Intracardiac electrogram showing under right ventricular pacing, atrial activation precocity in distal coronary sinus followed by His bundle.

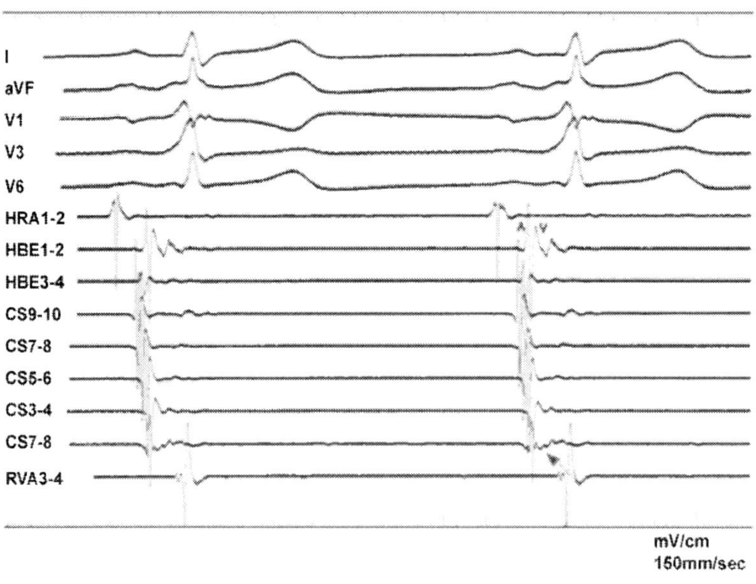

Cryptogenic Wolff-Parkinson-White

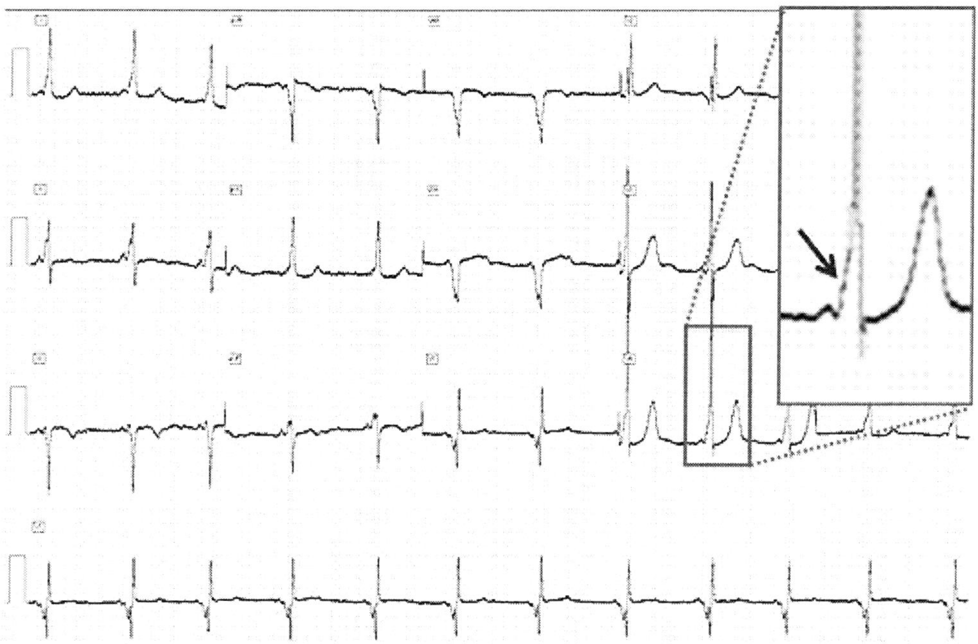

ECG 12 leads and RF ablation (Images)

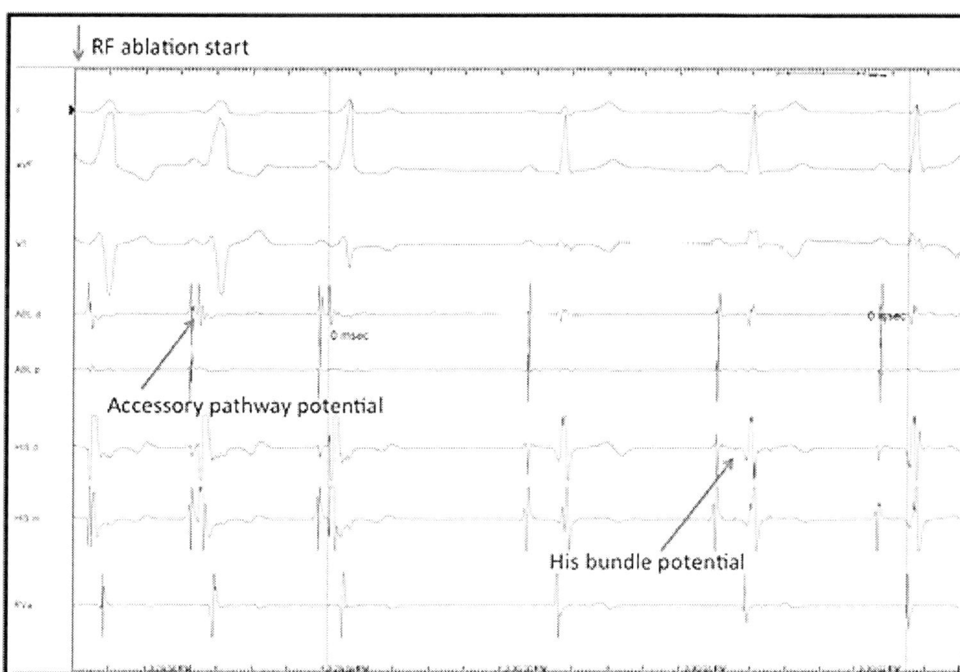

B. Lown-Ganong-Levine

This syndrome was described in 1952 by Lown, Ganong, and Levine; it is considered a pre-excitation syndrome [11]. Currently two types are the more known as preexcitation syndromes:

- The Wolf Parkinson White syndrome or ventricular preexcitation true.
- The Lown Ganong Levine or accelerated atrioventricular conduction.

This last is characterized by the association of a short PR interval (in adults, less than 0.12 sec) and various types of supraventricular tachyarrhythmias (regular tachycardia, atrial flutter, and atrial fibrillation). Etiology• acquired forms. • Congenital form: - Inheritable. - Not inheritable. The familial form is inherited as an autosomal dominant feature and has been associated with the gene encoding PRKAG2 AMP activated protein kinase, responsible for transporting and preserving the heart energy. A mutation in this gene could explain the susceptibility of the heart to the crises of tachycardia. Has been identified a mutation on the long arm of chromosome 7 (7q34-q36). Several structural abnormalities have been proposed as the possible base for Lown-Ganong-Levine, including the presence of James fibers, Mahaim fibers, and fibers of Brechenmacher [12] as well as an underdeveloped sinus node (hypoplastic). Each of these fibers can only be identified histologically. Thus, unless other studies can show structural or functional abnormalities, the definitive diagnosis of Lown-Ganong-Levine remains a clinical diagnosis. In the absence of significant structural heart disease, the mortality rate appears to be very low [13,14]. Many people can debut with an acute episode of tachycardia or a history of symptoms suggestive of paroxysmal tachycardia. For its diagnosis needs to be done at least:

1. A standard test for tachycardia, including an ECG to document the pace. 2. Serum electrolytes, calcium, magnesium levels, and levels of serum hormone thyroid-stimulating (TSH). Lithemy levels [10]. 3. History suggestive of recurrent paroxysms of tachycardia events. 4. A Holter monitor or an event recorder may be useful to document the rhythm during acute symptomatic episodes. 5. An ergometric study. 6. In rare cases, an implantable rhythm Monitor can be helpful. 7. Family History.

The diagnosis of Lown-Ganong-Levine syndrome, based on ECG interpretation:

- PR interval with duration of less than 0.12 seconds, with normal P waves.
- The QRS complex duration is normal.
- The absence of delta waves
- Episodes of paroxysmal supraventricular tachycardia.

Its anatomical substrate can be given by:

a) Accelerated nodal conduction.
b) Connections between the auricles and the His bundle that when inserted into the His bundle distal, also determine the existence of a short HV interval.

c) James fibers (posterior internodal tracts).

There is an accelerated nodal conduction when three conditions are met:

- An AH interval less than or equal to 60 msec.
- A persistence of conduction, 1 to 1, during atrial pacing cycle of 300 msec or less.
- A prolongation less than 100 msec in AH interval (with respect to baseline) performed during atrial pacing with a cycle of 300 msec. [15, 16]

In patients with nodal conduction accelerated, the nodal re-entry shows not significant differences in the cycle compared with patients whose PR interval is normal. This is because the tachycardia cycle is primarily determined by the speed from slow pathway conduction. Instead, may increase the incidence of supraventricular tachycardia, because the fast pathway has better drivability. But, this clinical entity has a small role for trigger off a sudden death.

Differential Diagnosis with Wolf-Parkinson-White

Despite apparently very similar, there are differences, in our opinion, which are critical with respect to drug treatment of choice.

The main differences are:

- The LGL has a shortened PR interval due to the presence of the accessory pathway which avoids the AV node, but the QRS complex is normal because the accessory pathway (James fibers) binds directly to the sinusal node and not depolarizes to the ventricles directly, if it does for the typical way conduction by His-Purkinje system.
- Are no "Delta Waves" by slurring of the ascending limb of QRS in D1, aVL, V5 and V6.
- The QRS complexes are narrows, because there is usually no interventricular conduction disturbance.
- Have not such frequent association of concomitant atrial fibrillation during crisis. [14-17]

Lown-Ganong-Levine (ECG 12 Leads)

(Courtesy of the Journal "The Heart")

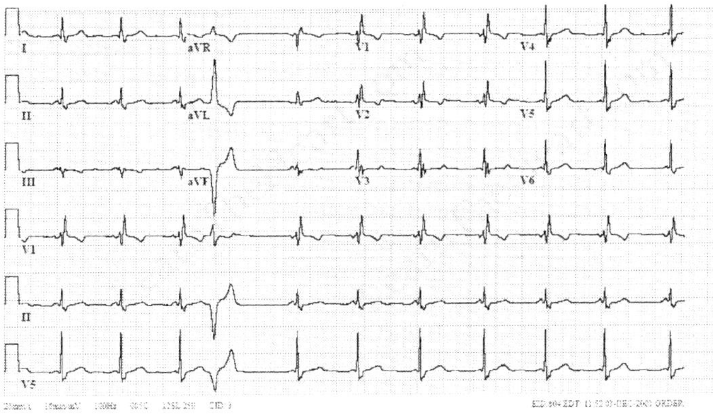

C. Mahaim Syndrome

Between 1938 and 1947 Mahaim and colleagues described a series of anatomical connections between the atrioventricular node and interventricular septum and between the fascicles of normal conduction system and ventricular myocardium [18]. It has been demonstrated that most patients with antidromic atrium-ventricular tachycardia with morphology of left bundle branch block bundles (LBBB) have the anatomical substrate in atriofascicular rights bundles [20-24].

It is not a frequent cause for paroxysmal atrioventricular tachycardia by re-entry and it is due to an accessory pathway as Mahaim fibers. These Mahaim fibers have anterograde conduction, with decreased properties in its proximal portion, and they have not conduction capability retrograde.

The related tachycardia has a typical left bungle branch block type QRS, due to preexcitation of the right ventricle through this pathway, closing the rentry circuit through the right bundle branch, His bundle, atrioventricular node and right atrium [21,23].

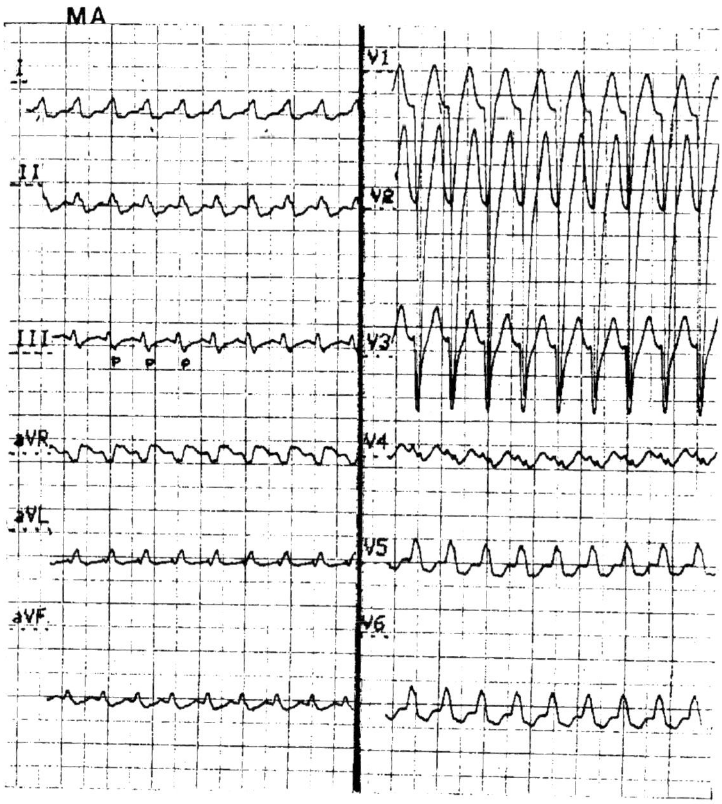

In 1988, in patients undergoing surgery for tachyarrhythmias, was identified this type of accessory pathway, by means of studying its histological substrate. The ventricular insertion is presumed to be in the same branch right, in its distal portion, or apex ventricular myocardium. Since then, the surgical process with catheter- ablation of Mahaim tachycardia has allowed us knows that tachycardia is conducted on the atrium right or on right ventricle free wall [24, 25]. The resulting tachycardia, to stimulate the ventricles through this beam anomalous (Mahaim fibers) , give us an image QRS with similar aspect of a left bundle branch block, closing the circuit to the atria by retrograde conduction through the right bundle, His bundle and atrioventricular node. With the development of surgery and radiofrequency ablation of supraventricular tachyarrhythmias has been determined this kind of Mahaim conduction is due, in most cases, to paths located in the right free of septum, which cross the ring tricuspid, joining the right atrium with the distal portion of the right branch of the His bundle [24,25]. Typical antidromic tachycardia with left bundle branch block image. In leads II and III, negative P waves can be observed immediately after the QRS complex (RP short, long PR).

Detail on V6

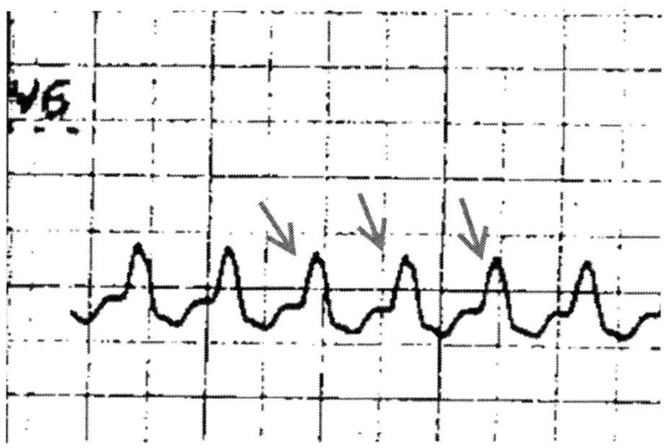

Mahaim (ECG 12 leads)

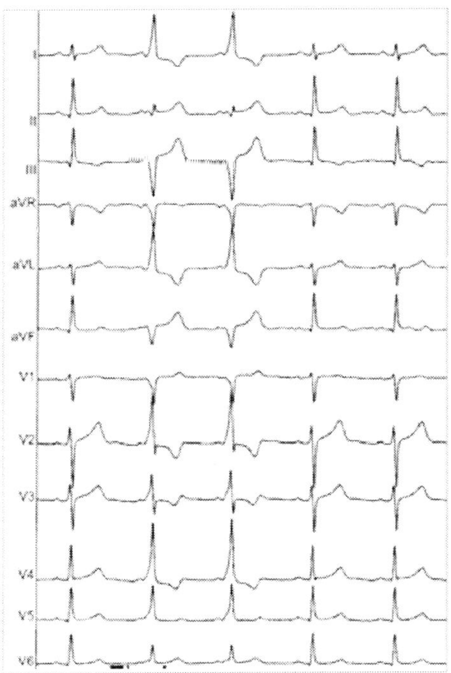

Short PR and QT Interval on the Same ECG Tracing: Breijo's Pattern

In 2006, Breijo-Marquez, Pardo Ríos et al [10,26] evaluated a series of young patients, who had had, since childhood, many episodes of nocturnal palpitations, chest pain, full loss of consciousness (syncope), and which were accompanied by tonic-clonic seizures. All had been diagnosed and treated as epileptic episodes. Treatment outcomes were null. They were always considered as normal in every cardiac studies performed absolutely. However, all these patients had an ECG recording common: A PR-interval lesser than 0,120 seconds with a QTc-interval equal or lesser than 0.350 seconds. That is, a pattern of short PR and QTc in the same person. The correct treatment was begun (beta-blockers and, in some cases, an implantable cardio defibrillator (ICD.). Was removed all treatment from epilepsy. The outcome to date is satisfactory. We do not know yet the exact etiology for this pattern: there are not positive genetic studies for a short QT-interval. That is, is negative for these genetic mutations of short QT types. This can say us that we are in front of a possible and little known syndrome new.

ECG to date, we know that there were two important misperceptions:

First. - The physicians mistook to syncopal episode, with an epileptic episode. Second. - The syncopal episodes are due to a cardiac disorder (was a cardiogenic syncope due to a cardiac electrical systole's alteration). This ECG recording may be easily confused with a Lown-Ganong-Levine, since both have a short PR-interval. Nevertheless, in this type of ECG pattern there is also a short QTc interval. Unfortunately, both entities are confused with epileptic episodes often. Most important clinical features are: Crises always occur at night during rest. The more frequent onset hours are between three and six in the morning.

- Patient wakes up suddenly with diaphoresis, severe palpitations (later, the ECG study reveals a crisis of paroxysmal tachycardia with a heart rate greater than 170-200 beats per minute).
- Feeling of impending doom.

It is by definition an emergency since of not taking treatment in time, a sudden death is almost certain. Unfortunately this cardiological entity is more frequent than that in principle may seem. It is an almost unknown entity.

Typical ECG Image of the "Short PR-Interval Alongside a Short QT-Interval" Intervals in the Same Person (during "Vigil Period"): Breijo's Pattern

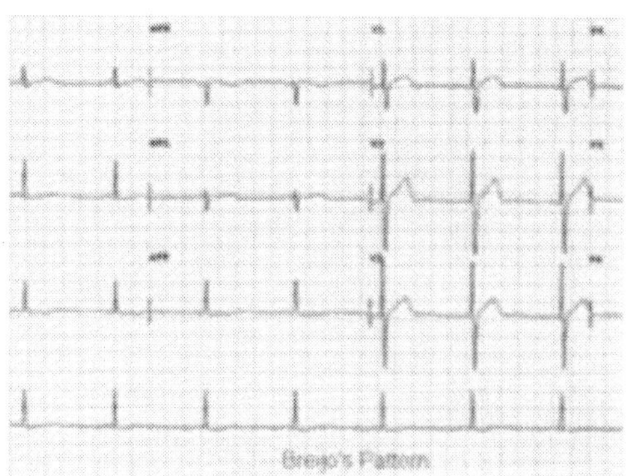

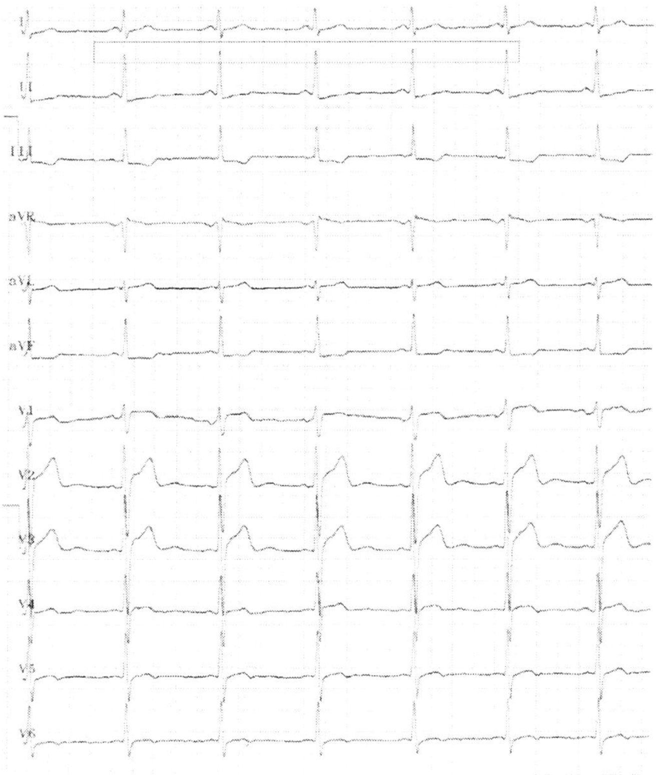

This ECG recording was the first with 12 leads that was obtained from our Hospital in Boston. MA. The patient was a 37 years-old male. We can see a shortening of the PR and QT intervals (Bazett), especially in inferior and left precordial leads. PR-interval length is lesser than 0.120 seconds and QTc length is lesser than 0.350 seconds. Patient had the symptoms exposed previously. He was also diagnosed for epileptic episodes. However, he had syncopal episodes by cardiological disturbances: a short PR-interval alongside a short QTc.

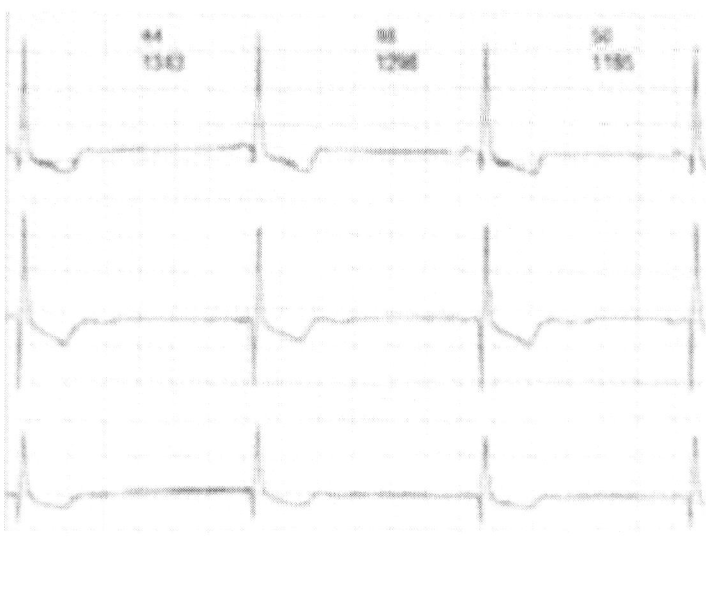

Detail on DIII

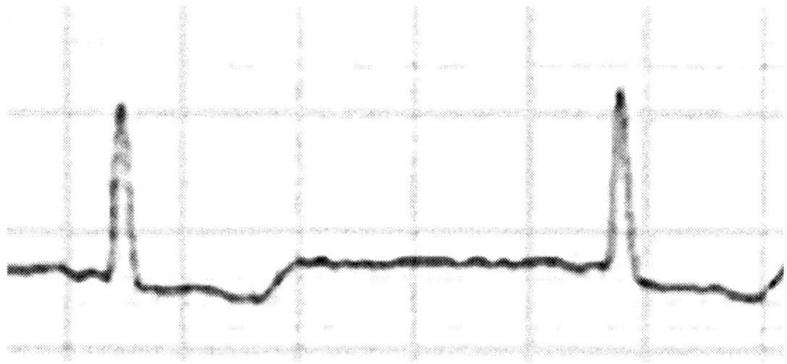

Differences among these Syndromes

ENTITY.	PR-interval	QRS complex	QTc -interval
W.P.W	Short.	Wide (δ-wave)	Normal
L.G.L	Short	Normal	Normal
Mahaim	Normal or Short	Normal or wide	Normal
Breijo's Pattern	Short	Normal	Short

2. Cardiac Blocks

The interruption of electrical conduction in the heart leads to what has been called: heart blocks [27, 28, 29]. They can occur anywhere in the conduction system. So, when atrial activation wave (P wave) takes more than 0.20 seconds to activate the AV node, we speak of first-degree AV block. This blockage, if isolated, can be considered as normal (particularly in elderly people). But there are already many studies linking its presence with increased episodes of atrial fibrillation and the need for a pacemaker. There may also be an electrical outage from the AV node to the Bundle of His. When this phenomenon occurs intermittently, we say that there is a second-degree AV block. We can consider that there are three types of second-degree block: When an atrial activation (P wave) does not reach the ventricles, the QRS complex does not occur. This event is called Mobitz type II [28]. There may be a progressive elongation of the PR interval until the stimulation wave can not reach the ventricles and therefore, is not followed by a QRS complex. This already has been prior described as Wenckebach Phenomenon. When atrial stimulation cannot reach the ventricles, the ventricular activation comes from some ventricular centres, with a slower ventricular rate. We speak of Complete AV block. This type of blockage is very dangerous and is indispensable pacemaker implantation. These three types of block, along with left bundle branch block, are the most dangerous at the time of, being able to produce sudden death. All other are called, blocks of bundle of His in its two branches, which may be Complete or Incomplete. At first, have not importance for Life. Excepting, the left bundle branch block of the His bundle. Normally, the electrical impulse travels down both the right and left branches at the same speed. Thus, both ventricles contract at the same time. Occasionally there's a block in one of the branches, so impulses must travel to the affected side by a detour that slows them down. That means one ventricle contracts a fraction of a second slower than the other. Usually if there's nothing else wrong, a person with bundle branch block shows no symptoms. But a bundle branch block shows up as an abnormality when the electrical impulses through the heart are recorded with an electrocardiogram (ECG). Usually no treatment is required, but your healthcare provider will want to see you regularly to be sure no other changes occur. It is important to have regular check-ups.

Summing up

Sometimes the electrical signal from the heart's upper chambers (atria) to lower chambers (ventricles) is impaired or doesn't transmit. There are several degrees of heart block. First-degree heart block occurs when the electrical impulse moves through the AV node more slowly than normal. The heart beat usually has a slower rate and may not cause noticeable symptoms such as light headedness and dizziness and may not require specific treatment. Certain drugs can cause first-degree heart block. These drugs include digitalis, beta-blockers, and calcium-channel blockers. Digitalis is one common drug that is used to slow down the heart rate. If it's taken in large amounts or for a long period of time, digitalis can cause first-degree heart block. Beta-blockers inhibit the part of the nervous system that speeds up the heart. This increases the conduction delay of the heart's electrical impulse and can cause first-degree heart block. Among its other effects, calcium-channel blockers have the ability to slow down the conduction of the AV node, resulting in heart block. People with this type of block along with regular assessment by a physician, should also be taught to take their pulse and monitor it regularly to detect changes.

Second-degree heart block occurs when some electrical signals from the atria do not reach the ventricles, resulting in "dropped beats." Second degree heart block can be classified as Mobitz Type 1 or Mobitz Type 2. Mobitz Type 1 is also commonly referred to as Wenckebach and may not cause noticeable symptoms. Symptoms associated with second degree heart block are chest pain, faintness (syncope), and palpitations, breathing difficulties, such as shortness of breath with exertion, rapid breathing, nausea, and fatigue. Second degree Type I may not require treatment but can be a forerunner for Type 2 and needs to be monitored on a regular basis as well as daily pulse checks by the patient. However, it can be a forerunner for Mobitz Type 2 and needs to be monitored by a physician. In Mobitz Type 2, the heart beat does not beat effectively and impacts the hearts' ability to pump blood to the rest of the body. Often times having a pacemaker inserted is necessary so the heart will beat effectively. Third-degree or complete heart block means that the heart's electrical impulse does not pass from the heart's upper to lower chambers at all. When this occurs, the heart does not beat correctly and cannot effectively move blood to the body. Secondary pacemaker cells in the lower chambers will take over, causing the ventricles to contract and pump blood, but at a slower rate than when signals come from the sinoatrial node. Complete heart block in adults is caused by heart conditions or as a side effect of drug toxicity. An injury to the electrical conduction system during heart surgery also may cause heart block. People with third-degree heart block experience irregular and unreliable heart beats, which requires immediate medical attention involving a temporary pacemaker because of the potential for having a cardiac arrest. A permanent pacemaker would be indicated to treat complete heart block.

IMAGES. Cardiac Blocks: first, second and complete degree.

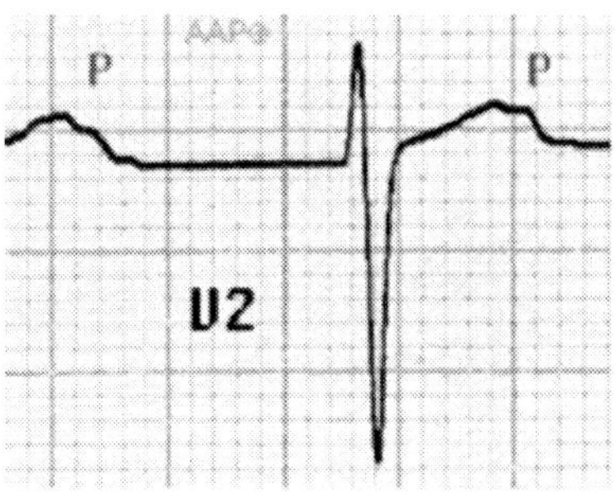

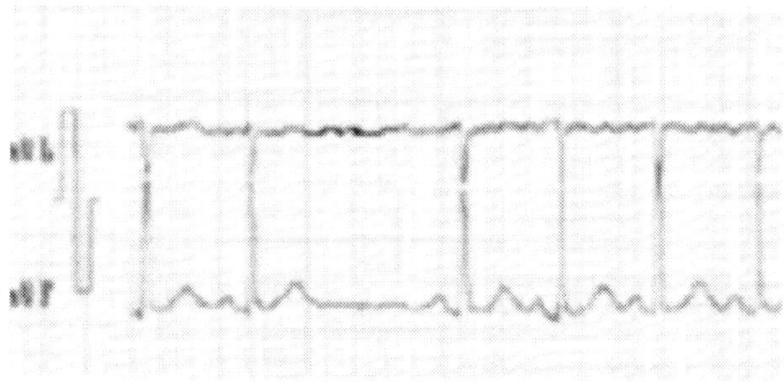

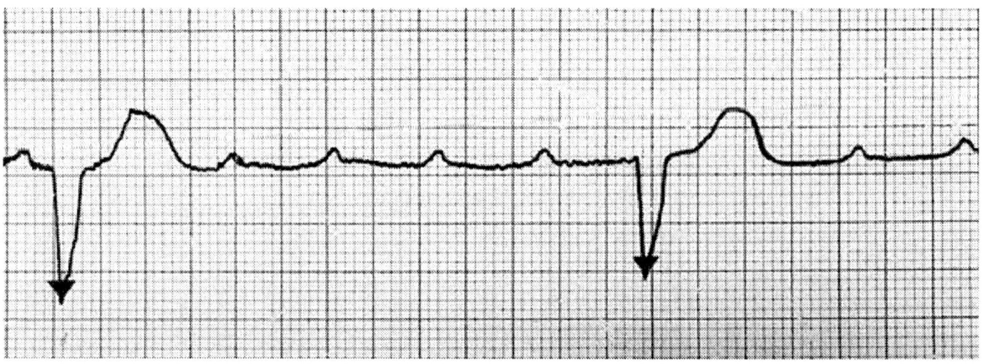

3. QRS-Complex Alterations

The **QRS complex** is one of the components of a typical electrocardiogram (ECG) tracing of a complete cardiac cycle, normally occurring after the P wave (atrial depolarization) and before the T wave (ventricular repolarization). It is a graphical representation of the cardiac impulse travelling into the ventricular myocardium. To further understand its morphological characteristics and clinical relevance, a brief discussion of the QRS complex is provided below. About 120 to 200 milliseconds (ms) after the generation of an action potential in the SA node, the cardiac impulse reaches the ventricles through the atrioventricular (AV) nodal/His bundle system. The cardiac impulse is conducted to the ventricular mass through the bundle branches and the Purkinje fibers. Normally, the QRS complex is seen as a "sharp" complex, resulting from the rapid depolarization of the ventricles via the fast conducting Purkinje fibers of the bundle branches. Compared to the intra-atrial conduction speed, the conduction speed of the bundle branches is high, averaging about 4 meters per second. The first deflection of the QRS complex is called a Q wave when it is negatively deflected (pointing downward) and an R wave when it is positively deflected (pointing upward). A positive deflection following a Q wave is called an R wave; and a negative deflection following an R wave is designated as an S wave. A second positive deflection after the R wave is called an R' (R prime).

A QRS complex may not always contain a Q, an R or a S. Many combinations of these deflections, as well as isolated deflections are generally referred to as QRS complexes. Upper case and lower case letters are used to describe not only the type of waves or deflections present but also the general orientation of the QRS complex. A prolonged duration of the QRS complex signifies a conduction delay in the ventricles. Being an important part of the ECG curve, the QRS complex is routinely analyzed when investigating cardiac pathologies. However, all the components of the ECG must be considered and correlated clinically to ensure an accurate diagnosis.

4. Long QT Syndrome

Since its discovery, much has been written about this cardiological entity.

Possibly this entity is the most studied alongside the atrial fibrillation (which, incidentally, should be included in this type of disorder). In 1856, Meissner described the sudden death of a young, deaf girl who was being berated at her school academy. Inadvertently, this was perhaps the first reported description of the Long QT Syndrome. A more detailed clinical characterization of deafness, prolonged QT interval on ECG and propensity to sudden cardiac death followed more than a century later when Jervell and Lange-Nielsen described a series of patients. A similar syndrome, but without deafness, was identified to run in families and was first described by Romano et al. in 1963 and later by Ward in 1964. The clinical spectrum of the Long QT Syndrome is now well characterized, with affected patients vulnerable to recurrent syncope or cardiac arrest from a polymorphic ventricular tachycardia known as torsade de pointes [30]. The hypothesis of the relationship between Long QT Syndrome and Sudden Infant Death was studied by Schwartz [31] by means of QTc measurements in the first week of life. In your follow-up, 34 children died, 24 of them from Sudden Infant Death.

Arnestad et al. studied 7 genes associated with Long QT Syndrome in 201 cases of sudden infant death, found that 9.5% of infants who died suddenly showed some of the mutations studied and showed that long QT is a cause which contributes significantly to sudden death in infants. Wang et al. studied the association between Sudden Infant Death and the presence of Long QT Syndrome, 5 variants (S216L, T1304M, F1486L, F2004L, and P2006A) had alterations in Na + channels, typical of SCN5A mutations associated with Long QT Syndrome. Authors speculated perform ECG screening programs in newborns, which has generated controversy despite the results obtained by several investigators. Incredible but true: a good management on an EKG study could save thousands of lives in the newborn. And however, there are many controversies yet. The fact that malignant forms of Long QT Syndrome are associated with a marked prolongation of the QTc interval could encourage the conduct of investigations by ECG and genetic screening in infants susceptible to suffer it, which would help not just to consider a good preventive therapy but also identify to all affected members in the same family (30). Long QT Syndrome can happen from mutation of one of several genes [30-35]. These mutations tend to prolong the duration of the ventricular action potential, thus lengthening the QT interval. LQTS can be inherited in an autosomal dominant or in an autosomal recessive manner. The autosomal recessive forms of Long QT

Syndrome have a propensity to have a more severe phenotype, with some variants having associated syndactyly (Long QT 8) or congenital neural deafness (Long QT 1). A number of specific gene loci have been identified that are associated with Long QT Syndrome. Genetic testing for Long QT Syndrome is clinically available and may help to direct appropriate therapies. The most common causes of Long QT Syndrome are mutations in the genes KCNQ1 (LQT1), KCNH2 (LQT2), and SCN5A (LQT3) [32]. According to expert consensus, the preventive and definitive treatment for sudden death by channelopathies is the implementation of an automatic implantable defibrillator in all patients with cardiogenic syncope, or sudden cardiac death recovered. But the prospects of new treatments are already being carried out. Conduction damage may cause arrhythmias, per example the Long QT, which are primarily treated pharmacologically or by medical device-based therapies, including defibrillation and tissue ablation. Nevertheless, drug therapies sometimes may not be effective or are associated with serious side effects. Device-based therapies for cardiac arrhythmias, even with well developed technology, still face inadequacies, limitations, hardware complications, and other challenges. Therefore, scientists are actively seeking other alternatives for antiarrhythmic therapy. In particular, cells and genes used for repairing cardiac conduction damage/defect have been investigated in various studies both in vitro and in vivo. Despite the complexities of the excitation and conduction systems of the heart, cell and gene-based strategies provide novel alternatives for treatment or cure of cardiac arrhythmias in general and of Long QT particularly. In addiction, there are peculiarities in some of them, in Long QT Syndrome are indicated changes in lifestyle, in the case of Long QT Syndrome 1 are contraindicated some sports, especially swimming, football . In the Long QT Syndrome 2, should avoid exposure to acoustic stimuli mainly during sleep. Beta blockers are the first line of treatment in all patients with a diagnosis of Long QT Syndrome, even in asymptomatic patients because it reduces the risk of events up to 60%. Implantation of pacemaker and left sympathetic ganglionic denervation are therapeutic options in Long QT Syndrome. Nevertheless, the current essays on this latter technique are still quite disappointing. There are still many discrepancies between different authors for to know which are the ranges for be considered as long (or prolonged) a QTc. We must also say that the LQT can be produced by external agents (non-genetic) as drugs and some systemic disorders, such as anemia. We believe that every person diagnosed with chronic anemia should be thoroughly assessed from the point of view electrocardiographic, and accurately measure the length of the QT interval [37,38].

5. Short QT Syndrome

It was first described in 2000 in a handful of patients, and since then 3 different genes associated with the disease and the biophysical basis have been described. Gussak, Brugada R. and associates have described for the first time what has now been defined as a clinical syndrome. They identified a short QT interval in three persons from the same family, one of whom had several episodes of paroxysmal atrial fibrillation [33-39]. The definitive link between short QT syndrome and sudden death on a family unit was described by Gaita and associates in 2003. In 2004, the genetic and biophysical bases, for this cardiological entity as well as a possible therapeutic approach were provided.

The short QT syndrome is characterized by a ventricular fibrillation in the absence of structural heart disease with presence of a QTc interval <350 msec. In most of the reported cases, there is a history of sudden death in the family and some affected individuals also have atrial fibrillation. The presence of a short QT interval in the ECG is associated with susceptibility to the ventricular arrhythmias, and it is linked to the ventricular refractoriness with the origin of this disorder. Confirmation of a ventricular effective refractory period significantly shortened (<150 msec) during programmed ventricular stimulation, supports this concept. As already we have said, this cardiological entity is a channelopathy and, in the particular case of short QT syndrome, it is postulated that the delivery of atrial and ventricular channels IKs, IKr, ICa-L determines a gain of function of potassium channels or the loss of calcium channel function , results in a reduction of atrial refractoriness and vulnerability to the onset of atrial fibrillation (three genes — KCNH2, KCNQ1 and KCNJ2 — encoding different potassium ion channels involved in repolarization have been linked to this syndrome).

Electrocardiogram. The QTc interval <350 msec in the absence of external involved factors, make to suspect the presence of this syndrome. The coexistence of acuminate T wave, alongside a high QRS voltage in precordial leads is not a consistent finding in all the reported cases.

Electrophysiological Study

During programmed ventricular stimulation from the right ventricle most of the patients had inducible ventricular fibrillation with 2 and 3 extra stimuli. Half of the patients also had atrial fibrillation inducibility. The ventricular effective refractory period was set at values below 150 msec, and the infusion of flecainide and other drugs of I-class determine a prolongation between 30 and 100 msec.

Short Qt-Interval (ECG 12 Leads)

Electrocardiogram of short QT syndrome. Observe the tall peaked T waves. (From article "short QT syndrome" by R. Brugada et al. in Journal CMAJ.)

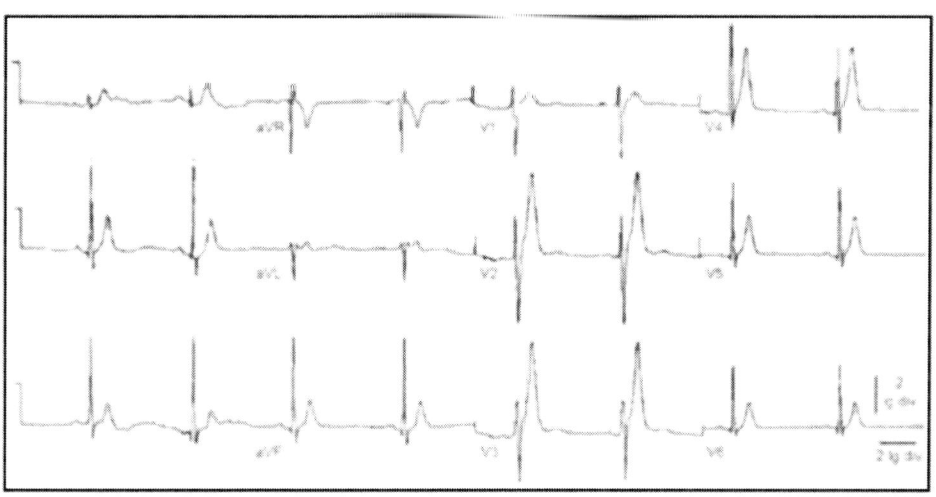

Summarizing

A prolonged QT interval has long been known to be a harbinger of life-threatening ventricular arrhythmias, and long QT syndrome is recognized as a hereditary condition with an increased risk of sudden cardiac death. A short QT interval, on the other hand, was not considered arrhythmogenic and was seen mostly in relation to hypercalcemia. This way of thinking changed after the first description in 2000 of a sporadic case of short QT interval and sudden cardiac death and of a family with short QT interval and paroxysmal atrial fibrillation. The short QT syndrome constitutes a new clinical entity that is associated with a high incidence of sudden cardiac death, syncope, and/or atrial fibrillation even in young patients and newborns. Patients with this congenital electrical abnormality are characterized by rate-corrected QT intervals lesser than 350 ms. The implantable cardioverter defibrillator is the therapy of choice in patients with syncope and a positive family history of sudden cardiac death. However, ICD therapy in patients with a short QT syndrome has an increased risk for inappropriate shock therapies due to possible T wave oversensing. In patients with a mutation in HERG, it turn into ventricular tachycardias/ventricular fibrillation non-inducible and restored the QT interval/heart rate relationship towards a normal range. It may serve as an adjunct to ICD therapy or as a possible alternative treatment, especially for children and babies (newborns).

6. Diversity on Electrical Cardiac Systole [10,26,37]

The authors of this chapter also have a considerable number of patients who have a variety of abnormalities in the heart's electrical systole. Combinations "short-long" "long-short" at different intervals are not uncommon. They need to be more valued. At first they may be overlooked. And however, they are also able to develop a sudden death.

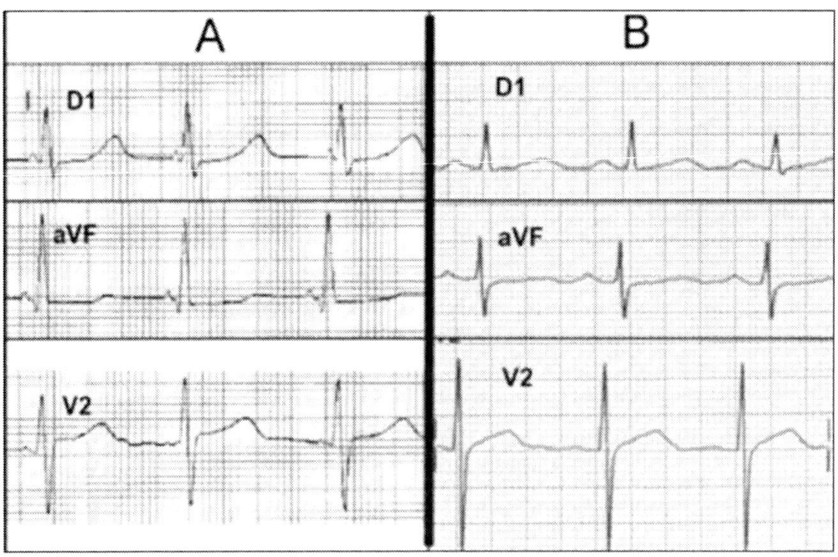

A. Short PR-interval alongside Long QT-interval.
B. Long PR-interval alongside Long QT-interval.

The association between structural and electrical challenges is not unusual. The author of this chapter, has highlighted associations such as a pattern of "PR and QT short" (Breijo's Pattern) with a pattern of Wellens (26,37), for example. (See the image below).

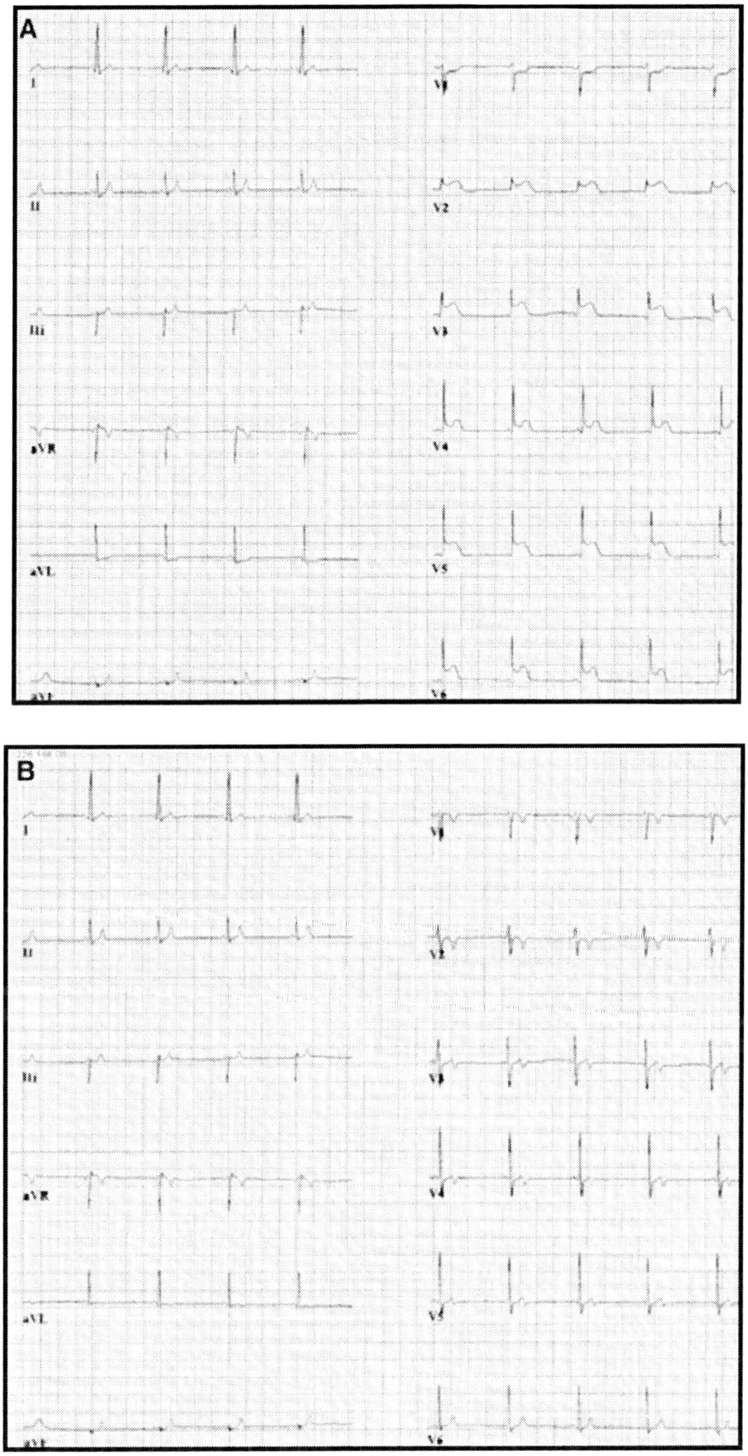

A: Inactive period. B: Recovered period.

References

[1] Wolff, L., Parkinson, J., White, PD. Bundle-branch block with short P-R interval in healthy young people prone to paroxysmal tachycardia. *American Heart Journal.* 1930/08;5:685-704.

[2] Durrer D, Schuilenburg RM, Wellens HJ. Pre-excitation revisited. *Am. J. Cardiol.* Jun 1970;25(6):690-7.

[3] Calkins H, Sousa J, el-Atassi R, et al. Diagnosis and cure of the Wolff-Parkinson-White syndrome or paroxysmal supraventricular tachycardias during a single electrophysiologic test. *N. Engl. J. Med.* Jun 6 1991;324(23):1612-8.

[4] Pappone C, Vicedomini G, Manguso F, et al. Risk of malignant arrhythmias in initially symptomatic patients with wolff-Parkinson-white syndrome: results of a prospective long-term electrophysiological follow-up study. *Circulation.* Feb 7 2012;125(5):661-8.

[5] Zhang Y, Wang L. Atrial vulnerability is a major mechanism of paroxysmal atrial fibrillation in patients with Wolff-Parkinson-White syndrome. *Med. Hypotheses.* 2006;67(6):1345-7.

[6] Fengler BT, Brady WJ, Plautz CU. Atrial fibrillation in the Wolff-Parkinson-White syndrome: ECG recognition and treatment in the ED. *Am. J. Emerg. Med.* Jun 2007;25(5):576-83.

[7] Derejko P, Szumowski LJ, Sanders P, Krupa W, Bodalski R, Orczykowski M, et al. Atrial Fibrillation in Patients with Wolff-Parkinson-White Syndrome:: Role of Pulmonary Veins. *J. Cardiovasc. Electrophysiol.* Oct 28 2011.

[8] Pappone C, Manguso F, Santinelli R, Vicedomini G, Sala S, Paglino G. Radiofrequency ablation in children with asymptomatic Wolff-Parkinson-White syndrome. *N. Engl. J. Med.* Sep 16 2004;351(12):1197-205.

[9] Jackman WM, Wang XZ, Friday KJ, et al. Catheter ablation of accessory atrioventricular pathways (Wolff- Parkinson-White syndrome) by radiofrequency current. *N. Engl. J. Med.* Jun 6 1991;324(23):1605-11.

[10] Breijo-Marquez FR, Pardo Ríos M (2011) Wolff-Parkinson-White and Prolonged "Q-T" Patterns in the Same Electrocardiographic Record. *J. Clinic Experiment Cardiol.* 2:118.

[11] Lown B, Ganong Wf, Levine Sa. The syndrome of short P-R interval, normal QRS complex and paroxysmal rapid heart action. *Circulation.* May 1952;5(5):693-706.

[12] Brechenmacher C, Laham J, Iris L, et al. [Histological study of abnormal conduction pathways in the Wolff-Parkinson-White syndrome and Lown-Ganong-Levine syndrome]. *Arch. Mal. Coeur. Vaiss.* May 1974;67(5):507-19.

[13] Moller P. Letter: Criteria for the LGL syndrome. *Am. Heart J.* Apr 1976;91(4):539-41.

[14] Josephson ME, Kastor JA. Supraventricular tachycardia in Lown-Ganong-Levine syndrome: atrionodal versus intranodal reentry. *Am. J. Cardiol.* Oct 1977;40(4):521-7

[15] Ward DE, Camm AJ, Spurrell RAJ. Dual AH pathways in patients with and without the Lown-Ganong-Levine syndrome. *Br. Heart J.* 1981;45:356.

[16] Benditt DG, Pritchett LC, Smith WM, et al. Characteristics of atrioventricular conduction and the spectrum of arrhythmias in lown-ganong-levine syndrome. *Circulation.* Mar 1978;57(3):454-65.

[17] Douglas JE, Mandel WJ, Danzig R, Hayakawa H. Lown-Ganong-Levine syndrome. *Circulation*. May 1972;45(5):1143-4.
[18] Mahaim I. Kent fibers and the A-V paraspecific conduction through the upper connections of the bundle of His-Tawara. *Am. Heart J.* 1947;33:651.
[19] Mahaim I, et al. Recherches d'lanatomic comparee et du pathologic experimentale sur les connexions hautes du faisceau de His-Tawara. *Cardiologia*. 1941;5:189–260.
[20] Gallagher JJ, et al. Role of Mahaim fibers in cardiac arrhythmias in man. *Circulation*. 1981;64:176–189.
[21] Gillette PC, et al. Prolonged and decremental antegrade conduction properties in right anterior accessory connections: wide QRS antidromic tachycardia of left bundle branch block pattern without Wolff-Parkinson-White configuration in sinus rhythm. *Am. Heart J.* 1982;103:66–74.
[22] Tchou P, et al. Atriofascicular connection or a nodoventricular Mahaim fiber? Electrophysiologic elucidation of the pathway and associated reentrant circuit. *Circulation* . 1988;77:837–848.
[23] Jose L. Serra. The related tachycardia has a typical left bungle branch block type. *QRS*. Fac..org.
[24] McClelland JH, et al. Radiofrequency catheter ablation of right atriofascicular (Mahaim) accessory pathways guided by accessory pathway activation potentials. *Circulation* . 1994;89:2655–2666.
[25] Haissaguerre M, et al. Catheter ablation of Mahaim fibers with preservation of atrioventricular nodal conduction. *Circulation*. 1990;82:418–427.
[26] Breijo-Marquez. FR. Decrease of electrical cardiac systole. *Int. J. Cardiol.* 2008. e124-126.
[27] Barold SS, Hayes DL. Second-degree atrioventricular block: a reappraisal. *Mayo Clin Proc*. Jan 2001;76(1):44-57.
[28] Silverman ME, Upshaw CB Jr, Lange HW. Woldemar Mobitz and His 1924 classification of second-degree atrioventricular block. *Circulation*. Aug 31 2004;110(9):1162-7.
[29] Lev M. Anatomic basis for atrioventricular block. *Am. J. Med.* Nov 1964;37:742-8.
[30] Morita H, Wu J, Zipes DP (August 2008). "The QT syndromes: long and short". *Lancet* 372 (9640): 750–63. doi:10.1016/S0140-6736(08)61307-0. PMID 18761222.
[31] Schwartz PJ, Moss AJ, Vincent GM, Crampton RS (1993). "Diagnostic criteria for the long QT syndrome. An update". *Circulation* 88 (2): 782–4.
[32] Hedley PL; Jorgensen P. et al. (2009). "The genetic basis of long QT and short QT syndromes: a mutation update". *Human Mutation* 30 (11): 1486–511.
[33] Ward OC (April 1964). "A new familial cardiac syndrome in children". *J. Ir. Med. Assoc.* 54: 103–6.
[34] Gussak I, Brugada P, Brugada J, et al. Idiopathic short QT interval: a new clinical syndrome? *Cardiology* 2000;94:99-102.
[35] Gaita F, Giustetto C, Bianchi F, et al. Short QT Syndrome: a familial cause of sudden death. *Circulation* 2003;108:965-70.
[36] Brugada R, Hong K, Dumaine R, et al. Sudden death associated with short-QT syndrome linked to mutations in HERG. *Circulation* 2004;109:30-5.
[37] Breijo-Marquez, FR. Cardiac Arrhythmias-New considerations. Riejeka. Croatia. In-Tech 2012: 236.

[38] Iona Mozos. Anemia and the QT interval in hypertensive patients. IJ of collaborative research on international and Public heath. 2012. Vol 4. 12.

[39] Priori SG, Pandit SV, Rivolta I, et al. A novel form of short QT syndrome (SQT3) is caused by a mutation in the KCNJ2 gene. *Circ. Res.* 2005;96:800-7.

[40] Cordeiro JM, Brugada R, Wu YS, et al. Modulation of I(Kr) inactivation by mutation N588K in KCNH2: a link to arrhythmogenesis in short QT syndrome. *Cardiovasc. Res.* 2005;67:498-509.

[41] Breijo-Marquez FR. Variability and diversity of the electrical cardiac systole. *BMJ Case Rep.*; 2009: bcr06.2008.0284.

[42] Breijo-Márquez FR, Ríos MP, Baños MA. Presence of a critical stenosis in left anterior descending coronary artery alongside a short "P-R" and "Q-T" pattern, in the same electrocardiographic record. *J. Electrocardiol.* 2010 Sep-Oct;43(5):422-4.

In: Sudden Death
Editors: Jiashin Wu and Jessica Wu

ISBN: 978-1-62618-825-9

Chapter VIII

Neoplasm-related Sudden Death: Causes and Clinicopathological Characteristics

Katsuya Chinen *

Department of Pathology, Nerima General Hospital,
Nerima, Tokyo, Japan

Abstract

Patients with neoplastic diseases, especially malignancies, are at greatly elevated risk of sudden death, because they may suffer from a variety of neoplasm-, and/or treatment-related clinical conditions including myelosuppression, immunosuppression, coagulation abnormalities, metabolic disorders, and malnutrition. Cancer patients die suddenly of miscellaneous etiologies, and about one third of sudden death in cancer patients is attributed to neoplasm-related complications.

In the literature, the majority of neoplasm-related sudden deaths (NSDs) are caused by neoplasms affecting critical organs such as the heart and brain. In addition, neoplasms damaging respiratory system or causing acute blood loss are responsible for sudden death. Mechanisms are miscellaneous and most are directly related to the anatomical location of the neoplasm. On the other hand, regardless of the site, specific types of neoplasm (e.g. hormone-producing tumors) sometimes cause sudden death by mechanisms which a pathophysiological function peculiar to the tumor induces critical manifestations of vital organs such as the heart.

As mentioned above, causes of NSD is classified as follows; (1) cardiac tumors, (2) brain tumors, (3) pulmonary tumor embolism, (4) asphyxia, (5) massive exsanguinations, and (6) sudden death due to neoplasm-specific pathophysiology. The latter includes amyloidosis, hyperviscosity syndrome, and hormone-induced complications, and these diseases can present with a variety of lethal clinical manifestations. In this chapter,

* Katsuya Chinen, MD, PhD, Department of Pathology, Nerima General Hospital, 1-24-1 Asahigaoka, Nerima, Tokyo 176-8530 Japan; Tel: 81-3-5988-2200; Fax: 81-3-5988-2250; E-mail; path.chinen@gmail.com.

clinical and pathological characteristics of NSDs are described based on this classification with a review of the literature.

Introduction

Patients with neoplastic diseases, especially malignancies, are at greatly elevated risk of sudden death, because they may suffer from a variety of neoplasm-, and/or treatment-related clinical conditions including myelosuppression, immunosuppression, coagulation abnormalities, metabolic disorders, and malnutrition. Cancer patients die suddenly of miscellaneous etiologies, and about one third of sudden death in cancer patients is attributed to neoplasm-related complications [1].

The cardiovascular and central nervous systems are crucial for life, and any damage affecting them can be life-threatening. In the literature, the majority of neoplasm-related sudden deaths (NSDs) are caused by neoplasms affecting critical organs such as the heart and brain. In addition, neoplasms damaging respiratory system or causing acute blood loss are responsible for sudden death. Mechanisms are miscellaneous and most are directly related to the anatomical location of the neoplasm. On the other hand, regardless of the site, specific types of neoplasm (e.g. hormone-producing tumors) sometimes cause sudden death by mechanisms which a pathophysiological function peculiar to the tumor induces critical manifestations of vital organs such as the heart.

An etiological classification of NSD is presented in Table 1. In this chapter, clinical and pathological characteristics of NSDs are described following this classification with a review of the literature.

Table 1. Etiological Classification of Neoplasm-Related Sudden Death

1) Cardiac tumors
2) Brain tumors
3) Pulmonary tumor embolism
4) Asphyxia
5) Massive exsanguination
6) Sudden death due to neoplasm-specific pathophysiology
    a) Amyloidosis
    b) Hyperviscosity syndrome
    c) Hormone-induced complications

1. Cardiac Tumors

Cardiac tumors, regardless of their nature (i.e., primary or metastatic, benign or malignant) constitute risks for sudden death by themselves. The pathophysiology is miscellaneous, including cardiac ischemia, arrhythmia, pump failure, outflow obstruction, valvular dysfunction, and cardiac tamponade.

1.1. Primary Cardiac Tumors

In the literature, there have been a large number of cases of sudden death attributed to primary cardiac neoplasms. Cina et al. [2], in their review, indicated that in most cases the tumors are histologically benign but their intracardiac location precipitates conductive and hemodynamic abnormalities.

1.1.1. Cystic Tumor of the Atrioventricular (AV) Node

The cystic tumor of the AV node is a benign, congenital, cystic mass located at the base of the atrial septum. The size ranges from 2 to 20 mm [3], and microscopically ductular structures, cysts, and solid nests of epithelial-like cells within loose fibrous stroma are characteristic (Figure 1). Occasionally, cysts are filled with proteinaceous debris. Previously the cystic tumor of the AV node was regarded as a mesothelioma, but it is now considered to be a developmental abnormality of epithelial nature and endodermal origin [4, 5]. It is well known as a cause of AV block or sudden death [5,6], and has been called the "smallest tumor causing sudden death" [7]. In fact, this tumor is the most common neoplasm of cardiac origin that causes sudden death [2]. Since the gross findings may be minimal, a lesion may not be discovered unless the AV node is microscopically examined [2]. Therefore, a histopathological examination of AV node is essential in order to clarify the etiology of cardiac sudden death.

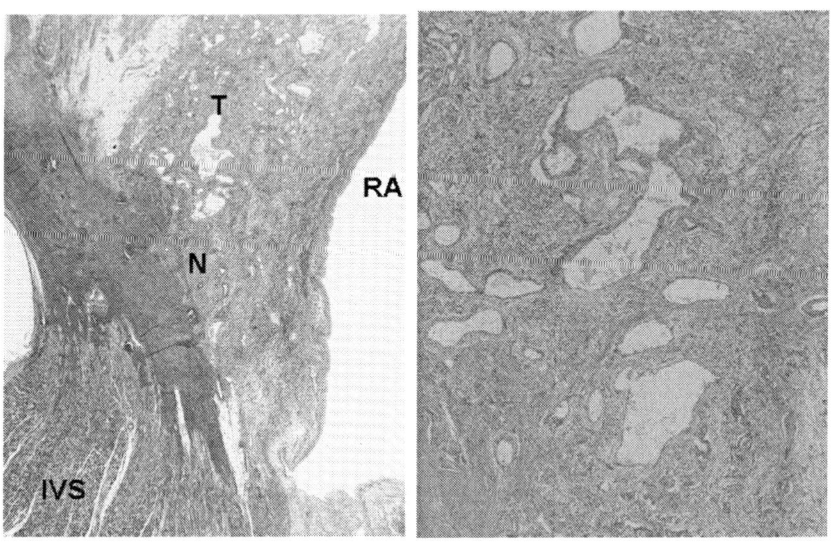

(A) **(B)**

Figure 1. Microscopic findings of a cystic tumor of the atrioventricular (AV) node. **A**) The tumor (T) is located in the lower right atrium (RA) and has reached to the AV node (N). (IVS: interventricular septum) (Azan stain). **B**) Multiple microcysts lined by columnar and cuboidal cells are apparent within loose fibrous stroma (hematoxylin-eosin). (Courtesy by Dr. Tomio Arai, Tokyo Metropolitan Geriatric Hospital).

1.1.2. Fibroma

Fibroma, the most commonly resected cardiac tumor of children, constitutes the second most frequent causing sudden death [2]. The cardiac sites of fibromas are, in order of decreasing frequency, the interventricular septum, left ventricular free wall, right ventricle, and atria [3].

The location has been noted as a determining factor in the presentation and outcome of affected patients. Fibromas arising in the interventricular septum are inoperable, but those of the ventricular free wall may be removed surgically.

It seems that sudden death occurs due to compression of the conducting system (bundle of His) or triggering of ventricular fibrillation. In one study [8], more than half of the cases presenting with sudden death had tumors in the interventricular septum, where compression of the conduction system is more likely.

1.1.3. Myxoma

Among primary cardiac tumors, myxoma is the most common in adults and is the third most frequent neoplasm causing sudden death [2].

It usually develops in the atria; about 75% originate in the left atrium, and 15 to 20 % in the right atrium.

If the tumor is sufficiently large, soft, and easily deformable, and if it has a long stalk, obstruction of the orifice of the mitral or tricuspid valve may occur [9]. Sudden death may be the result of either acute disturbance in cardiac hemodynamics or systemic embolization by tumor fragments.

The lethal potential of this tumor can be attributed to both its location (usually in the left atrium) and its configuration [2].

1.1.4. Rhabdomyoma

Rhabdomyoma is the most common primary cardiac tumor in children. It may occur as solitary, multiple or diffuse lesions of the myocardium, and is considered to be a malformation tumor (hamartoma), rather than a true neoplasm [10]. Sudden cardiac death may result from rhythm disturbance, outflow obstruction and valvular distortion [11]. Cardiac rhabdomyoma is also frequently associated with tuberous sclerosis, an autosomal dominant inherited disease.

If a cardiac rhabdomyoma is identified in patients presenting with sudden death, other lesions characteristic of this syndrome such as adrenal angiomyolipoma and subependymal giant cell astrocytoma, may further be present and mortality may in fact be due to complications of tuberous sclerosis [2, 11-13].

1.1.5. Papillary Fibroelastoma

The papillary fibroelastoma is a benign endocardial papilloma predominantly affecting the cardiac valves, especially the aortic valve (Figure 2), where it has been implicated in sudden death because of obstruction of the ostium of the right or left coronary artery. In one review of reported cases of papillary fibroelastoma [14], sudden death was found in 21 of 725 patients (2.9%).

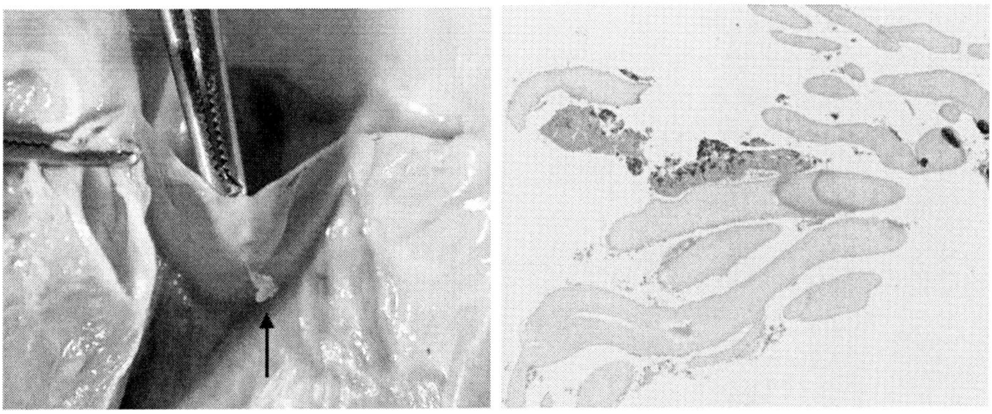

(A) (B)

Figure 2. Papillary fibroelastoma of the aortic valve. **A**) Macroscopically, an expophytic tumor with thin stalk, measuring 5 mm in diameter, is apparent on the right coronary cusp of the aortic valve (arrow). **B**) Microscopic examination shows a papillary endocardial tumor with hyalinized central core. Fibrin clot and bacterial colonization are also evident. (hematoxylin-eosin, original magnification x40).

1.1.6. Hemangioma

Hemangiomas are proliferations of endothelial cells forming vascular channels of variable size. The cardiac hemangioma occurs in patients of all ages and there is a male predominance [15]. It appears most lethal when disrupting the conducting system or involving the atrioventricular node. Very rarely, this tumor can induce cardiac tamponade resulting in sudden death [16, 17].

1.1.7. Angiosarcoma

Angiosarcoma is the most frequent primary malignant cardiac neoplasm and most commonly arises in the right atrium [18]. Extension into the pericardial sac or atrial chamber often leads to hemopericardium, cardiac tamponade, or obstruction of blood flow. Widespread metastasis (especially pulmonary) is common and may be related to causes of death [19]. However, the number of patients with cardiac angiosarcoma presenting with sudden death is limited [2, 20, 21].

1.1.8. Miscellaneous Primary Cardiac Tumors

Many other kinds of primary cardiac tumors have been reported as causes of sudden death, although their incidences are very low. They include the rhabdomyosarcoma, malignant lymphoma, undifferentiated sarcoma, fibrosarcoma, malignant nerve sheath tumor, teratoma, lipoma, angiomyoma, cardiac inflammatory myofibroblastic tumor, low-grade myofibroblastic sarcoma, and coronary artery intimal sarcoma [2, 22-25].

1.2. Metastatic Cardiac Tumors

Metastatic tumors in the heart are far more frequent than primary neoplasms, by at least a 30 to 1 ratio [26]. The most common lesions with cardiac metastatic potential are carcinomas of the lung, breast, esophagus and thyroid gland, leukemia and malignant lymphomas [27]. Metastatic cardiac tumors also cause sudden death due to impaired cardiac function, including cardiac tamponade, conduction disturbance and outflow obstruction [28-30]. In the literature, metastatic cardiac tumors responsible for sudden death have been derived from a variety of organs, such as the lung [30], esophagus [31], thyroid gland [32], pancreas [33] and colon [28], as well as soft tissue [34]. T-cell lymphomas, when compared with B-cell lymphomas, metastasize more frequently and are more likely to give rise to cardiac manifestations, including sudden death (Figure 3) [35].

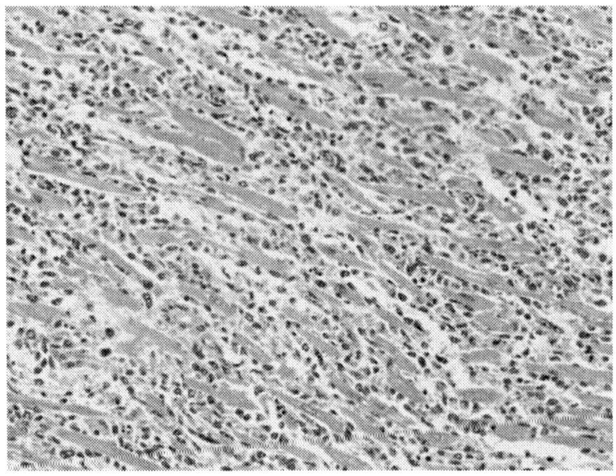

Figure 3. An example of cardiac involvement by malignant lymphoma in a 74 year-old man presenting with sudden death. Note diffuse interstitial infiltration of lymphoma cells (hematoxylin-eosin, original magnification x200).

2. Brain Tumors

Brain tumors, like cardiac tumors, are etiological factors for NSD. Although the actual proportion of sudden deaths from this cause is very low (0.02% to 2.1%) [36], many anecdotal cases have been reported. Any kind of brain tumors, regardless of their nature (i.e. primary or metastatic, benign or malignant), can cause sudden death. In the literature, however, the astrocytoma-glioblastoma category has predominated [37]. Other examples include oligodendroglioma, medulloblastoma, subependymoma, microglioma, meningioma, colloid cyst, lymphoma, teratoma, hemangiopericytoma and metastatic brain tumors [37-45]. Of the metastatic intracranial tumors, bronchial carcinoma, choriocarcinoma and melanoma are the most common [46].

Sudden death in patients with brain tumors is caused mainly by rapid functional deterioration of a vital focus, such as the brainstem, which controls circulatory or respiratory functions. Mechanisms of sudden death have been explained as detailed below.

2.1. Raised Intracranial Pressure

The most common mechanism is raised intracranial pressure as a result of an intracranial expanding (space-occupying) lesion. Hemorrhage from a tumor often causes rapid increase of the tumor mass. Raised intracranial pressure finally causes cerebral herniation and brainstem compression with a fatal outcome.

2.2. Acute Obstructive Hydrocephalus

Tumors that can obstruct cerebrospinal fluid flow are responsible for acute hydrocephalus. It is the site of tumor, rather than its nature, that is of importance. If there is a small tumor in a crucial site adjacent to a ventricular foramen, then it is of much greater importance than a large expanding tumor in a frontal or occipital lobe. For example, tumors of the third ventricle can cause acute obstructive hydrocephalus by blocking the foramen of Munro or the posterior third ventricle and cerebral aqueduct. Primary third-ventricle tumors include colloid cysts (the most frequent type), astrocytomas, ependymomas, and choroid plexus papillomas, and these tumors have been reported as causes of sudden death [47]. Leptomeningeal seeding of tumor cells, such as lymphoma cells, may also be responsible for acute obstructive hydrocephalus [48]. Most patients with acute hydrocephalus are not diagnosed antemortem as having brain tumors, because clinical manifestations of acute hydrocephalus, including vomiting, headache and lethargy, often lead to a misdiagnosis as a viral illness such as gastroenteritis [47].

2.3. Neoplastic Involvement of the Respiratory and/or Cardiac Centers

In infratentorial tumors, direct involvement with the respiratory and/or cardiac centers in the brainstem can cause sudden death. In the literature, oligodendroglioma [42,43], ganglioglioma [49,50], and mycosis fungoides [51] have been reported as responsible lesions. Mechanical compression, without direct invasion, caused by tumors neighboring the brainstem may be involved [39].

2.4. Epilepsy

The incidence of epileptic seizures for all intracranial tumors is about 20-50%, but sudden death caused by epilepsy is rare [52]. In one review article [52], tumors causing fatal epilepsy were miscellaneous, including low-grade astrocytoma, anaplastic astrocytoma, oligodendroglioma, meningioma, subependymal giant cell astrocytoma, anaplastic oligodendroglioma, gangliocytoma, ependymoma, subependymoma, and teratoma. The most common localization was the frontal lobe and the thalamus. It is interesting that there was no tumor solely in the parietal lobe, which is reported to be the most common location for tumors causing seizures. The mechanism of epilepsy-induced sudden death remains controversial. The most widely accepted theory proposes that seizure activity results in autonomic nervous system discharge, which ultimately triggers lethal cardiac arrhythmias or respiratory arrest [12, 52].

2.5. Neurogenic Pulmonary Edema

Some patients with brain tumor die suddenly of neurogenic pulmonary edema [45]. Not only brain tumors but also subarachnoid and intraventricular hemorrhage may be responsible.

The exact pathophysiology is unclear, but it may feature an adrenergic response induced by cerebral insult, which leads to increased pulmonary hydrostatic pressure and lung capillary permeability. It is known that an increase of cerebrospinal fluid pressure, infusion of thrombin and fibrinogen into the cistern magna, and intravenous or intrathecal infusion of massive amounts of catecholamines can cause neurogenic pulmonary edema [45].

3. Pulmonary Tumor Embolism

Autopsy studies estimate that the incidence of pulmonary tumor embolism (PTE) is between 3% and 26% among patients with solid tumors. Primary tumors for PTE have been reported to be, in order of decreasing frequency, carcinomas of the breast, stomach, lung, liver, prostate, and pancreas [53]. Pulmonary hypertension due to PTE is considered a major contributory cause of death, which may occur in as much as 8% of cases [54]. Although comprehensive studies are still lacking, many anecdotal case reports dealing with PTE-induced sudden death have been published. Sudden deaths are caused by tumors that have high angioinvasive potential, such as renal cell carcinomas (Figure 4) [1], hepatocellular carcinomas [55], testicular germ cell tumors [56], and Wilms tumors [57,58]. Primary tumors causing PTE are often undiagnosed before sudden death, which is the first clinical presentation in many cases. Tumors originating from the vessel wall of large veins or pulmonary artery can also obstruct the pulmonary arterial system and cause mortality, for example with leiomyosarcoma of the pulmonary artery [59] and intravenous leiomyoma [60]. Strictly speaking, when tumors in the pulmonary artery are contiguous with the original tumor site, they are not "PTE" because PTE is defined as "the presence of isolated cells or clusters of tumor cells within the pulmonary arterial system, which are not contiguous with primary or metastatic foci" [61]. However, because these types of tumors can cause sudden death by the same mechanism as true "PTE", it may be reasonable to describe here as "sudden death due to tumorous obstruction of the pulmonary circulation system."

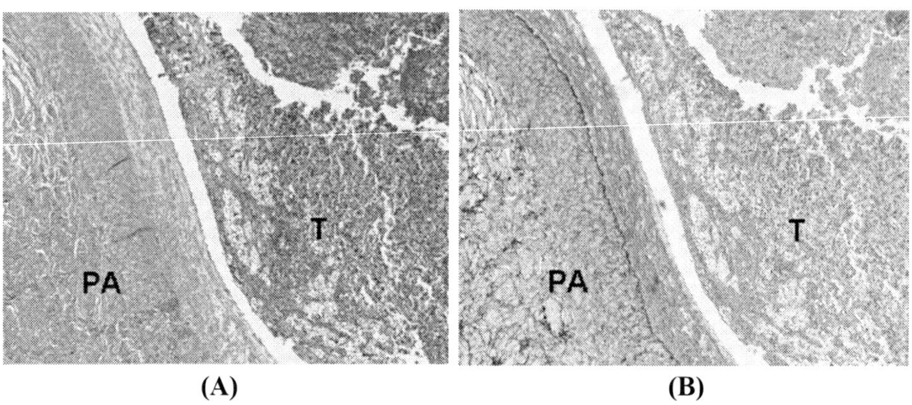

Figure 4. Microscopic findings of a neoplastic pulmonary embolus from a renal cell carcinoma in a 54-year-old man. The pulmonary artery (PA) is occupied by tumor cells (T). A small amount of thrombus is also observed. (hematoxylin-eosin (**A**) and elastic van Gieson stain (**B**), original magnification x40). This patient was found in the state of cardiopulmonary arrest. Neoplastic involvement of the right renal vein, inferior vena cava, right atrium, and pulmonary truncus was grossly observed.

3.1. Pulmonary Tumor Thrombotic Microangiopathy

Recently, a distinct form of PTE, designated as "pulmonary tumor thrombotic microangiopathy (PTTM)", has become recognized as a cause of sudden death.

Clinicopathological characteristics of PTTM are quite different from those of conventional PTE in many points, therefore it seems better to document PTTM as a single disease entity. PTTM is in fact a rare clinicopathologic condition that causes severe clinical manifestations including pulmonary hypertension, right-sided heart failure and sudden death. It is characterized by wide spread tumor emboli in the small arteries and arterioles of the lung, associated with thrombus formation and fibrocellular and fibromuscular intimal proliferation [62]. It differs from conventional PTE in that metastatic tumors do not cause simple mechanical obstruction of the pulmonary vasculature but rather stimulate vessel reactions (Figure 5). Apparent clinicopathologic features [63,64] include:

1) adenocarcinomas as the predominant histology, especially of poorly differentiated type including the signet-ring cell carcinoma;
2) the stomach as the most frequent primary site, PTTM often being due to clinically undetected, occult gastric carcinoma;
3) no age dependence, both the old and young being affected; and
4) a difficult antemortem diagnosis with frequent misdiagnosis as primary pulmonary hypertension.

In cases of sudden death with unexplained pulmonary hypertension or cor pulmonale, the possibility of PTTM should be considered and special attention should be paid in postmortem examination. Since gross findings of the lung are often unremarkable, microscopic examination of the lung is required for the diagnosis. Although neoplasms of various organs can cause PTTM [65], the most frequent neoplasm is, as mentioned above, the gastric carcinoma [62]. Therefore, in cases of PTTM with obscure primary neoplasm, the stomach should be examined carefully. Many serial step sections of the stomach may be necessary for detection of the primary lesion because PTTM is sometimes caused by a tiny early cancer limited to the mucosal or submucosal layer [66, 67].

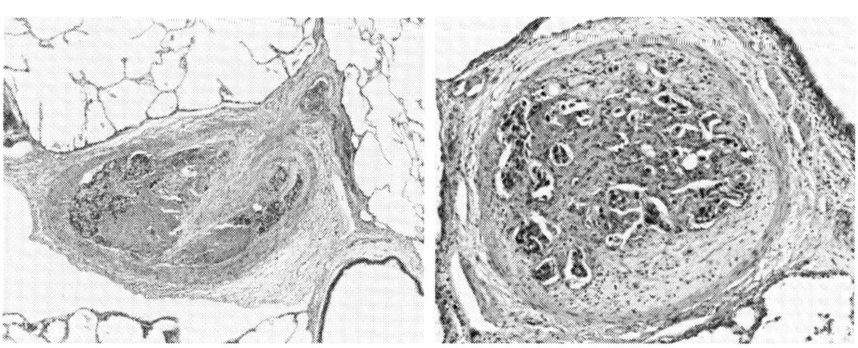

(A) (B)

Figure 5. (Continued).

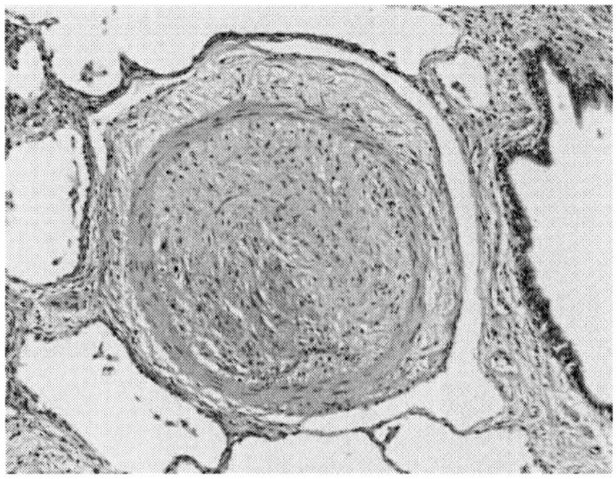

(C)

Figure 5. Histologic findings of pulmonary tumor thrombotic microangiopathy (PTTM) in a 62 year-old male patient with gastric cancer, who died suddenly of pulmonary hypertension. **A**) Characteristic findings of PTTM showing a tumor embolism associated with thrombus formation and fibrocellular intimal proliferation in a small pulmonary artery (hematoxylin-eosin, original magnification x40). **B**) A small pulmonary artery is occluded by proliferated intima and cancer cells. A small amount of fibrin thrombus is also apprarent (hematoxylin-eosin, original magnification x100). **C**) Complete vascular occlusion of a small pulmonary artery due to fibrocellular intimal proliferation. Note that no tumor cells are identiable within this arterial lesion (hematoxylin-eosin, original magnification x100).

4. Asphyxia

Asphyxia is one mechanism of NSD. Neoplasms affecting the upper airway can cause lethal airway obstruction. In the literature, lesions arising in the larynx causing sudden death include schwannoma [68], lymphoma [69], papillomatosis [70, 71], basosquamous carcinoma [72], and hemangioma [73]. Prolapsed tumors originating from the esophagus (fibrolipoma) [74] or hypopharynx (lipoma) [75] are also reported causes. In addition, lethal asphyxia may occur as a result of external compression of the trachea or bronchus caused by mediastinal tumors such as lymphoma [76], paraganglioma [77], and esophageal leiomyoma [78].

5. Massive Exsanguination

Massive exsanguination can be a lethal complication in neoplastic diseases. The anatomical environment around neoplasms is very important in this context and neoplasms in the body cavity may cause hemoperitoneum or hemothorax. Examples originating from or neighboring great vessels present an obvious risk for vessel rupture.

5.1. Hemoperitoneum

Intraperitoneal bleeding is a common etiology for massive exsanguination. Hemoperitoneum due to spontaneous hepatic rupture is a well-known fatal complication of hepatocellular carcinoma (Figure 6), with a reported incidence of 3% [79]. Metastatic liver tumors can also cause spontaneous rupture [80]. Extrahepatic neoplasms causing hemoperitoneum and sudden death include mesenteric malignant hemangioendothelioma [81], Wilms tumor [76] and chronic myelogenous leukemia with splenic rupture [82]. Even a uterine leiomyoma, a very common benign neoplasm, can be a cause of fatal intraperitoneal bleeding [13].

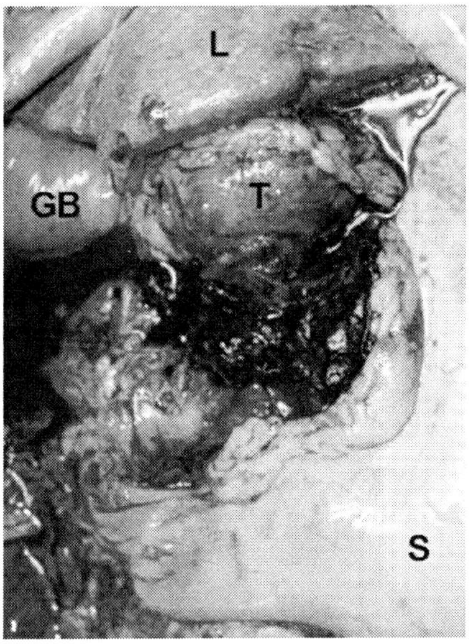

Figure 6. A case of sudden death in a 77-year-old man with hepatocellular carcinoma. Autopsy reveals a protruding tumor (T), measuring 6.5 x 5.0 x 4.0 cm, of the left lobe of the liver (L). The tumor has ruptured and was associated with 2000 mL of hemoperitoneum. (GB; gallbladder, S; stomach)

5.2. Hemothorax

Intrapleural bleeding from tumors may also cause massive exsanguination and the negative pressure in the intrapleural cavity may exacerbate bleeding from a pleural tumor. Many lethal cases have been documented with hepatocellular carcinomas [83]. In von Recklinghausen's disease or neurofibromatosis, bleeding in the pleural cavity has been reported as a result of rupture of friable vasculature by either vascular invasion or arterial dysplasia [84, 85].

5.3. Alimentary Tract Hemorrhage

Alimentary tract hemorrhage is another cause of massive exsanguination. Rupture of esophageal varices often induces sudden death in patients with hepatocellular carcinoma and liver cirrhosis [86]. Fistula formation caused by tumor invasion between great vessels and the alimentary canal may also be responsible for fatal blood loss (Figure 7) [1].

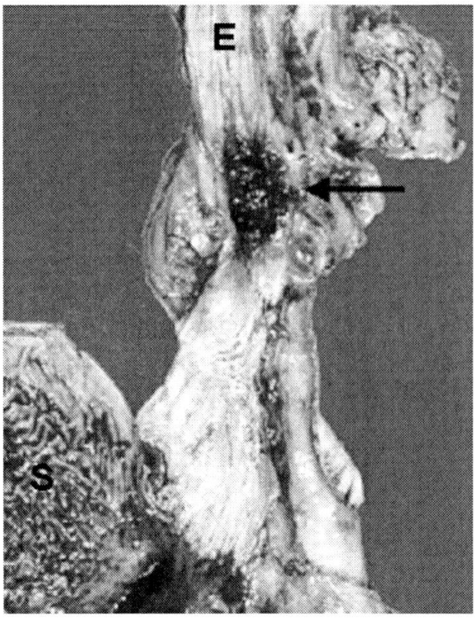

Figuure 7. An autopsy finding of a 66-year-old man, who received radiotherapy for an esophageal cancer, presenting with sudden death after acute onset of hematomesis. An esophago-aortic fistula (arrow) is apparent in the middle portion of the esophagus (E). The stomach (S) is full of fresh blood.

5.4. Bleeding from Superficial Vessels

Primary and metastatic tumors existing in the subcutaneous tissue may invade large vessels, such as the femoral artery, and destroy the vessel wall, leading to fatal bleeding [87].

6. Sudden Death Due to Neoplasm-Specific Pathophysiology

Specific types of neoplasm sometimes cause sudden death by mechanisms which pathophysiological function peculiar to the neoplasm induces critical manifestation of vital organs.

6.1. Amyloidosis

Amyloidosis sometimes occurs as a complication of some neoplastic diseases, including multiple myeloma and thyroid medullary carcinoma. The heart is one of the target organs for amyloid deposits and cardiac amyloidosis can cause lethal arrhythmia and/or pump failure leading to sudden death [88]. Another mechanism of amyloidosis-induced sudden death is hepatic or splenic rupture as a result of amyloid deposition in these organs [89].

6.2. Hyperviscosity Syndrome

The hyperviscosity syndrome is one of the lethal complications in patients with hematological malignancies. Embolic events due to hyperviscosity have been documented as a cause of sudden death in multiple myeloma [90] and leukemia [76].

6.3. Hormone-Induced Complications

6.3.1. Hypercalcemia

Hypercalcemia is one critical complication in cancer patients. Metastatic bone tumors destroy bony structures and induce hypercalcemia. In addition, over-production of parathyroid hormone (PTH) or PTH-related peptide (PTH-rP) by specific types of neoplasm can cause a lethal clinical condition as a result of hypercalcemia. Adult T-cell leukemia/lymphoma (ATLL) is a well-known malignancy inducing lethal hypercalcemia. Metastatic calcification of the heart is reported as a cause of sudden death in patients with ATLL [91] and parathyroid adenoma [92].

6.3.2. Hypokalemia

Hypokalemia may cause severe clinical symptoms such as cardiac arrhythmia and respiratory failure due to muscle weakness. Hypokalemia and consequent lethal arrhythmia are documented to constitute a fatal pathophysiology in patients with primary aldosteronism [93] and Cushing syndrome [94].

6.3.3. Pheochromocytoma

Pheochromocytoma can cause miscellaneous severe clinical symptoms. In addition to critical arterial hypertension, severe cardiac arrhythmia must be recognized as a life-threatening associated complication [95-97]. Catecholamine-induced cardiomyopathy due to pheochromocytoma may also elevate the risk of cardiac sudden death [98].

6.3.4. Insulinoma

Hypoglycemia is itself a lethal clinical condition, and increased sympathetic nerve activity followed by hypoglycemia can be responsible for lethal cardiac arrhythmia. In the literature, sudden death due to hypoglycemia-induced cardiac arrhythmia has been reported in a patient with a duodenal insulinoma [99].

References

[1] Chinen, K., Kurosumi, M., Ohkura, Y., et al (2006) Sudden unexpected death in patients with malignancy: A clinicopathologic study of 28 autopsy cases. *Pathol Res Pract* 202:867-875.

[2] Cina, S.J., Smialek, J.E., Burke, A.P., et al (1996) Primary cardiac tumors causing sudden death: a review of the literature. *Am J Forensic Med Pathol* 17:271-281.

[3] Burke, A. & Virmani, R. Tumors of the heart and the great vessels. Atlas of Tumor Pathology, Third series, Fascicle 16. Washington DC, Armed Forces Institute of Pathology, 1996.

[4] Duray, P.H., Mark, E.J., Barwick, K.W., et al (1985) Congenital polycystic tumor of the atrioventricular node: autopsy study with immunohistochemical findings suggesting endodermal derivation. *Arch Pathol Lab Med* 109:30-34.

[5] Burke, M.A,P., Anderson, P.G., Vermani, R., et al (1990) Tumor of the atrioventricular nodal region: a clinical and immunohistochemical study. *Arch Pathol Lab Med* 114:1057-1062.

[6] Law, K.B., Feng, T., Nair, V., et al (2012) Cystic tumor of the atrioventricular node: rare antemortem diagnosis. *Cardiovasc Pathol* 21: 120-127.

[7] Wolf, P.L. & Bing, R. (1965) The smallest tumor which causes sudden death. *JAMA* 194:204-205.

[8] Amr, S.S., Al-Ragheb, S.Y.A., Soleiman, N.A., et al (1987) Sudden, unexpected death due to cardiac fibroma: report of a case and review of the literature. *Am J Forensic Med Pathol* 8:142-147.

[9] Reynen, K. (1995) Cardiac myxomas. *New Engl J Med* 333:1610-1617.

[10] Böhm, N. & Krebs, G. (1980) Solitary rhabdomyoma of the heart: clinically silent case with sudden, unexpected deatn in an 11-month-old boy. *Eur J Pediatr* 134:167-172.

[11] Byard, R.W., Blumbergs, P.C., James, R.A. (2003) Mechanisms of unexpected death in tuberous sclerosis. *J Forensic Sci* 48:172-176.

[12] Prahlow, J.A., Teot, L.A., Lantz, P.E., et al (1995) Sudden death in epilepsy due to an isolated subependymal giant cell astrocytoma of the septum pellucidum. *Am J Forensic Med Pathol* 16:30-37.

[13] Ihama, Y., Miyazaki, T., Fuke, C. (2008) Hemoperitoneum due to rupture of a subserosal vein overlying a uterine leiomyoma. *Am J Forensic Med Pathol* 29:177-180.

[14] Gowda, R.M., Khan, I., Nair, C.K., et al (2003) Cardiac papillary fibroelastoma: a complihensive analysis of 725 cases. *Am Heart J* 146:404-410.

[15] Burke, A.P., Johns, J.P., Virmani, R. (1990) Hemangiomas of the heart: a clinicopathologic study of ten cases. *Am J Cardiovasc Pathol* 3:283-290.

[16] Kaminsky, R.A. (2001) Pathologic quiz case: an exceedingly rare cause of sudden cardiac death. *Arch Pathol Lab Med* 125:573-574.

[17] Patel, J. & Sheppard M.N. (2011) Sudden death owing to right atrial hemangioma. *J Forensic Sci* 56: 529-530.

[18] Burke, A.P., Cowan, D., Vermani, R. (1992) Primary sarcomas of the heart. *Cancer* 69:387-395.

[19] Herrmann, M.A., Shankerman, R.A., Edwards, W.D., et al (1992) Primary cardiac angiosarcoma: a clinicopathologic study of six cases. *J Thorac Cardiovasc Surg* 103:655-664.

[20] Yoshida, A., Kanda, T., Sakamoto, H., et al (1999) Sudden death with malignant hemangioendothelioma originating in the pericardium: a case report. *Angiology* 50:607-611.

[21] Kamiyoshihara, M., Ishikawa, S., Morishita, Y. (2001) Sudden death due to rupture of an omental metastatic tumor arising from cardiac angiosarcoma: a case report. *J Cardiovasc Surg* 42:495-497.

[22] Burke, A., Li, L., Kling, E., et al (2007) Cardiac inflammatory myofibroblastic tumor: a "benign" neoplasm that may result in syncope, myocardial infarction, and sudden death. *Am J Surg Pathol* 31:1115-1122.

[23] Eisenstat, J., Gilson, T., Reimann, J., et al (2008) Low-grade myofibroblastic sarcoma of the heart causing sudden death. *Cardiovasc Pathol* 17:55-59.

[24] Jurek, T., Czuba, M., Smigiel, R., et al (2011) Giant heart tumors in infants leading to sudden, unexpected death: description of two cases. *Pediatr Int* 53: 1090-1093.

[25] Jiang, W.X., Gao, C.R., Sun, J.H., et al (2009) Sudden cardiac death caused by a primary intimal sarcoma of the left coronary artery. *Int J Legal Med* 123: 503-506.

[26] Roberts, W.C. (1997) Primary and secondary neoplasms of the heart. *Am J Cardiol* 80:671-682.

[27] Reynen, K., Köckeritz, U., Strasser, R.H. (2004) Metastases to the heart. *Ann Oncol* 15:375-381.

[28] Norell, M.S., Sarvasvaran, R., Sutton, G.C. (1984) Solitary tumor metastasis: a rare cause of right ventricular outflow tract obstruction and sudden death. *Eur Heart J* 5:684-688.

[29] Ottaviani, G., Matturri, L., Rossi, L., et al (2003) Sudden death due to lymphomatous infiltration of the cardiac conduction system. *Cardiovasc Pathol* 12:77-81.

[30] Altun, G., Bilgi, A., Altun, A. (2005) Sudden death due to cardiac tamponade caused by metastasis of squamous cell carcinoma of the lung. *Cardiology* 103:53-54.

[31] Kataoka, M., Shigemitsu, K., Tanabe, S., et al (2005) Sudden death from metastatic esophageal cancer to the ventricular septum. *Jpn J Thorac Cardiovasc Surg* 53:365-368.

[32] Fukuda, A., Saito, T., Imai, M., et al (2000) Metastatic cardiac papillary carcinoma originating from the thyroid in both ventricles with a mobile right ventricular pedunculated tumor. *Jpn Circ J* 64:890-892.

[33] Ottaviani, G., Rossi, L., Matturri, L. (2002) Histopathology of the cardiac conduction system in a case of metastatic pancreatic ductal adenocarcinoma. *Anticancer Res* 22:3029-3032.

[34] Hallahan, D.E., Vogelzang, N.J., Borow, K.M., et al (1986) Cardiac metastases from soft-tissue sarcomas. *J Clin Oncol* 4:1662-1669.

[35] Chinen, K. & Izumo, T. (2005) Cardiac involvement by malignant lymphoma: a clinicopathologic study of 25 autopsy cases based on the WHO classification. *Ann Hematol* 84:498-505.

[36] Vougiouklakis, T,, Mitselou, A., Agnantis, N.J. (2006) Sudden death due to primary intraclanial neoplasms: a forensic study. *Anticancer Res* 26:2463-2466.

[37] DiMaio, S.M., DiMaio, V.J.M., Kirkpatrick, J.B. (1980) Sudden, unexpected death due to primary intracranial neoplasms. *Am J Forensic Med Pathol* 1:29-45.

[38] Abu Al Ragheb, S.Y., Koussous, K.J., Amr, S.S. (1986) Intracranial neoplasms associated with sudden death: a report of seven cases and a review of the literature. *Med Sci Law* 26:270-272.

[39] Mørk, S.J., Morild, I., Giertsen, J.C. (1986) Subependymoma and unexpected death. *Forensic Sci Int* 30:275-280.

[40] Schwarz, K.O., Perper, J.A., Rozin, L. (1987) Sudden, unexpected death due to fourth ventricular subependymoma. *Am J Forensic Med Pathol* 8:153-157.

[41] Byard, R.W., Bourne, A.J., Hanieh, A. (1991-1992) Sudden and unexpected death due to hemorrhage from occult central nervous system lesions. *Pediatr Neurosurg* 17:88-94.

[42] Rajs, J., Råsten-Almquvist, P., Nennesmo, I. (1997) Unexpected death in young infants mimics SIDS: autopsies demonstrate tumors of medulla and heart. *Am J Forensic Med Pathol* 18:384-390.

[43] Ozkul, A., Meteoglu, I., Tataroglu, C., et al (2007) Primary diffuse leptomeningeal oligodendrogliomatosis causing sudden death. *J Neurooncol* 81:75-79.

[44] Sanchez-Hermosillo, E., Sikirica, M., Carter, D., et al (1998) Sudden death due to undetected mediastinal germ cell tumor. *Am J Forensic Med Pathol* 19:69-71.

[45] Bunai, Y., Akaza, K., Tsujinaka, M., et al (2008) Sudden death due to undiagnosed intracranial hamagiopericytoma. *Am J Forensic Med Pathol* 29:170-172.

[46] Black, M. & Graham, D.I. (2002) Sudden unexplained death in adults caused by intracranial pathology. *J Clin Pathol* 55:44-50.

[47] Shemie, S., Jay, V., Rutka, J., et al (1997) Acute obstructive hydrocephalus and sudden death in children. *Ann Emerg Med* 29:524-528.

[48] Chen, H.S., Shen, M.C., Tien, H.F., et al (1996) Leptomeningeal seeding with acute hydrocephalus – unusual central nervous system presentation during chemotherapy in Ki-1-positive anaplastic large-cell lymphoma. *Acta Haematol* 95:135-139.

[49] Nelson, J., Frost, J.L., Schochet, S.S. Jr. (1987) Sudden, unexpected death in a 5-year-old boy with an unusual primary intracranial neoplasm: ganglioglioma of the medulla. *Am J Forensic Med Pathol* 8:148-152.

[50] Gleckman, A.M. & Smith, T.W. (1998) Sudden unexpected death from primary posterior fossa tumors. *Am J Forensic Med Pathol* 19:303-308.

[51] Downs, A.M.R., Love, S., Kennedy, C.C.T. (1999) Sudden death secondary to mycosis funoides of the midbrain. *Acta Derm Venereol* 79:475.

[52] Büttner, A., Gall, C., Mall, G., et al (1999) Unexpected death in persons with symptomatic epilepsy due to glial brain tumors: a report of two cases and review of the literature. *Forensic Sci Int* 100:127-136.

[53] Roberts, K.E., Hamela-Bena, D.. Saqi, A., et al (2003) Pulmonary tumor embolism: a review of the literature. *Am J Med* 115:228-232.

[54] Shields, D.J. & Edwards, W.D. (1992) Pulmonary hypertension attributable to neoplastic emboli: an autopsy study of 20 cases and a review of literature. *Cardiovasc Pathol* 1:279-287.

[55] Chan, G.S.W., Ng, W.K., Ng, I.O.L., et al (2000) Sudden death from massive pulmonary tumor embolism due to hapatocellular carcinoma. *Forensic Sci Int* 108:215-221.

[56] Dada, M.A. & van Velden, D.J.J. (1995) Sudden death caused by testicular germ cell tumor. *Med Sci Law* 35: 357-359.

[57] Zakowski, M.F., Edwards, R.H., McDonough, E.T. (1990) Wilms' tumor presenting as sudden death due to tumor embolism. *Arch Pathol Lab Med* 114:605-608.

[58] van den Heuvel-Eibrink, M.M., Lankhorst, B., Egeler, R.M., et al (2008) Sudden death due to pulmonary embolism as presenting symptom of renal tumors. *Pediatr Blood Cancer* 50: 1062-1064.

[59] Marchetti, D., La Monaca, G., Ranalletta, D. (1996) Death due to a leiomyosarcoma of the pulmonary artery. *Am J Forensic Med Pathol* 17:315-318.

[60] Roman, D.A. & Mirchandani, H. (1987) Intravenous leiomyoma in intracardiac extension causing sudden death. *Arch Pathol Lab Med* 111:1176-1178.

[61] Bassiri, A.G., Haghighi, B., Doyle, R.L., et al (1997) Pulmonary tumor embolism. Am J Respir Crit Care Med 155: 2089-2095.

[62] von Herbay, A., Illes, A., Waldherr, R., et al (1990) Pulmonary tumor thrombotic microangiopathy with pulmonary hypertension. *Cancer* 66:587-592.

[63] Chinen, K., Kazumoto, T., Ohkura, Y., et al (2005) Pulmonary tumor thrombotic microangiopathy caused by a gastric carcinoma expressing vascular endothelial growth factor and tissue factor. *Pathol Int* 55: 27-31.

[64] Chinen, K., Tokuda, Y., Fujiwara, M., et al (2010) Pulmonary tumor thrombotic microangiopathy in patients with gastric carcinoma: an analysis of 6 autopsy cases and review of the literature. *Pathol Res Pract* 206: 682-689.

[65] Chinen, K., Fujino, T., Horita, A., et al (2009) Pulmonary tumor thrombotic microangiopathy caused by an ovarian cancer expressing tissue factor and vascular endothelial growth factor. *Pathol Res Pract* 205: 63-68.

[66] Igarashi, S., Kawaguchi, T., Hoshi, N. (1997) Early gastric carcinoma with widespread metastasis and pulmonary tumor thrombotic microangiopathy (PTTM): report of an autopsy case. I to Cho (Stomach and Intestine) 32:861-865 (in Japanese with English abstract).

[67] Hara, A., Ichinoe, M., Ogawa, T., et al (2005) A microscopic adenocarcinoma of the stomach with pulmonary tumor thrombotic microanigopathy in a 17-year-old male. *Pathol Res Pract* 201:457-461.

[68] Gardner, P.M., Jentzen, J.M., Komorowski, R.A., et al (1997) Asphyxial death caused by a lanynegal schwannoma: a case report. *J Laryngol Otol* 111:1171-1173.

[69] Donnelly, S.C., Hogan, J.M., Bredin, C. (1991) Sudden death from primary B-cell non-Hodgkin's lymphoma of the larynx. *Respir Med* 85:77-79.

[70] Sperry, K. (1994) Lethal asphyxiating juvenile laryngeal papillomatosis: a case report with human papillomavirus in situ hybridization analysis. *Am J Forensic Med Pathol* 15:146-150.

[71] Balažic, J., Masera, A., Poljak, M. (1997) Sudden death caused by laryngeal papillomatosis. *Acta Otolaryngol Suppl* 527:111 113.

[72] Belding, R.C. & Sabet, Z. (2002) Basosquamous carcinoma of the supraglottic larynx with sudden death from asphyxia. *South Med J* 95:765-767.

[73] Porzionato, A., Macchi, V., Rodriguez, D., et al (2007) Airway obstruction by laryngeal masses in sudden and homicidal deaths. *Forensic Sci Int* 171:e15-e20.

[74] Taff, M.L., Schwartz, I.S., Boglioli, L.R. (1991) Sudden asphyxia death due to a prolapsed esophageal fibrolipoma. *Am J Forensic Med Pathol* 12:85-88.

[75] Fyfe, B. & Mittleman, R.E. (1991) Hypopharyngeal lipoma as a cause for sudden asphyxial death. *Am J Forensic Med Pathol* 12:82-84.

[76] Somers, G.R., Smith, C.R., Perrin, D.G., et al (2006) Sudden unexpected death in infancy and childhood due to undiagnosed neoplasia: an autopsy study. *Am J Forensic Med Pathol* 27:64-69.

[77] Hutchins, K.D., Dickson, D., Hameed, M., et al (1999) Sudden death in a child due to an intrathoracic paraganglioma. *Am J Forensic Med Pathol* 20:338-342.

[78] Peacock, J.A., Saleem, S.R., Becker, S.M. (1985) Sudden asphyxia death due to an esophageal leiomyoma. *Am J Forensic Med Pathol* 6:159-161.

[79] Kaczynski, J., Hansson, G., Wallerstedt, S. (2005) Clinical features in hepatocellular carcinoma and the impact of autopsy on diagnosis: a study of 530 cases from a low-endemicity area. *Hepatogastroenterology* 52:1798-1802.

[80] Mittleman, R.E. (1987) Hepatic rupture due to metastatic lung carcinoma. *Am J Clin Pathol* 88:506-509.

[81] Perrot, L.J. (1997) Malignant hemanigioendothelioma: a rare case of sudden unexpected death in infancy. *Am J Forensic Med Pathol* 18:96-99.

[82] Nestok, B.R., Goldstein, J.D., Lipkovic, P. (1988) Splenic rupture as a cause of sudden death in undiaghosed chronic myelogenous leukemia. *Am J Forensic Med Pathol* 9:241-245.

[83] Sohara, N., Takagi, H., Yamada, T., et al (2000) Hepatocellular carcinoma complicated by hemothorax. *J Gastroenterol* 35:240-244.

[84] Griffiths, A.P., White, J., Dawson, A. (1998) Spontaneous haemothorax: a cause of sudden death in von Recklinghausen's disease. *Postgrad Med J* 74:679-681.

[85] Baldó, X., Ortiz, M.R., Sebastián, F., et al (2003) Fatal right spontaneous haemothorax in Von Recklinghausen's disease. *Interact Cardiovasc Thorac Surg* 2:35-37.

[86] Tsokos, M. & Türk, E.E. (2002) Esophageal variceal hemorrhage presenting as sudden death in outpatients: a study of 45 medicolegal autopsy cases. *Arch Pathol Lab Med* 126:1197-1200.

[87] Türk, E.E., Lockemann, U., Tsokos, M. (2007) Fatal bleeding from major femoral vessels: three case reports. *Int J Legal Med* 121:220-222.

[88] Skadberg, B.T., Bruserud, Ø., Karwinski, W., et al (1988) Sudden death caused by heart block in a patient with multiple myeloma and cardiac amyloidosis. *Acta Med Scand* 223:379-383.

[89] Okazaki, K., Moriyasu, F., Shiomura, T., et al (1986) Spontaneous rupture of the spleen and liver in amyloidosis: a case report and review of the literature. *Gastroenterol Jpn* 21:518-524.

[90] Arai, N., Nakata, M., Yamazaki, J., et al (1992) Sudden death due to bilateral pulmonary thromoboembolism in a patient with multiple myeloma: an autopsy case report. Nihon Kyobu Shikkan Gakkai Zasshi 30:1756-1760 (in Japanese with English abstract).

[91] Furukawa, Y., Tanaka, K., Hasuike T et al (1991) Adult T-cell leukemia lymphoma with metastatic calcification. *Rinsho Byori* 39:886-890 (in Japanese with English abstract)

[92] Al-Daraji, W.I, & Prescott, R.J. (2005) Heterotopic cardiac calcification: a rare presentation of multiple endocrine neoplasia. *Histopathology* 47:643-652.

[93] Geist, M., Dorian, P., Davies, T., et al (1996) Hyperaldosteronism and sudden cardiac death. *Am J Cardial* 78:605-606.

[94] Scott, B.D. & Friday, K.J. (1988) Cushing's syndrome presenting as sudden death. *Am Heart J* 115:487-488.

[95] Primhak, R.A., Spicer, R.D., Variend, S. (1986) Sudden death after minor abdominal trauma: an unusual presentation of phaemochromocytoma. *Br Med J* 292:95-96.

[96] Preuβ, J., Woenckhaus, C., Schwesinger, G., et al (2006) Non-diagnosed pheochromocytoma as a cause of sudden death in a 49-year-old man: a case report with medico-legal implications. *Forensic Sci Int* 156:223-228.

[97] Methe, H., Hinterseer, M., Wilbert-Lampen, U., et al (2007) Torsades de Pointes: a rare complication of an extra-adrenal pheochromocytoma. *Hypertens Res* 30:1263-1266.
[98] Kassim, T.A., Clarke, D.D., Mai, V.Q., et al (2008) Catecholamine-induced cardiomyopathy. *Endocr Pract* 14:1137-49.
[99] Iscovich, A.L. (1983) Sudden cardiac death due to hypoglycemia. *Am J Emerg Med* 1:28-29.

In: Sudden Death
Editors: Jiashin Wu and Jessica Wu

ISBN: 978-1-62618-825-9

Chapter IX

Sudden Death Related to Myocardial Tuberculosis

Valentina Gabbolini*[*], *Anna Laura Santunione and Enrico Silingardi
Department of Legal medicine, University of Modena and Reggio Emilia, Emilia-Romagna, Italy

Abstract

Sudden death is currently described as natural unexpected death occurring within 1h of new symptoms. A frequent cause of sudden death in adults is related to cardiovascular disease. Sudden cardiac death is defined as death due to cardiac causes, and preceded by an abrupt and unexpected loss of consciousness within one hour of the onset of acute symptoms, in an individual who may have or not known pre-existing heart disease. In the young adults, myocarditis is the major cause of sudden unexpected death. Tuberculosis (TB) is still a serious problem for public health, even in highly developed countries. In the latest World Health Organization (WHO) report, TB was responsible for 8.5–9.2 million cases and 1.2–1.5 million deaths (including deaths from TB among HIV-positive people). TB is also more common among men than women, and around 2/3 of cases are estimated to occur among people aged 15–59 years. Tuberculosis has a predilection for the pulmonary system; extrapulmonary manifestation is rare, but around 1-2% of TB patients have cardiovascular involvement (MTB). MTB can present in a miliary or nodular form, occasionally with aneurysm. The infection can reach the myocardium through the blood or the lymphatic system, or as a result of contiguity from pericardium or pulmonary cavity. In the past MTB was hardly ever diagnosed while the person was alive, but now the advancement in cardiac imaging and imaging guided biopsy techniques, lead to a more frequent antemortem diagnosis. Clinically, MTB may be asymptomatic or presenting with different manifestations including intractable ventricular arrhythmias, long QT syndrome, complete heart block and in some rare cases right atrial obstruction, right ventricular outflow tract obstruction, superior vena cava obstruction,

[*] Correspondence: Valentina Gabbolini, MD, valegabbolini@hotmail.it.

left ventricular aneurysm, aortic regurgitation and heart failure. The MTB average incidence on the total number of autopsies is < 0.3%. A systematic study relative to 13.658 autopsies reported a frequency of 0.14%. MTB represents up to 4% of all TB related deaths and the majority of TB related sudden death. Cases of sudden death from previously undiagnosed MTB have rarely been reported in the literature, and they refer frequently to male subjects. According to the clinical symptoms observed in living patients, the most probable mechanism for sudden cardiac death is cardiac arrhythmias. The autopsy diagnosis of MTB depends largely on the microscopic detection of acid-fast bacilli (AFB) and on mycobacterial culture, but the demonstration of AFB within foci of necrotizing granulomatous inflammation is rare. In recent years, polymerase chain reaction (PCR) amplification for the detection of mycobacterial DNA in formalin-fixed, paraffin-embedded archival tissues has been widely demonstrated in various tissue specimens, including heart, lung, lymph nodes, and other tissues. Differential diagnosis is from other forms of granulomatous inflammations including sarcoidosis and large cell idiopatic granulomatous myocarditis. A proposal of diagnostic criteria may comprise positive TB PCR, positive bacterial culture or acid-fast bacilli isolation from myocardium, since these tests provide definitive diagnosis.

Keywords: Sudden death, tubercular myocarditis, autopsy diagnosis

Introduction

Sudden death is currently described as natural unexpected death occurring within 1h of new symptoms.

In particular sudden cardiac death is defined as death due to cardiac causes, preceded by an abrupt loss of consciousness within one hour of the onset of acute symptoms, in an individual who may have known pre-existing heart disease, but in whom the time and the manner of death are unexpected.

The underlying pathology is usually coronary heart disease in middle-aged and elderly. However, it can also be one of the familial well-defined cardiomyopathies, such as hypertrophic or dilated cardiomyopathy, arrhythmogenic right ventricular dysplasia or long QT syndrome. In the young adults, myocarditis is the major cause of sudden unexpected death. Myocarditis is an inflammatory disease of the myocardium caused by various infections, autoimmune disorders and toxic agents.

Tuberculosis (TB) is still a serious problem for public health, even in highly developed countries. In the latest World Health Organization (WHO) report, TB was responsible for 8.5–9.2 million cases and 1.2–1.5 million deaths (including deaths from TB among HIV-positive people). TB is also more common among men than women, and around 2/3 of cases are estimated to occur among people aged 15–59 years.

The disease is spread in the air when people who are sick with pulmonary TB expel bacteria, for example by coughing. Only few patients infected with Mycobacterium tuberculosis will go on to develop TB disease. The probability of develop TB is much higher among people infected with the human immunodeficiency virus (HIV).

Tuberculosis has the ability to infect any part of the human body, but it has a predilection for the pulmonary system (pulmonary TB); extrapulmonary TB is commonly found in the pleura, lymph nodes, abdomen and central nervous system. Around 1-2% of TB patients have cardiovascular involvement (MTB).

Cardiac involvement is usually secondary to lesions elsewhere in the body, the pericardium is most commonly involved in cardiac tuberculosis, and according to Rooney et al., tuberculous pericarditis accounts for 11% of all types of pericarditis. Pericardial involvement may result either from direct extension from a mediastinal, pulmonary, or osseous lesion or from retrograde lymphatic spread. Endocardial and coronary artery tuberculosis is exceedingly rare.

Myocardial involvement is rare. The earliest report of myocardial tuberculosis was in 1664 by Maurocordat, a Turkish physician. As late as 1865, Virchow denied the existence of tuberculous nodules in the myocardium. The specific findings of TB in the myocardium are rarely seen and are postulated to be related to a low affinity of *M. tuberculosis* for the myocardium. The incidence of myocardial tuberculosis in patients died of tuberculosis was <0.3% in a 1935 study and 0.44% in a 1939 study. For the most part, it affects subjects in their youth and it is generally asymptomatic; for this reason, is usually an autopsy diagnosis.

Horn and Saphir described three histological patterns of cardiac TB:

- a nodular type (also known as tuberculoma), varying "from pea to egg size" with central caseation usually affecting the right side of the heart, particularly the right atrium;
- a miliary type of the myocardium complicating generalized miliary disease;
- the uncommon diffuse infiltrative type, usually associated with tuberculous pericarditis, in which the myocardium is diffusely infiltrated by granulation tissue containing giant cells, endothelial cells and lymphocytes.

Three possible routes of spread were postulated: firstly via direct extension from the pericardium or the pulmonary cavity, secondly via lymphatic spread, and thirdly by haematogenous seeding.

The common sites are the right atrium and left ventricle. Right atrial involvement is considered to be related to frequent involvement of the right mediastinal lymph nodes.

The differential diagnosis of myocardial tuberculosis includes granulomatous diseases such as sarcoidosis, idiopathic granulomatous and giant-cell myocarditis, syphilitic gummata, fungal infection, rheumatic fever, rheumatoid arthritis, and metastatic tumors containing giant cells, e.g., Hodgkin disease and osteosarcoma.

Symptomatology and Diagnosis

The increasing rates of immigration from countries where tuberculosis and multidrug-resistant variants are endemic emphasize the importance of making a prompt diagnosis in cases of tubercular myocarditis.

MTB is hardly ever diagnosed while the person is alive. Clinically, tuberculoma may be asymptomatic or presenting with varied manifestations including intractable ventricular arrhythmias, long QT syndrome, complete heart block, right atrial obstruction, right ventricular outflow tract obstruction, superior vena cava obstruction, left ventricular aneurysm, aortic regurgitation and heart failure.

Outflow obstruction is an important cause of sudden death in hypertrophic obstructive cardiomyopathy, in particular the obstruction of superior vena cava and the right atrium lead to a progressive deterioration of cardiac function that are detectable with echocardiograms.

The valvular dysfunction tends to present with chronic symptoms such as prostration and dyspnoea and is not been reported to cause sudden cardiac death. Cardiac murmurs may be heard on auscultation. Echocardiograms often demonstrate impaired cardiac output and this usually signifies gradual deterioration of cardiac function.

Although there is an association between pulmonary tuberculosis and venous thromboembolism, in fact deep vein thrombosis and pulmonary emboli have been reported to occur in TB patients without underlying coagulation disorders but the mechanism is not known.

Once the condition is suspected, relevant investigations must be undertaken to exclude viral illnesses, sarcoidosis and malignancies such as lymphoma. Definitive diagnosis of the condition relies on the detection of characteristic histological changes using Ziehl-Nielsen staining.

The cardiac MRI diagnostic imaging is the most important for diagnosis; it is a technique to identify non-invasively and accurately the extension of the interest infarction by this pathology. The myocardial inflammation in fact induces an abnormal signal intensity mode T2 and analysis of sequences late after injection of gadolinium allows to highlight the areas later collection, with localization preferably sub-epicardial or intra-myocardial median. Breton et al. have emphasized the diagnostic importance of MRI in cardiac myocardial TB in the observation of 3 cases. The examination has allowed to highlight a contrast late one or more nodules disseminated without vascular distribution.

Some authors, for the patients with intra-cardiac masses, suggest transthoracic and transesophageal echocardiography as a method of choice to perform myocardial guiding biopsy safe and easy, especially if the right atrium wall, the predominant location of tuberculoma is involved. Endomyocardial biopsy is not a procedure without risk. It is therefore appropriate to reserve it in the event that the other diagnostic procedures have been inconclusive.

Cases Reports of Sudden Death from MTB

There are very few cases described in the literature of sudden cardiac death rate from MTB and the first to describe this association was Behr et al. in 1977.

In the first case the authors described a case of young man (21 years old) physically fit that died after an episode of syncope. The histological sections showed a caseating granulomas of myocardium and mediastinal lymph nodes, while other organs were not involved, specially the lungs. Because the tubercular bacilli were not demonstrated from the granulomas, the authors made the diagnosis of MTB with mediastinal lymph node involvement based on characteristic histological findings. In this case the mechanism of death was not specified. The second case is another young man who died to ventricular fibrillation and the post-mortem examination showed a MTB. This patient was found in ventricular tachycardia, treated with drugs and electrical cardioversions but he developed ventricular fibrillation and asystole. The patient was treated 5 years prior for tuberculous tenosynovitis. Because the cardiac enzymes were raised, was suspected a myocarditis or infarction and the diagnosis was confirmed at autopsy. In fact were observed two large areas of myocardial necrosis, in the left ventricular wall and in the inter-ventricular septum. Also it was found granulomas in the lymph nodes and the porta hepatis. The other organs were not involved, specially lungs and coronary vessels. Though this case was not classify as sudden cardiac death because the cause of death was known and the death was not unexpected, it suggested that ventricular tachycardia (VT) was induced by MTB or myocardial necrosis. Although it was known that a damage of interventricular septum caused the VT, however the authors didn't specify which of the two foci of necrosis played a more important role. Finally they showed that the MTB is possible without co-morbid pulmonary or miliary TB, which was not thought possible previously.

In 1984 Wallis at al. described a case of 31 years old Asian man who collapsed and died unexpectedly at work. The postmortem examination showed miliary tubercles in the choroid, lungs, liver, kidneys, lymph nodes and heart. In particular the heart was enlarged and the microscopic examination of the interventricular septum revealed an extensive granulomatous infiltration surrounding but not destroying the conducting tissue. For the authors, the MTB was the most likely cause of death for the abrupt onset of death and for the lack of pulmonary symptoms, and the cause of the sudden death was probably a fatal ventricular arrhythmia or a conduction defect due to extensive disease surrounding the conducting tissue of the heart.

Chan and Dickens reported in 1992, a case of 71 years old Chinese male, who died unexpectedly during a recovery for haematuria. The autopsy showed active caseating tuberculosis with intrapulmonary miliary spread, also the liver and the spleen showed multiple whitish miliary nodules. The histology also showed multiple caseating granulomas in the kidneys, in the bone marrow and also in the heart. The abruptness of death and in the excellent premorbid state justified a sudden death. The authors recognized the cause of death in a fatal arrhythmia due to the position of the granulomas in atrial wall near the sino-atrial node.

In 2000 Dada et al. described a 25 years old fit man who died suddenly during a soccer match. The autopsy demonstrated a fibrinous pericarditis with pericardial effusion. The pericardial fluid was rich in neutrophils, protein and gram-positive bacilli, which were considered to have caused by postmortem contamination. No acid fast bacilli were seen. The heart show a firm, white, well demarcated nodular lesion with the appearance of an infiltrative tumor involving the posterior wall of the left ventricle; no pathological changes were observed in the valves and coronary arteries. The histological examination showed necrotizing granulomatous inflammation involving the myocardium associated with a fibrinous pericarditis; the acid fast bacilli were not demonstrated. The authors demonstrated the presence of TB from the myocardial specimens using a proteinase K ligase chain reaction technique. This was important because it was the second case demonstrating sudden cardiac death secondary to MTB without evidence of miliary TB and it also highlighted the importance of using molecular techniques to detect TB in samples stained negative for acid fast bacilli.

Biedrzychi et al. described in 2006 a case of 20 years old Asian female that getting off a bus and collapsed to the ground and died. The autopsy showed a single area of fibrosis in the myocardium in the anterior wall of the left ventricle. Endocardium, coronary vessels and cardiac valves are unremarkable. The histologic examination of the myocardium revealed an area of fibrosis with lymphocytic infiltrate and the Ziehl-Nielsen stain confirmed the presence of acid-fast bacilli in the sections from the myocardium. Lungs, kidneys and liver contained multiple noncaseating granulomas confirming the presence of miliary TB. The authors did not comment on the possible mechanism of sudden cardiac death, but they point out that unlike the other cases, the patient was asymptomatic.

In the same year Silingardi et al. reported a case of sudden cardiac death in a 33 years old Italian woman, in good health, that died suddenly at home. At autopsy the surface of incision of the left ventricular myocardium showed nodules, localized throughout the antero-septal wall and posterior wall and they extended longitudinally from the atrio-ventricular groove toward the apex. Nothing was found in endocardium, valves, coronary tree and pericardium. Also lymph nodes and spleen are infiltrated by nodular formations and pale nodules of small dimension were observed on the surface of the liver. The histological exams of the myocardium showed large cell granulomas, epithelial cells and lymphocites immersed in a wide context of dense fibrous replacement tissue. The nodules at the hepato-splenic and lymphonodal level showed similar aspects. Some microscopic granulomas were observed in the lungs and the remaining organs were negative. The test for alcohol-acid resistant bacilli was negative. Given the probable tubercular nature of the granulomatous inflammation, the mycobacterial DNA was examined using the nested polymerase chain reaction method that carried out with specific oligonucleotides and was positive for Mycobacterium avium in all samples examined and also for tubercular complex in left ventricle, liver, spleen and kidneys. We postulated that ventricular arrhythmia was the underlying mechanism leading to sudden cardiac death. This was supported by the rapid onset of death and the extensive TB infiltration of the septal conduction system and also by the absence of coronary and valvular pathologies.

In 2009, Amonkar et al. described a case of a 65 years old woman, who was admitted to hospital for diabetic foot and oliguria and died suddenly after 48 h. At autopsy the heart showed multiple lesions measuring 2x2 cm in the postero-septal wall of both ventricles; also the liver showed tiny whitish lesions, the other organs were unremarkable. Histological analysis demonstrated extensive necrosis of the myocardium with surrounding lymphocytes, macrophages and multinucleate giant cells of both Langhans type and also pericardial mononuclear infiltrations and caseating granulomas in the liver. Stains for acid-fast bacilli and fungi were negative; however the authors diagnosed MTB based on the characteristic histological appearance.

The final report was by Kanchan et al. in 2010. They reported a case of a 58 years old diabetic Indian man, who developed sudden onset of chest pain and died on the way to hospital. The internal examination didn't show lesions of the organs, but the histopathology of the heart revealed a single granuloma of the left ventricular apex. It comprised a central area of caseous necrosis surrounded by epithelioid cells, lymphocytes, plasma cells and Langhans giant cells. Sections from the ascending aorta showed grade III atherosclerosis with narrowing of the coronary ostia. Acid fast bacilli were not demonstrated. The other organs did not show any significant histopathology, and no primary site of infection was demonstrated. The authors excluded the possibility of cardiac sarcoidosis based on the absence of systemic involvement and a non-necrotic granuloma. Also other conditions were excluded based on the medical history. Based on the histopathological findings, the authors postulated that the cause of death could be ventricular arrhythmia originating from either the apical granuloma or from the underlying coronary artery disease.

Pathogenetic Mechanisms

The causes of death resulting from MTB include arrhythmias, cardiac rupture, coronary occlusion, obstruction to pulmonary blood flow leading to fatal hemorrhage, heart failure and impaired myocardial contractility.

Heart failure, an important cause of sudden cardiac death, is most commonly caused by hypertension or ischemic heart disease and frequently occurs in patients with congestive heart failure and dilated cardiomyopathy. For this reason these are possible causes of sudden cardiac death in MTB. However, the link between ischemic heart disease and TB related sudden cardiac death is not clear. In all reported cases the coronary arteries were intact but a minor coronary inflammation or spasms are possible causes of ischemic heart disease.

The most probable mechanism for sudden cardiac death is cardiac arrhythmias because MTB may causes heart blocks and ventricular tachyarrhythmias. Ventricular arrhythmias capable to causing cardiac death are broadly divided into ventricular tachycardia or ventricular fibrillation, which can be caused by asystole. Case reports which demonstrated extensive septal involvements of MTB indicate aberrant conduction as the cause of ventricular tachycardia. Other cases showing ventricular wall necrosis suggest electro-mechanical uncoupling as the source of ventricular tachycardia.

Autopsy Diagnostic

The diagnosis of MTB depends largely on the microscopic demonstration of acid-fast bacilli (AFB) and on mycobacterial culture, but the demonstration of AFB within foci of necrotizing granulomatous inflammation is rare. Methods for the diagnosis of MTB have improved in recent years, and several molecular techniques have been introduced for clinical use. Of these, polymerase chain reaction (PCR) amplification for the detection of TB in formalin-fixed, paraffin-embedded archival tissues has been widely demonstrated in various tissue specimens, including lung, lymph nodes, and other tissues.

The histopathological diagnosis of TB is defined as *'a chronic granulomatous inflammation, suggestive of tuberculosis'*, but histopathologic features of chronic granulomatous inflammation can be found in various conditions and diseases other than TB, such as foreign body reaction, fungal infection, sarcoidosis, leprosy and brucellosis. For this reason AFB stain, TB tissue culture and TB-PCR should be performed to enable a definitive diagnosis of TB.

In terms of the speed of diagnosis, the TB-PCR method is advantageous because sensitivity of the Ziehl-Nielsen stain for AFB is low and bacterial culture for TB is protracted.

A Proposal of Diagnostic Criteria

In the diagnosis of myocarditis, a big step forward was made with the advent of the Dallas criteria in 1986 that the demonstration of lymphocyte or monocyte infiltrates with or without necrosis of myocytes would be sufficient to make the diagnosis of myocarditis, there isn't equally consent for the diagnosis of tuberculosis myocarditis. For this reason it is important defined a common set of criteria in order to make diagnosis of MTB. Liu et al. have recently proposed a system of diagnostic criteria, divided into major and minor, as is showed in the following table.

Table 1.

MAJOR CRITERIA
PCR identification of tuberculous DNA extracts from myocardial samples
Positive tuberculous culture from myocardial samples
Positive acid-fast bacilli from myocardial samples
MINOR CRITERIA
Positive inflammatory cell infiltrates or necrosis in myocardial samples
Positive granulomas in myocardial samples
Military tubercolosis in one or more extra-cardiac organs
Imaging evidence of myocardial tubercolosis, e.g cardiac magnetic resonance

Modified from Liu et al.

Major criteria would comprise of positive TB PCR, positive TB culture or acid-fast bacilli isolation from myocardium, since these tests provide definitive diagnosis. The presence of any one of these criteria would demonstrate the presence of TB in the myocardium thus suggest definitive diagnosis. Minor criteria may include inflammatory cell infiltration and granuloma within the myocardium, each of these is suggestive but non diagnostic of TB myocardium.

The importance of MRI has recently been pointed out by Khurana et al. However, although CMR is a useful tool at demonstrating evidence of myocardial inflammation, this is not specific to TB myocardium, and for this reason, CMR imaging of myocardial inflammation is a suitable minor criterion.

Conclusion

Although there are only a few cases reported in the literature, MTB is associated with sudden cardiac death. The majority of patients were asymptomatic before death.

MTB can present in a miliary or a nodular forma, occasionally with aneursysm and the infection can reach the myocardium thorough the blood or the lymphatic system, or as a result of contiguity with mediastinic lymph nodes.

The diagnosis of TB is favored by the histologic demonstration of central caseation, evidence of typical tuberculous lesions in other organs and, infrequently presence of acid-fast bacilli. This emphasizes the role of applying molecular biology techniques to diagnose MTB. In particular, DNA amplification (PCR) on formalin-fixed paraffin-embedded histological samples is currently considered a more sensitive and specific method.

The underlying mechanism of these sudden cardiac deaths was probably cardiac arrhythmias. The absence of coronary and valvular pathologies and the typical circumstances of death in the cases reported, supported this diagnosis.

The diagnosis antemortem of MTB is difficult and rare but it should be suspected in patients presenting with arrhythmias who could have been exposed to tubercolosis.

If the clinical suspicion is strong and the adjunctive imaging, such as a serial late gadolinium-enhanced cardiac magnetic resonance imaging, is suggestive, an early endomyocardial biopsy is indicated. Some authors suggest a transesophageal echocardiography can be a superior method to make biopsy safe and easy, especially if the right atrial wall (the predominant location of tuberculoma) is involved.

References

Agarwal, R., Malhotra, P., Awasthi, A., Kakkar, N., Gupta, D., (2005). Tuberculous dilated cardiomyopathy: an under-recognized entity? *BMC Infect. Dis.* 5, 29.

Amonkar, G., Rupani, A., Shah, V., Parmar, H., (2009). Sudden death in tubercolosis myocarditis. *Cardiovasc. Pathol.* 18, 247-248.

Ashizawa, N., Yano, K., (1998). Tuberculosis in circulation system. *Jap. J. Clin. Med.* 56, 3114-3117.

Basso, C., Corrado, D., Thiene, G., (1999). Cardiovascular causes of sudden death in young individuals including atlete. *Cardio. Rev.* 7, 127-35.

Behr, G., Palin, H.C., Temperly, J.M., (1977). Myocardial tubercolosis, *Br. Med. J.* 1, 951.

Brisson-Noel, A., Gicquel, B., Lecossier, D., Levy-Frebault, V., Nassif, X., Hance, A. J., (1989). Rapid diagnosis of tuberculosis by amplification of mycobacterial DNA in clinical samples. *Lancet* 2,1069–1071.

Breton, G., Leclerc, S., Longuet, P., Leport, C., Vildè, J.L., Laissy, J.P., (2005). Localisation myocardique de la tubercolose: interet diagnostique del L'IRM cardiaque. *Presse Med.* 34 (4), 293:296.

Chan, A.C.L., Dickens, P., (1992) Tuberculous myocarditis presenting as sudden cardiac death. *Forensic Sci. Int.* 57,45-50.

Custer, E.W., Charr, R., (1939). Tuberculosis of the myocardium. *JAMA* 112,1333-1334.

Dada, M.A., Lazarus, N.G., Kharsany, A.B., Sturm, A.W., (2000). Sudden death caused by myocardial tubercolosis: case report and review of the literature. *Am. J. Forensic Med. Pathol.* 21, 385-388.

Fanning, A., (1999). Tubercolosis: Extrapulmonary disease. *CMAJ* 160,1597-603.

Horn, H., Saphir, O., (1935). The involvement of the myocardium in tuberculosis: a review of the literature and report of three cases. *Am. Rev. Tuberc.* 32, 492-506.

Kanchan, T., Nagesh, K.R., Lobo, F.D., Menezes, R.G., (2010). Tubercular granuloma in the myocardium: an autopsy report. *Singapore Med. J.* 51 (1): e15.

Kapoor, O.P., Mascarenhas, E., Rananaware, M.M., Gadgil, R.K., (1973). Tuberculoma of the heart: report of 9 cases. *Am. Heart J.* 86,334-340.

Khurana, R., Shalhoub, J., Verma, A., Assomuli, R., Prasad, S.K., Kooner, J.S., Sethi, A., (2008). Tubercular myocarditis presentingwith ventricular tachycardia. *Nat. Clin. Pract. Cardiovasc. Med.* 5, 169-174.

Krishnaswami, H., Cherian, G., (1984). Right atrial tuberculoma: report of a case with complete recovery. *Thorax* 39,550-551.

Licht, J. et al., (2009). Tubercoloma of the myocardium: a rare case of intra-vitam diagnosis. *Clin. Res. Cardiol.* 98,331-333.

Liu, A., Hu, Y., Coates, A., (2012). Sudden cardiac death and tubercolosis-How much do we know? *Tubercolosis* 92, 307-313.

Menon, T.B., Rao, C.K., (1945). Tubercolosis of the myocardium causing complete heart block. *Am. J. Pathol.* 21,1193-1197.

Myeburg, R.J., Castellanos, A., (2005). Cardiovascular collapse, cardiac arrest, and sudden cardiac death. *In Braunwald, E., Fauci, A.S., Kasper, D.L., et al. (2005). Harrison's Principles of internal medicine:16th ed. New York Mcgraw Hill,* 1618-824.

Naithani, R., Agrawal, N., Choudhary, V.P., (2007). Deep venous thrombosis associated with tubercolosis. *Blood coagul. Fibrinolysis.* 18, 377-380.

Rawls, W.J., Shuford, W.H., Logan, W.D. et al., (1968). Right ventricular outflow tract obstruction produced by a myocardial abscess in a patient with tubercolosis. *Am. J. Cardiol.* 21,738-745.

Rooney, J.J., Crocco, J.A., Lyons, H.A., (1970). Tuberculous pericarditis. *Ann. Intern. Med.* 72,73-78.

Rose, A.G., (1987). Cardiac tuberculosis: a study of 19 patients. *Arch. Pathol. Lab. Med.* 111, 422-426.

Schnitzer, R., (1947). Myocardial tubercolosis with paroxysmal ventricular tachycardia. *Br. Heart. J.* 9, 213-219.

Silingardi, E., Rivasi, F., Santunione, A.L., Garagnani, L., (2006). Sudden death from tubercular myocarditis. *J. Forensic Sci.* 51 (3), 667-669.

Soyer, R., Brunet, A., Chevallier, B., Leroy, J., Morere, M., Redonnet, M., (1981). Tubercolous aortic insufficiency. Report of a case with successful surgical treatment. *J. Thorac. Cardiovasc. Surg.* 82,254-256.

Wallis, P.J.W, Branfoot, A.C., Emerson, P.A., (1984). Sudden death due to myocardial tubercolosis. *Thorax* 39,155-156.

WHO report 2011, Global tubercolosis control.

In: Sudden Death
Editors: Jiashin Wu and Jessica Wu
ISBN: 978-1-62618-825-9

Chapter X

Bath-Related Sudden Death

Takahisa Okuda[1,2*] and Seiji Shiotani[3]
[1] Department of Legal Medicine, Nippon Medical School, Tokyo, Japan
[2] Department of Legal Medicine, Nippon Medical School,
Office of the Chief Medical Examiner, Tsukuba Medical Center, Tsukuba City, Japan
[3]Department of Radiology, Tsukuba Medical Center, Tsukuba City, Japan

Abstract

Bath-related sudden death (BRSD) occurs commonly in elderly people without notice, especially in Japan. In Japan, there are an estimated greater than 14,000 cases of BRSD every year. The number of victims of BRSD is more than twice the number of traffic-related deaths in recent years in Japan. The high number of cases may be due to Japanese bathing practices, which involve spending long periods of time in hot water in a deep bathtub. Epidemiologically, this type of death is reported most often in the winter season and in people aged 65 years or older, particularly those with a medical history of diabetes or hypertension. The cause of death is generally reported as drowning or cardiovascular disease; however, an autopsy is rarely performed. A major problem is that it is often unknown whether the cause of death is accidental drowning or sudden unexpected natural death. It is difficult to accurately diagnose BRSD at this time.

In the course of taking a bath, the body is subjected to several changes in the thermal environment. The major cause of bathtub fatalities is inappropriate physiological adjustment in response to environmental variations. The substantial difference in the temperature of a heated living room and an unheated dressing room may increase blood pressure (BP) due to the cold pressor response while disrobing, especially in the cold season. Hot bath temperatures (40-43°C) first contribute to increasing BP due to sympathomimetic effects and then contribute to decreasing BP due to a decrease in the resistance of peripheral blood vessels. Several papers have noted that elderly people may not be able to achieve the appropriate cardiovascular response because of a lower compensatory ability. Sudden BP elevation may present risks of cerebral hemorrhage or aneurysm rupture. Rapid BP reduction may lead to ischemic damage of the brain or heart

[*] Correspondence: Takahisa Okuda, takahisa.okuda@gmail.com.

and trigger cardiac events or transient cerebral ischemic attack, resulting in bathtub drowning.

In terms of preventive medicine, the most appropriate measures for preventing BRSD is to avoid overlapping the factors that decrease BP. Consuming alcohol, having orthostatic hypotension, and taking a long bath in extremely hot water are individual risk factors. Other preventive measures include not taking BP drugs before a bath and setting the same room temperature in dressing rooms as in living rooms during the winter. Additionally, bathtubs should be filled only halfway to prevent drowning if a person becomes unconscious while sitting in the bathtub.

Japanese People Like Taking a Bath as Much as the Romans -Termae Romae

On February 11, 2012, the famous American pop singer Whitney Houston was found unresponsive in her hotel room in Beverly Hills, submerged in a bathtub that contained extremely hot water. She was pronounced dead at the scene by paramedics. An autopsy was performed by the Los Angeles County coroner's office. The cause of death was ruled to have been 'drowning contributing effects of atherosclerotic heart disease and cocaine use' [1]. Her sudden death shocked the world. However, sudden death in the bathtub frequently takes place in Japan, especially in the elderly. The Japanese thoroughly enjoy their baths. More than 14,000 cases of bath-related sudden death (BRSD) are estimated each year in Japan [2], much higher than the number of cases in other countries. The number of victims of BRSD in Japan is more than twice the number of traffic-related deaths, which accounted for under 5000 deaths in 2009 [3]. Epidemiologically, in Japan, BRSD is reported most often in the winter season and in the homes of elderly people aged 65 years or older who live alone, particularly in those with a medical history of adult lifestyle-related diseases, such as diabetes or hypertension [2, 4-7]. Despite the high number of incidents, BRSD is not very familiar to the Japanese population. The subject was seriously debated in the Health, Labour and Welfare Committee at the House of Councilors of the National Diet of Japan on March 22, 2012, where the Minister of Health, Labour and Welfare promised to construct a framework for research on BRSD [8].

Bathing culture varies by country. The Japanese take a bath almost every night, preferring a relaxing time in a bathtub filled with water to a cleansing shower. Figure 1 shows a typical Japanese bath module. The Japanese bathtub is narrow in width but deep in depth; a shower area, in which a shower is installed, is situated around the bathtub; there is a window and a tiled shower floor in the bathroom that becomes very cold during the winter; a dressing room is located outside the bathroom. In the process of taking a bath, Japanese people first remove their clothes in the dressing room and enter the shower area. They take a shower for approximately 1 minute, and then enter a deep bathtub filled with hot water (40-43°C) up to shoulder level. They spend 5 to 15 minutes sitting in the bottom of the bathtub with their knees up. Following the bath, they enter the shower area to cleanse their body and then again soak in the bathtub for several more minutes. People in other countries usually take a shower to cleanse their bodies. Recently, soaking in a tub filled with lukewarm water and bath oils has become popular in Western countries for its health and beauty benefits. In Scandinavian countries, it is customary to use a sauna before a shower. The temperature in the sauna is usually 80-100°C and humidity is approximately 10-15%. They spend 5-20 minutes in the sauna and then enter a cold-water bath [9].

Although BRSD can occur worldwide, most fatalities reported are from Japan [2, 5, 7, 10] and Scandinavian countries [11-13]. The reason BRSD is more prevalent in these countries is due to their bathing style [4, 6, 14]. In Japan, it is important to consider the effects of an increasing elderly population. In recent years, postmortem computed tomography (PMCT) has been utilized as a tool to screen the cause of death including BRSDs [15]. In this chapter, common features associated with BRSD in Japan are discussed along with case studies of BRSDs.

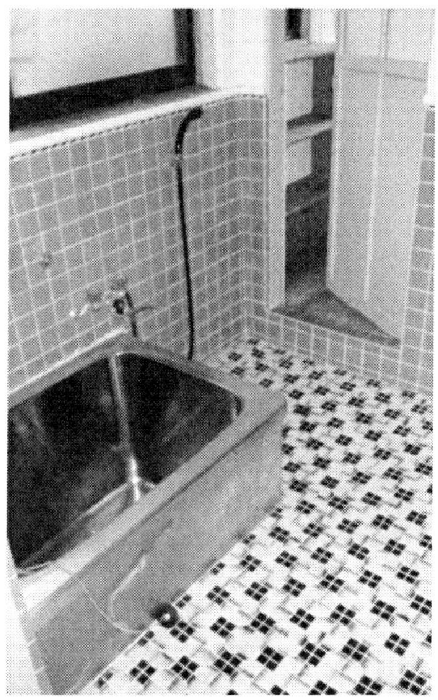

Figure 1. A typical Japanese bath module. This bathtub is 0.9 meters long, 0.6 meters wide and 0.53 meters deep. A shower area contains a shower, where wraps around the bathtub. A window is positioned in the bathroom and a dressing room is located outside the bathroom.

Causes and Risk Factors

1. Thermal Environmental Changes

In the course of taking a bath, the body is subjected to several changes in the thermal environment. The major cause of bathtub fatality is an inappropriate physiological adjustment to environmental variation [4-7, 16]. The substantial difference in the temperatures of a heated living room and an unheated dressing room may increase blood pressure (BP) due to the cold pressor response while disrobing, especially in the cold season. Hot bath water temperatures first contribute to increasing BP due to sympathomimetic effects and then contribute to decreasing BP due to a decrease in resistance of peripheral blood vessels. Several papers have suggested that elderly people may not be able to achieve an appropriate cardiovascular response under environmental variations because of a lower compensatory ability. A dull cardiovascular response causes a drastic BP change. Sudden BP elevation may present some practical risks of cerebral hemorrhage or aneurysm rupture. Rapid BP reduction may lead to ischemic damage of the brain or heart and trigger a cardiac event or transient cerebral ischemic attack (TIA), resulting in the person drowning in the bathtub.

Case 1 (Figure 2)

A 76-year-old woman with unknown medical history was found lying face down in a bathtub filled with water 10 minutes after starting a bath. She was brought to the emergency room in a state of cardiopulmonary arrest (CPA) and was pronounced dead shortly after admission, despite cardiopulmonary resuscitation (CPR) attempts. Body examination revealed there was no external injury on the surface skin. Whole body PMCT was performed soon after her death. PMCT of the abdomen displayed a ruptured abdominal aortic aneurysm (AAA) with a maximum diameter of 6 cm and a retroperitoneal hematoma. PMCT of the brain and heart provided no additional information. The cause of death was defined as massive retroperitoneal hemorrhage due to AAA rupture.

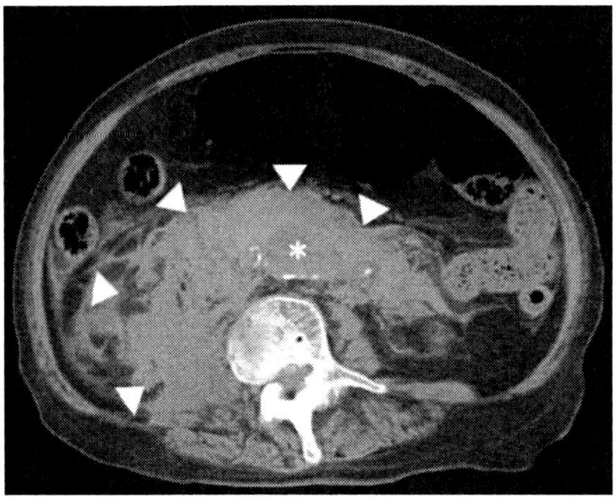

Figure 2. **A** 76-year-old woman who died of abdominal aortic aneurysm (AAA) rupture. PMCT of the abdomen exhibits ruptured AAA *(asteresk)* and retroperitoneal hematoma *(arrowheads)*.

Case 2 (Figure 3)

A 58-year-old drinker who lived alone was found in the right lateral recumbent position in the bathtub at the beginning of cold season. The bath water was filled to the height of 28 cm. His mouth and nostrils were submerged in the bath water. The deceased body had already started decomposing. Investigation at the scene revealed a half-finished bottle of distilled spirits, an unfinished glass on a table, and several empty bottles scattered around. PMCT of the thorax disclosed bilateral diffuse ground-grass attenuation and endotracheal air-fluid level. The pneumothorax at the left thoracic cavity, regarded as a postmortem change, and pleural effusion at the right thoracic cavity were observed. PMCT of the abdomen displayed swallowed water in a distended stomach with air-fluid level. Hepatic intravascular gas, known to be putrefaction, was observed. Autopsy revealed that the lungs (left, 505 g; right, 745 g) were overinflated and extremely edematous. Dark red color pleural effusion was accumulated in bilateral thoracic cavities (left, 50 ml; right, 400 ml). The stomach contained 250 ml of light-brown water. A histological section of the lung shows that the capillaries were congested and the alveoli were filled with eosinophilic fluid, suggesting emphysema aquosum. Other viscera did not exhibit any significant pathological changes. Chemical analysis of the blood showed an alcohol level of 2.4 mg/ml, suggesting that he was moderately to heavily intoxicated. The cause of death was reported as accidental drowning due to intoxication.

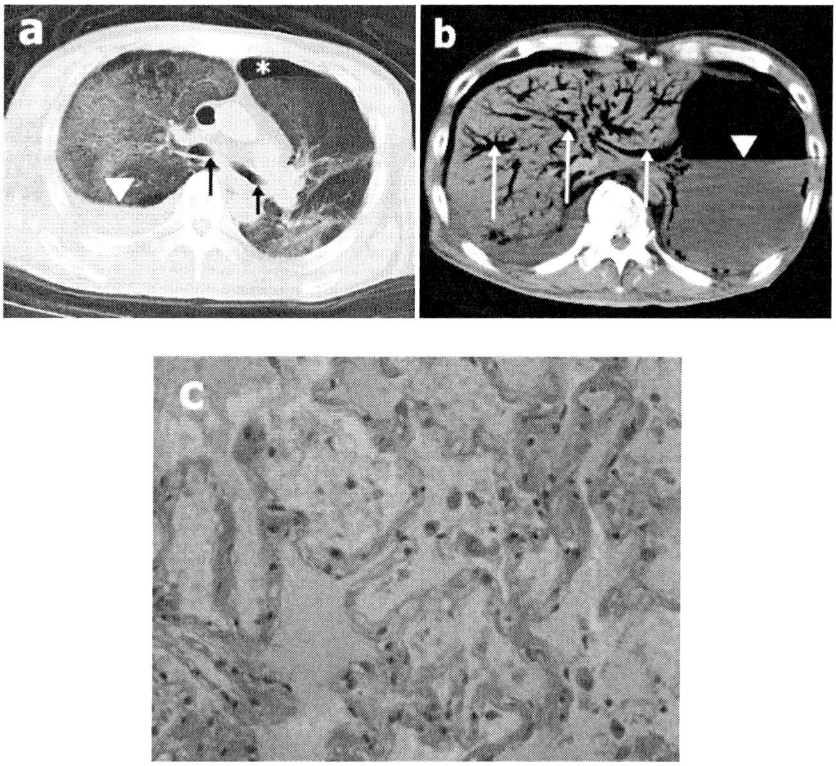

Figure 3. **A** 58-year-old drinker who was home alone who died of accidental drowning due to intoxication. a) PMCT of the thorax at lung window setting exhibits bilateral diffuse ground-grass attenuation and endotracheal air-fluid level *(arrows)*. Pneumothorax in the left thoracic cavity *(asterisk) and pleural effusion at the right thoracic cavity (arrowhead) are observed.* b) PMCT of the abdomen exhibits swallowed water in a distended stomach with air-fluid level *(arrowhead)* and hepatic intravascular gas *(arrows)*. c) Histological section of the lung reveals that the alveoli are filled with eosinophilic fluid (Hematoxylin-Eosin stain 40 ×).

Case 3 (Figure 4)

An 85-year-old pensioner with a history of hypertension and cerebral infarction was found dead in the bathtub in the cold season. The water level reached just above his nose and mouth. He had normal activity until day before his death. He lived with his family and took care of himself. Interestingly, his wife died of BRSD in the same bathtub a month before. The body examination revealed that the skin did not have seriously trauma but was peeling and detached. PMCT was performed at 17 hours after certification of death. PMCT of the thorax at the lung window setting disclosed bilateral diffuse ground-glass attenuation and a severe calcification of the coronary arteries. Autopsy was performed at 30 hours after certification of death. The lungs (left, 470 g; right, 535 g) were mildly edematous, but not overinflated, denoting that the lungs did not exhibit a 'drowning appearance'. The stomach contained no water. Coronary arteries were severely calcified and the left coronary arteries were over 80% stenosed. Acute ischemic changes, such as contraction band necrosis, were observed histologically at the left ventricular myocardium. The pathologic examination of other organs ruled out any life-threatening lesions. Blood concentration of carbon monoxide-hemoglobin was 1.5%, indicating that carbon monoxide intoxication was negative. The cause of death was defined as natural, caused by acute left heart failure due to ischemic heart disease.

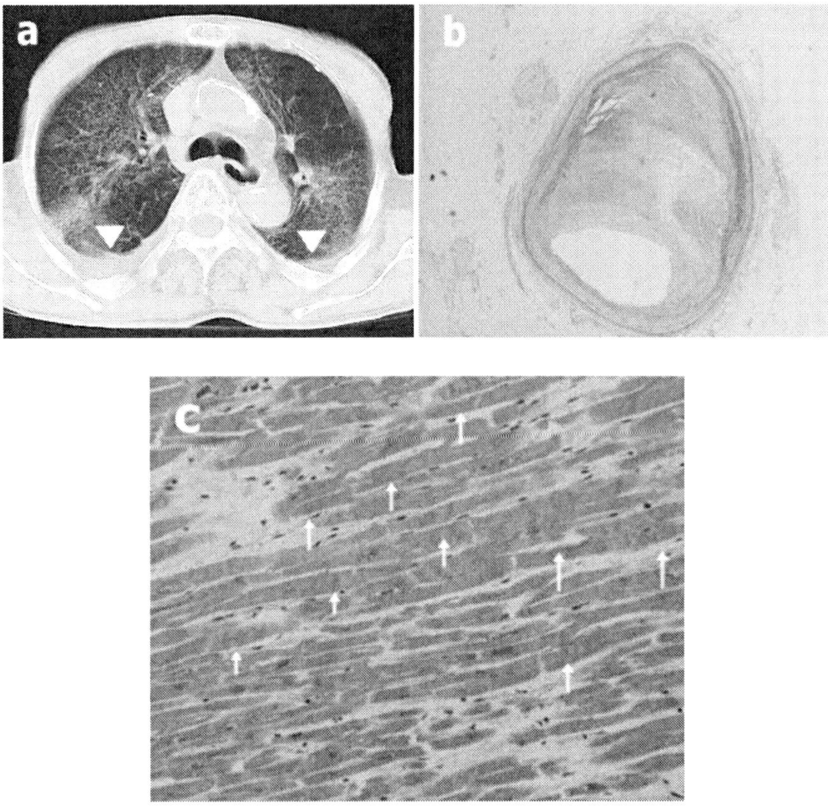

Figure 4. An 85-year-old pensioner who died of acute left heart failure due to ischemic heart disease. a) PMCT of the thorax at the lung window setting exhibits bilateral diffuse ground-glass attenuation and pleural effusion (arrowheads). b) A cross section of proximal left anterior descending coronary artery. The lumen is narrowed by fibro-lipid plaque, representing severe atherosclerosis (Elastica van Gieson stain 4 ×).c) Histological section of the left ventricular myocardium reveals contraction band necrosis (arrows), representing acute ischemic changes (Masson trichrome stain 20 ×).

2. Syncope due to Drastic BP Reduction

BP reduction depends on bath water temperature. According to 'Tameshite-Gatten' which is the Japanese science television program created by NHK (Japan Broadcasting Corporation) (Figure 5) [17], at a bath water temperature of 42°C, systolic BP is first elevated after soaking in the bathtub. At a bath water temperature of 38°C, systolic BP does not change at the beginning of soaking. Both temperatures decrease BP after 1 minute. Subsequently, systolic BP at a bath temperature of 38°C reaches equilibrium, whereas systolic BP at a bath temperature of 42°C continuously decreases for 8 minutes. BP volatility at a bath temperature of 42°C is approximately 30 mmHg, which is much higher than BP at a bath temperature of 38°C. The result indicates that extremely hot bath water causes a drastic BP reduction during soaking. Elderly people in Japan generally prefer spending long periods soaking in an extremely hot bath. This preference increases the risk for a cardiac event or syncope, resulting in an increase of bath accidents.

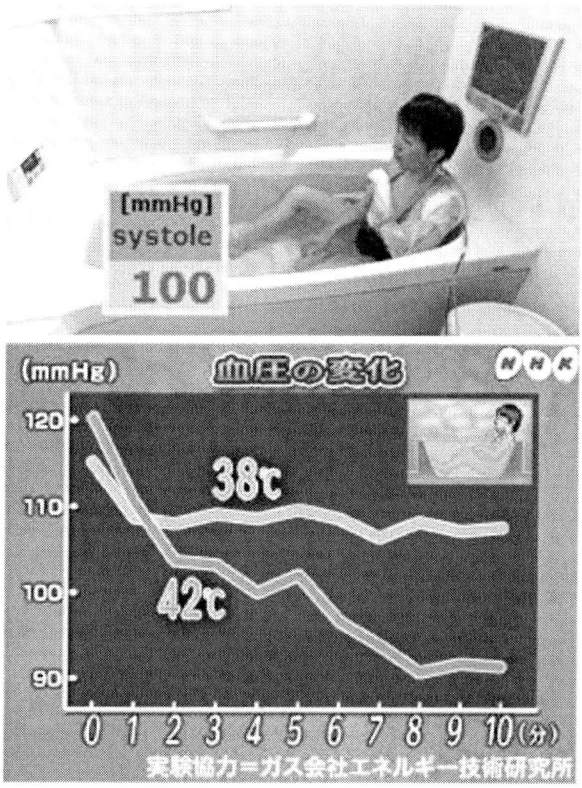

Figure 5. The data cited from NHK. http://www9.nhk.or.jp/gatten/pdf/ program/P20090128.pdf A) A young man takes part in the experimental trial (above). B) Effects of bath temperature and bath time on change in blood pressure (below).

Case 4

The deceased was a 61-year-old cleaner living with his family that was found lying unconscious, face submerged in a water-filled bathtub after walking around in the evening in the winter season. He was found within 40 minutes after he started the bath and was brought to the hospital in a state of CPA and pronounced dead shortly after admission despite CPR attempts. He had a medical history of cerebral infarction 5 years earlier and took benzodiazepines for dementia associated with cerebral vascular disease. The bath temperature was set at approximately 40°C, but it was reported that he preferred a hotter bath. Autopsy was performed at 36 hours postmortem. A light red foam appeared in the bronchial tubes. The overinflated lungs (left, 670 g; right, 885 g) were markedly edematous. Large amounts of fluid and foam were exuded from the pulmonary cut surface. The mildly dilated stomach contained a light-brown watery fluid (200 ml), and the heart (330 g) was morphologically normal. The coronary arteries exhibited slight atherosclerosis but no narrowing or occlusion.

The brain had no signs of edema and no pathological lesions associated with sudden death. Other viscera did not show any significant pathology. Toxicological analysis of blood and urine revealed that the concentration of nitrazepam, diazepam, gabapentine, and valproic acid in the serum and urine were all within therapeutic range, indicating that the cause was unlikely drug overdose. Thus, the death was declared to be by natural causes: drowning due to unknown cause of loss of unconsciousness.

3. Hydrostatic Pressure

Soaking up to the shoulders in an extremely hot bath directly increases cardiac load [6, 16]. Heart rate elevation due to an extremely hot bath may increase myocardial oxygen requirement, and therefore increase the risk of ischemic heart disease. Hydrostatic pressure placed on the thoracoabdominal region or lower part of the body affects venous compression and increases venous return to the right atrium (RA). Increasing venous return causes cardiac preload, inducing congestive heart failure and cardiac arrhythmia, such as bradycardia, ventricular tachycardia, and in the worst case, ventricular fibrillation. Sudden removal of the body from the bathtub, such as by standing rapidly, reduces hydrostatic pressure. Cardiac output decreases with reducing venous return to the RA, which may lead to TIA or myocardial ischemia, resulting in accidental drowning.

Case 5

A 68-year-old pensioner living with his son was found lifeless in the bathtub. The water level only reached the submental region, thus his mouth and nostrils were not submerged in bath water. He had a medical history of untreated depression, hypertension, and diabetes. He had been unable to articulate properly for the past few weeks but had not been to a clinic. Autopsy was performed 26 hours after certification of death. Abundant frothy fluid appeared in the airways. The lungs (left, 655 g; right, 680 g) were overinflated, and a light red fluid pleural effusion was accumulated in the bilateral thoracic cavities (left, 250 ml; right, 500 ml). Cardiac examination revealed a heart weight of 545 g and a thick ventricular wall (left, 1.5 cm; right, 0.5 cm), indicating cardiomyopathy. Multiple histologic sections of the myocardium revealed that there was no evidence of fibrosis or necrosis. Additional autopsy findings included small multiple infarct areas in the surrounding basal ganglia, pons, and medulla oblongata. Diabetic alteration was observed in the renal mesangial region. Instant toxicological examination results were negative. The cause of death was defined as congestive heart failure due to hypertensive cardiac hypertrophy.

4. Dehydration

Hyperthermia is a side effect caused by sitting in a hot bath for long periods of time. Elderly people generally have dulled central nerve functions that elicit thirst. Whole blood viscosity and hematocrit is considerably increased and blood perfusion to vital organs is decreased due to dehydration during a bath [18]. Hyperviscosity may produce a thrombus, which may cause cerebral stroke or ischemic heart events, resulting in cardiopulmonary arrest.

5. Epilepsy

Additional risk factors for BRSD include epilepsy for children aged 5 years or older and adolescents. Previous reports on submersion injury in children have disclosed that the incidence of submersion injury in children with epilepsy is 4-10 times greater than that in children without epilepsy [10, 19-20]. It should be noted that some epileptic seizures are easily induced by a hot bath [6]. Furthermore, low medication compliance may occasionally induce a convulsion while bathing [10].

Case 6

The deceased was a 16-year-old high school student found lying face down in a water-filled bathtub 30 minutes after starting a bath. He was taken to the hospital and was pronounced dead despite CPR attempts. He had been treated for epilepsy since he developed limbic encephalitis at age of 5. He took phenytoin, zonisamide, and clobazam; however, epileptic seizures still occurred approximately once a year. His final epileptic attack had been a year prior. At autopsy, abundant frothy light red fluid in the airways was observed. The lungs (left, 695 g; right, 765 g) were markedly congested and edematous. The heart (330 g) showed no macroscopic or microscopic abnormality. The brain (1535 g) had signs of edema but no pathological legions. Toxicological analysis of the blood showed that the serum concentrations of phenytoin, zonisamide, and clobazam were 3.0 μg/ml (10-20 μg/ml in therapeutic range), 9.5 μg/ml (10-30 μg/ml), and 22 μg/ml (100-400 μg/ml), respectively, indicating that the convulsion was uncontrolled. The cause of death in this case was reported to be accidental drowning most likely due to an epileptic seizure.

Is It Accidental Drowning due to TIA or Sudden Unexpected Natural Death?

Although there are some possible causes and risk factors for BRSD, our knowledge of the events is incomplete. BRSD is commonly not witnessed, so BRSD as a cause of death in the previous cases is unclear. In some cases, victims are found dead with their face immersed or completely submerged in the bath water. A major problem is that it is often unknown whether the cause of death is accidental drowning due to TIA or sudden unexpected natural death while bathing.

A body examination often shows that light brown liquid has leaked from the mouth and nostrils in all face positions, regardless of cause of death. The foam can be observed exuding from the mouth and nostrils when pressure is applied to the chest. Abundant foam is usually a sign of drowning [21]; however, foam is commonly found in deaths that occurs during acute pulmonary edema due to left cardiac failure or neurogenic pulmonary edema due to brain hemorrhage. Although the presence of foam in the airway indicates that a victim was alive at the time of submersion for drowning in a river or the sea, this correlation is not applicable to bathtub drowning.

PMCT of the drowning victim usually displays fluid accumulation in the airways, bilateral diffuse ground-grass attenuation of the lungs, swallowed water in the stomach, and water accumulation in the paranasal sinus [22-23]; however, these are not necessarily specific to drowning. Fluid accumulation in the airways and lung edema is also observed in deaths due to acute left heart failure due to ischemic heart disease [24] and also if a long period of time has elapsed since death, regardless of the cause [25]. Water accumulation in the paranasal sinus can also be observed as a postmortem change [26].

At autopsy, the lungs of a drowning victim are commonly wet and heavy, similar to those in deaths associated with acute pulmonary edema. The absence of water in the bronchi may not always indicate natural death because drowning without aspiration of fluid in the bronchi due to a laryngospasm occasionally occurs [27]. On the other hand, the presence of water in the stomach is noteworthy because a victim of drowning often swallows water during the drowning process. Large amounts of water in the stomach may suggest that the cause of death was accidental drowning. Lung histology often shows engorged capillaries and a granular pink precipitate that fills the intra-alveolar air space in drowning victims. There is no significant difference between bathtub drowning and acute lung edema, unless bacterial mass derived from bath water appears in the airway.

It is difficult to ascertain the cause of unconsciousness that leads to drowning, even when an autopsy or PMCT is performed for medicolegal investigation of death. There is usually no morphological abnormality particularly in cases of accidental drowning due to syncope. For these reasons, it is difficult to accurately diagnose BRSD at this time.

Present Issues

The diagnosis of BRSD often presents some considerable medicolegal problems. In all BRSD cases, the police perform scene investigation and explore the circumstances surrounding the incident to rule out suspicious criminal activity. Forensic autopsies are performed in limited cases, such as deaths with external injuries, deaths of the young, or deaths in a hotel room. Except for the autopsy cases, medical examiners or police surgeons perform the body examinations and report according to their inspections. The cause of death is typically treated as drowning or cardiovascular disease, and the manner of death is ruled as accident or natural. Under the current situation, one of the problems is that no exact statistics exist for the number of BRSDs in a year in Japan. It would be helpful for medical examiners or police surgeons to write down 'bath-related sudden death' in the comment section on death certificates.

Another problem relates to the payment of the insurance claim. If the cause of death is reported as drowning, the death is categorized as an exogenous death. On the other hand, if the cause of death is reported as cardiovascular disease in the bathtub, the death is categorized as a sudden unexpected natural death. The amount payable to a beneficiary varies according to whether the manner of death is an 'accident' or 'natural'. However, it is difficult to provide the accurate cause of death to insurance companies under the current situation where an autopsy or PMCT is not performed in every case.

Prevention

Japanese bathing practices drastically affect the bather's blood circulation. In terms of preventive medicine, the most appropriate measures for preventing BRSD are to avoid overlapping risk factors. Consuming alcohol, spending a long time in an extremely hot bath, and orthostatic hypotension due to the release of hydrostatic pressure are individual risk factors. Consuming alcohol is contraindicated before taking a bath. Bath temperature should remain lower than 40°C. Emerging from the bathtub slowly may not induce orthostatic hypotension. Soaking up the shoulders in a full bathtub increases the risk of drowning. Therefore, bathtubs should be filled only halfway to prevent drowning in the case of unconsciousness in the bathtub. A hip bath should be promoted as the ideal relaxing bathing style. In addition, the bathtub should be made wider and shallower. Other preventive measures include not taking BP drugs before bathing, setting the dressing room at the same temperature as the living rooms during the winter, and using a bath heater. Elderly people should refrain from taking a bath at midnight or early in the morning because of changes in the thermal environment. Ensuring the sufficient intake of water before taking a bath is an important to avoid acute dehydration. Epileptic patients and their families must understand the risk of bathtub drowning while bathing alone, and epileptics should take regular medication to avoid an unexpected epileptic attack. All persons at risk for BRSD should avoid taking a bath if signs of physical disorder are present.

The number of elderly people who live alone is increasing in Japan so rapidly that first aid and lifesaving measures are often delayed for bath accidents. Elderly people should live with their families and announce when they start a bath so that family members may watch over them. It is important for scene investigators, medical examiners, and citizens to share the common hazards associated with BRSDs. If BRSD is avoided, lives can be saved from unexpected death.

Acknowledgments

The authors thank Dr. Hideyuki Hayakawa of Office of the Chief Medical Examiner, Tsukuba Medical Center and Hiroki Takanari of the Department of Medical Physiology, Division of Heart & Lungs University Medical Center Utrecht for useful comments on the paper.

References

[1] Los Angeles Times (April 04, 2012), Whitney Houston: Final coroner's report. Available from: http://documents.latimes.com/whitney-houston-coroners-report-final/ (cited Octover 29, 2012)

[2] Kaneko T, Hibi M, Ishibashi M, Nakatsuka A, Omori Y, Ishikura K, et al. Postmortem computed tomography is an informative approach for prevention of sudden unexpected natural death in the elderly. *Risk Manag Healthc Policy*. 2010;3:13-20.

[3] The Japanese National Police Academy, Annual 2009 report on traffic accident fatalities. Available from: http://www.npa.go.jp/toukei/kouki/ 0102_H21dead.pdf (cited October 29, 2012 in Japanese)
[4] Kanda K, Ohnaka T, Tochihara Y, Tsuzuki K, Shodai Y, Nakamura K. Effects of the thermal conditions of the dressing room and bathroom on physiological responses during bathing. *Appl Human Sci.* 1996;15(1):19-24.
[5] Yoshioka N, Chiba T, Yamauchi M, Monma T, Yoshizaki K. Forensic consideration of death in the bathtub. *Leg Med.* 2003;5 Suppl 1:375-81.
[6] Chiba T, Yamauchi M, Nishida N, Kaneko T, Yoshizaki K, Yoshioka N. Risk factors of sudden death in the Japanese hot bath in the senior population. *Forensic Sci Int.* 2005;149(2-3):151-8.
[7] Hayashi T, Ago K, Ago M, Ogata M. Bath-related deaths in Kagoshima, the southwest part of Japan. *Med Sci Law.* 2010;50(1):11-4.
[8] Congressional Record of the House of Councilors on the National Diet of Japan. 180-Health, Labour and Welfare Committee-3rd (March 22, 2012), Available from: http://www.sangiin.go.jp/japanese/joho1/ kaigirok/kaigirok.htm
[9] Helamaa E, Aikäs E. The secret of good 'löyly'. *Ann Clin Res.* 1988;20(4):224-9.
[10] Osamura T, Fushiki S, Yoshioka H, Yamanaka T, Mizuta R. An autopsy case of bathtub drowning in epilepsy. *Brain Dev.* 1997;19(7):499-501.
[11] Ylikahri R, Heikkonen E, Soukas A. The sauna and alcohol. *Ann Clin Res.* 1988;20(4):287-91.
[12] Kenttämies A, Karkola K. Death in sauna. *J Forensic Sci.* 2008 May;53(3):724-9.
[13] Rodhe A, Eriksson A. Sauna deaths in Sweden, 1992-2003. *Am J Forensic Med Pathol.* 2008;29(1):27-31.
[14] Hannuksela ML, Ellahham S. Benefits and risks of sauna bathing. *Am J Med.* 2001;110(2):118-26.
[15] Okuda T, Shiotani S, Sakamoto N, Kobayashi T. Background and current status of postmortem imaging in Japan: Short history of "Autopsy imaging (Ai)". *Forensic Sci Int.* 2013;225(1-3):3-8.
[16] Hashiguchi N, Ni F, Tochihara Y. Effects of room temperature on physiological and subjective responses during whole-body bathing, half-body bathing and showering. *J Physiol Anthropol Appl Human Sci.* 2002;21(6):277-83.
[17] NHK (Japan Broadcasting Corporation). 'Tameshite-Gatten', a program report on January 28, 2009. Available from: http://www9.nhk.or.jp/gatten/pdf/program/ P20090128.pdf (cited Octover.29, 2012 in Japanese)
[18] Satoh F, Fujita M, Misawa S, Nakajima Y, Takeuchi S, Yamamura M. Elevation of blood viscosity as a putative risk factor for sudden death during bathing. *J Jpn Soc Biorheology.* 2006:20(1):44-50.
[19] Saxena A, Ang LC. Epilepsy and bathtub drowning. Important neuropathological observations. *Am J Forensic Med Pathol.* 1993;14(2):125-9.
[20] Kemp AM, Sibert JR. Epilepsy in children and the risk of drowning. *Arch Dis Child.* 1993;68(5):684-5.
[21] Spitz UW. Drowning, in: Spitz UW (Eds.), Spitz and Fisher's Medicolegal Investigation of Death: Guidelines for the Application of Pathology to Crime Investigation, 3rd ed., CHARLES C THOMAS, Springfield, 1993, pp. 498-515.

[22] Levy AD, Harcke HT, Getz JM, Mallak CT, Caruso JL, Pearse L, et al. Virtual autopsy: two- and three-dimensional multidetector CT findings in drowning with autopsy comparison. *Radiology*. 2007;243(3):862-8.

[23] Christe A, Aghayev E, Jackowski C, Thali MJ, Vock P. Drowning--post-mortem imaging findings by computed tomography. *Eur Radiol*. 2008;18(2):283-90.

[24] Shiotani S, Kohno M, Ohashi N, Yamazaki K, Nakayama H, Watanabe K, et al. Non-traumatic postmortem computed tomographic (PMCT) findings of the lung. *Forensic Sci Int*. 2004;139(1):39-48.

[25] Shiotani S, Kobayashi T, Hayakawa H, Kikuchi K, Kohno M. Postmortem pulmonary edema: a comparison between immediate and delayed postmortem computed tomography. *Legal Med*. 2011;13(3):151-155.

[26] Shiotani S, Yamamoto S, Guidebook for Interpretation of Ai, 1st ed., Bunkodo, Tokyo, 2008 (in Japanese).

[27] Aghayev E, Thali MJ, Sonnenschein M, Hurlimann J, Jackowski C, Kilchoer T, et al. Fatal steamer accident; blunt force injuries and drowning in post-mortem MSCT and MRI. *Forensic Sci Int*. 2005;152(1):65-71.

In: Sudden Death
Editors: Jiashin Wu and Jessica Wu
ISBN: 978-1-62618-825-9

Chapter XI

Sudden Death and the Effects of Particulate Matter Air Pollution

Na Zheng[*]
Department of Forensic Science, Shantou University Medical College, Guangdong, China

Abstract

Exposure to air pollution poses a significant health risk. The present review focuses on the adverse effects of particulate matter air pollution on sudden death. Long-term and short-term studies both clearly indicate that relative exposures to particulate matter in the ambient air are associated with increased mortality of sudden death for the susceptible populations, such as infants, the elderly, and the subjects with preexisting cardiovascular diseases, or respiratory diseases. A variety of biological mechanisms responsible for the direct pathways of the cardiovascular outcomes of sudden death associated with particulate matter exposure have been described, including ion channel dysfunction, vascular epithelium, and increased generation of reactive oxygen species followed by the release of pro-oxidative and pro-inflammatory mediator. The indirect pathways of particulate matter linked to particulate matter exposure have been demonstrated to be associated with pulmonary inflammation, autonomic nervous system and central nervous system imbalance, and pulmonary oxidative stress. For the effects on respiratory system, it is also confirmed that fine particulate matter can increase the number and severity of asthma attacks, cause or aggravate bronchitis and other lung diseases, and reduce the body's ability to fight infections. The current knowledge on the particulate matter develops a new pharmacological strategy aimed at decreasing adverse effect during daily and extreme episodes, and provides early guidance to prevent future mortality of sudden death.

Keywords: Sudden death, particulate matter, air pollution, cardiovascular effects, respiratory effects

[*] Corresponding author: Xinling Road 22#, Shantou, Guangdong Province, PR China. Email: nana96069@163.com.

Introduction

As it is well-known, exposure to air pollution poses a significant health risk, both for the healthy populations and the susceptible populations. Until the 1990s, particulate matter was recognized mostly as a nuisance pollutant, and airborne particulate matter became a public concern in recent years, not only in the developed countries, but also in the developing countries. "Particulate matter,' is also known as particle pollution or PM. There are several frequently used classifications for the particulate matter, mainly depending on the diameters or the sources. The questions of which type of the particulate matter would be more harmful and how they work becomes more of a concern in many societies, such as public health society, pediatric society, cardiovascular society, and respiratory society. Concurrently, more about the hypothesis have arisen, such as the adverse effects of particulate matter in sudden infant death syndrome or sudden death syndrome. For these syndromes, which role would the particulate matter act, the incentive cause, the direct cause, or just the false alarm? Plenty of studies have confirmed the adverse effects of airborne particulate matter on the general populations; therefore, they there isare still a lot of work that needs to be done by the government and the general populations to reduce the particulate matter level.

What is the Particulate Matter and How to Classify?

Particulate matter becomes has become a more concerned concerning topic all over the world, but about the definition, it is different in various countries.

The United States Environmental Protection Agency (EPA) defines particulate matter as a complex mixture of extremely small particles and liquid droplets. It is made up of a number of components, including acids (such as nitrates and sulfates), organic chemicals, metals, and soil or dust particles. Environment Canada describes that particulate matter consists of airborne particles in solid or liquid form. United Kingdom Air Quality Strategy for England, Scotland, Wales and Northern Ireland (AQEG) explains that airborne particulate matter is made up of a collection of solid and/or liquid materials of various sizes that range from a few nanometers in diameter (about the size of a virus) to around 100 micrometers (100 μm, about the thickness of a human hair) [1]. Ministry of Environmental Protection of the People's Republic of China represents total suspended particle matters as the general designation of solid and liquid particulate matter in the atmosphere, with the size ranging from 0. 1 -to 100 μm.

Whatever, no matter what the exact definition of particulate matter is, there are three key points about the particulate matter. First, particulate matter is a monomer or a mixture of solid and/or liquid particles. Second, the sources of particulate matter are extensive. Last, the diameter of particulate matter is small, and some are particularly tiny.

Particulate matter is often classified depending on its size and this classification is used in concentration measurements, because the size of particulate matter largely determines the extent of environmental and health damage.

U. S. EPA classifies particulate matter as super coarse particles ($d_{pa} \geq 10$ μm), coarse particles (2. 5 μm$\leq d_{pa} \leq$10 μm), fine particles (0. 1 μm$\leq d_{pa} \leq$2. 5μm), and ultrafine particles ($d_{pa} \leq$0. 1 μm). Although the dividing line between two groups seems so tiny, there is a substantial difference in size of these particles, all of which are considered moderate-to-large in air pollution control. Depending on the adverse effects on health, EPA also groups particle pollution into two categories: "Inhalable coarse particles," such as those found near roadways and dusty industries, are larger than 2. 5 micrometers and smaller than 10 micrometers in diameter; "Fine particles," such as those found in smoke and haze, are 2. 5 micrometers in diameter and smaller. These particles can be directly emitted from sources such as forest fires, or they can be formed when gases emitted from power plants, industries and automobiles react in the air.

Environment Canada divides particulate matter into three groups: Total particulate matter (TPM)-airborne particulate matter with an upper size limit of approximately 100 micro meter (μm) in aerodynamic equivalent diameter; Particulate matter < 10 microns (PM_{10}) -airborne particulate matter with a mass median diameter less than 10 μm; Particulate matter <2. 5 microns ($PM_{2.5}$) -airborne particulate matter with a mass median diameter less than 2. 5 μm. In this classification, aerodynamic equivalent diameter is the diameter of unit-density sphere having the same gravitational setting velocity as the particle, meanwhile mass median diameter is defined as the diameter at which 50 % of the particles by mass are larger and 50 % are smaller.

Particulate matter also could be classified as primary component and secondary component, depending on the compounds and processes involved during its formation. Primary particulate matter is released directly from the source into the atmosphere in particle form, for example, the smokestack of an electrical power plant or a recently tilled field subject to wind erosion. Secondary particulate matter are is formed in the atmosphere by a series of chemical and physical reactions involving different precursor gases, such as sulphur oxides and nitrogen oxides, and ammonia reacting to form sulphate, nitrate and ammonium particulate matter. Table 1 lists some of the leading components of particulate matter with different sources based on this classification.

Due to the special boundary of the size of particulate matter, at present, most routine air quality-monitoring systems generate data based on the measurement of PM_{10} as opposed to other particulate matter sizes. Consequently, the majority of epidemiological studies use PM_{10} as the exposure indicator.

The U. S. EPA defines PM_{10} as particulate matter with a diameter of 10 micrometers collected with 50 % efficiency by a PM_{10} sampling collection device. PM_{10} is a mixture of materials that can include smoke, soot, dust, salts, acids, and metals. PM_{10} is also forms formed when gases emitted from motor vehicles and industry undergoes chemical reactions in the atmosphere. In the western United States, there are sources of PM_{10} in both urban and rural areas. Major sources include: motor vehicles, wood burning stoves and fireplaces, dust from construction, landfills, and agriculture, wildfires and brush/waste burning, industrial sources, and windblown dust from open lands. Moreover, the source and composition of PM_{10} varies vary greatly by region. For example, coarse particulate matter is highly correlated with PM_{10} in desert and some agricultural regions, but not in urban areas. For the coastal area, during the sea/land breeze season near Venice, the elemental composition and water-soluble inorganic ions content of PM_{10} are mainly mineral dust, road traffic, fossil fuels and marine aerosol [2].

Table 1. Components of Particulate Matter [1]

Primary components	Sources
Sodium chloride	Sea salt.
Elemental carbon	Black carbon (soot) is formed during high temperature combustion of fossil fuels such as coal, natural gas and oil (diesel and petrol) and biomass fuels such as wood chips.
Trace metals	These metals are present at very low concentrationsand include lead, cadmium, nickel, chromium, zinc and manganese. They are generated by metallurgical processes, such as steel making, or by impurities found in or additives mixed into fuels used by industry. Metals in particles are also derived from mechanical abrasion processes, e. g. during vehicle motion and break and tyre wear.
Mineral components	These minerals are found in coarse dusts from quarrying, construction and demolition work and from wind-driven dusts. They include aluminum, silicon, iron and calcium.
Secondary components	Sources
Sulphate	Formed by the oxidation of sulphur dioxide (SO_2) in the atmosphere to form sulphuric acid, which can react with ammonia (NH_3) to give ammonium sulphate.
Nitrate	Formed by the oxidation of nitrogen oxides (NOx) – which consists of nitric oxide (nitrogen monoxide, NO) and nitrogen dioxide (NO_2) in the atmosphere to form nitric acid, which can react with NH_3 to give ammonium nitrate. Also present as sodium nitrate.
Water	Some components of the aerosol form of particulate matter, such as ammonium sulphates and ammonium nitrates, take up water from the atmosphere.
Primary and secondary components	Sources
Organic carbon	Primary organic carbon comes from traffic or industrial combustion sources. Secondary organic carbon comes from the oxidation of volatile organic compounds (VOCs). There may be several hundred individual components. Some of these trace organic compounds, such as certain polycyclic aromatic hydrocarbons, are highly toxic.

Except forBesides PM_{10}, $PM_{2.5}$ is another crucial indicator to assess the air quality. As aniconic fine matter particulate, the organic carbon component of ambient $PM_{2.5}$ is a complex mixture of hundreds or even thousands of organic compounds, which organic carbon component influenced by the regions. In Toronto, the four main sources are coal combustion related to regional transport and secondary sulfate, secondary nitrate related to both local and upwind sources of NO_X and NH_3, secondary organic aerosols formed from a variety of precursor organic emissions, and motor vehicle traffic. The other detectable sources were road salt and three types of primary $PM_{2.5}$ hypothesized to be associated with smelters, coal and oil combustion, industry, and local construction [3]. Moreover, the source and composition of $PM_{2.5}$ varies vary greatly by season. For example, the road salt is just represented in winter; sulfate levels are higher in summer than in autumn or winter. In addition, a source exceeding these major source thresholds for any pollutant determined to be a $PM_{2.5}$ precursor in a given area is also major for $PM_{2.5}$. $PM_{2.5}$ precursors are regulated as follows: sulfur dioxide (SO_2) —regulated in all areas; nitrogen oxides (NO_X) — regulated unless a State demonstrates that NO_X is not a significant precursor; volatile organic compound sand ammonia - not regulated unless a State demonstrates they are a significant precursor [4].

How Does Particulate Matter Cause Adverse Effects?

The sources and components of particulate matter are diverse and complex, therefore, scientists have hypothesized that the toxic or adverse health effects of ambient particulate matter are varying depending on the components. Table 2 lists some of the leading candidates that have been associated with biologic responses observed in a variety of studies and experimental systems.

The epidemiological evidence shows adverse effects of particulate matter following both short-term and long-term exposures [6]. The ranges of health effects linked to particulate matter exposure are board, but the predominantly affected parts are the cardiovascular and respiratory systems.

Table 2. Chemical components of particulate matter and their biologic effects on populations [5]

Components	Major Subcomponents	Biologic Effects
Metals	Iron, vanadium, nickel, copper, platinum, and others	Can trigger inflammation, cause DNA damage, and alter cell permeability by inducing production of reactive oxygen species (particularly hydroxyl free radicals) in tissues
Organic compounds	Many are adsorbed onto particles; some volatile or semivolatile organic species form particles themselves	Some may cause mutations, some may cause cancer; others can act as irritants and can induce allergic reactions
Biologic origin	Viruses, bacteria and their endotoxins (lipopolysaccharides), animal and plant debris (such as pollen fragments), and fungal spores	Plant pollens can trigger allergic responses in the airways of sensitive individuals; viruses and bacteria can provoke immune defense responses in the airways
Irons	Sulfatea (usually as ammonium sulfate), nitrateb (usually ammonium or sodium nitrate), and acidity (H+)	Sulfuric acid at relatively high concentrations can impair mucociliary clearance and increase airway resistance in people with asthma; acidity may change the solubility (and availability) of metals and other compounds adsorbed onto particles
Reactive gases	Ozone, peroxides, aldehydes	May adsorb onto particles and be transported into lower airways, causing injury
Particle core	Carbonaceous material	Carbon induces lung irritation, epithelial cell proliferation, and fibrosis after long-term exposure

The initial studies on particulate matter exposure were about work-related disease, e. g. asbestosis. Following the first assessed adverse effects on respiratory diseases and lung cancer, a large body of epidemiological and clinical studies definitely documented an even stronger association of lower aerodynamic diameter particulate matter exposure with acute cardiovascular events, particularly related to coronary and cerebrovascular disease, which was the main cause of sudden death.

Adverse cardiovascular events such as coronary artery disease, cerebrovascular disease, venous thromboembolism, vascular dysfunction, and disturbance in cardiac autonomic control were thought to link with particulate matter. Recently, an association has also been found between cardiac hypertrophy and particulate matter [7]. The mechanisms leading to these harmful effects on the cardiovascular system are still on debate, but several supposed pathways have been proposed that elucidate the direct and indirect effects of particulate matter displaying in Figure 1.

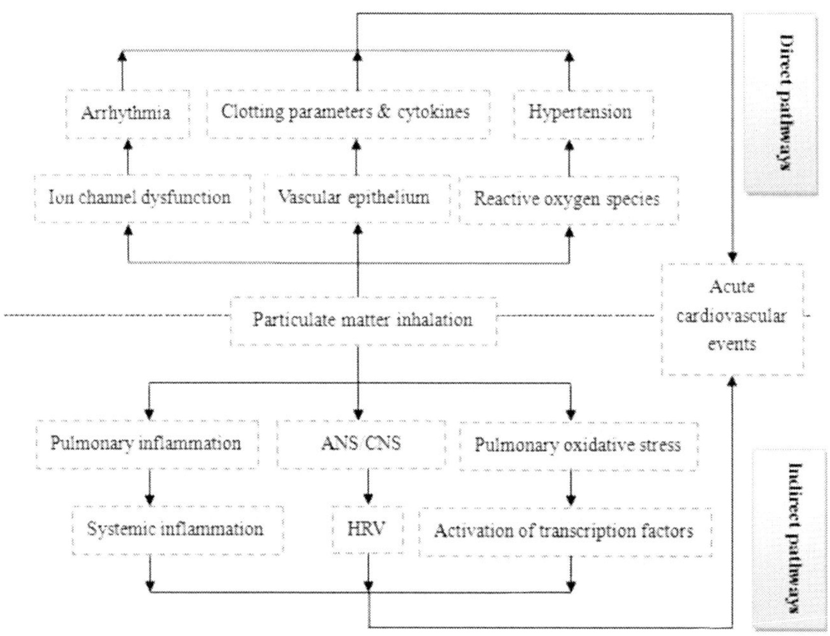

Figure 1. The direct and indirect effects of particulate matter on acute cardiovascular events.

Direct effects of particulate matter on the cardiovascular system started at the fine particles inhalation penetrating beyond the upper respiratory tract into the parenchymal region of the lung. Recent works demonstrated that particulate matter affected the cardiovascular system directly by entry into the systemic circulation. This process caused acute cardiovascular events through mechanisms of ion channel interference, vascular dysfunction, and accumulation of reactive oxygen species production [8].

The mechanistic links between exposure to airborne particulate matter pollution and the associated increases in cardiovascular morbidity and mortality showed a tendency in the people with congestive heart failure. In the animal experiment, the genetically engineered mice (CREBA133), which displayed aberrant cardiac physiology and anatomy reminiscent of human congestive heart failure, with particulate matter exposure via aspiration, exhibited significantly reduced heart rate variability (HRV), respiratory dyssynchrony, and increased ventricular arrhythmias. The genome-wide expression analyses of CREBA133 left ventricular tissues demonstrated prominent Na+ and K+ channel pathway gene dysregulation. The following research results suggested a multi-organ pathobiology inherent to the CHF phenotype that was exaggerated by particulate matter exposure via heightened carotid body sensitivity and cardiac Na+ channel dysfunction [9].

Numerous studies indicated that the direct toxic effects of particulate matter exposure on vascular epithelium to cause vascular dysfunction mediated by affecting vascular smooth muscle function, and more were about the aortic rings. After the particulate matter inhalation, total suspended particulate matter (TSP) effects were inhibited by Trolox, suggesting a role of oxidants. Nudation of aortic rings showed that effects of TSP were only partly endothelium-dependent, while preincubation with L-NAME increased TSP-induced relaxation. It was concluded that both the particle core and soluble components of TSP could affect the smooth muscle function, leading to changes in the vascular contractile response [10].

Multiple studies have been postulated to cause the increase inatherothrombotic and thromboembolic events, mainly pointed at the production of reactive oxygen species through the oxidative stress pathway. Studies have suggested that the association at the reaction of reactive oxygen species by fines particulate matter exposure and hypertension, especially in short-term exposure. Recently research found that the associations of short-term increases in particulate matter with aerodynamic diameters <10 μm with higher nighttime blood pressure and blunted systolic blood pressure dipping were preceded by associations with reduced ability of the kidney to excrete sodium during daytime. The underlying mechanism linking air pollution to increased cardiovascular risk might include disturbed circadian rhythms of renal sodium handling and blood pressure [11].

Fewer and conflicting data also suggested an association with venous thromboembolism. Although not completely elucidated, a series of mechanisms have been hypothesized and tested in experimental settings. These phenomena, including vasomotor and cardiac autonomic dysfunction, hemostatic unbalance, oxidative stress and inflammatory response, have been shown to change over time and differently contributed to the short-term and long-term adverse effects of pollution exposure. Recently epidemiological research suggested that the short-time exposure to high concentrations of fine particulate matter might favor an increased rate of emergency department accesses for venous thromboembolism through the induction of a prothrombotic state [12]. Beyond environmental health policies, crucial for improving air quality and reducing the impact of such an elusive threat to public health, the recognition and assessment of the individual risk, together with specific advice, should be routinely implemented in the strategies of primary and secondary cardiovascular prevention.

Indirect effects of particulate matter on the cardiovascular system are mediated through the autonomic nervous system or central nervous system, which controls HRV, inflammatory responses and reactive oxygen species, moreover, the pulmonary oxidative stress, which augment acute cardiovascular events and atherosclerosis.

A decreased HRV is a powerful marker with heart disease and in the general population, and it is a predictor of sudden cardiac death and arrhythmias. The underlying mechanisms responsible for the association between fine particulate matter exposure and impaired HRV are not yet fully understood. Two main candidate mechanisms are release of pro-thrombotic and inflammatory cytokines from the lung, and effects on the electrical activity and autonomic function of the heart [5]. As an indicator, HRV represents the physiological responses of the autonomic nervous system, of the combined sympathetic and parasympathetic activity. Alterations in autonomic control of the heart may represent a major pathophysiological mechanism by which air pollution leads to cardiac mortality. Two possible pathways can lead to changes in neural control of the heart affecting HRV by particulate matter exposure. Inhaled particles can promote a systemic sympathetic stress response that leads to decreased HRV measurements and may cumulate in ventricular tachyarrhythmia. On the other hand, the inhaled particles can stimulate irritant receptors in the lung parenchyma and respiratory airways, which leads to the opposite, an increased parasympathetic vagal response and decreased HRV [13].

After particulate matter inhalation, the lung releases locally and into the systemic circulation pro-oxidative, e. g. reactive oxygen species, or proinflammatory, such as cytokines mediators, such as interleukin 1-beta, IL-6, and TNF-α, or both and vasoactive hormones, such as endothelins [14,15]. Acute-phase reactions take place and lead to the increase in plasma of such reactants as C-reactive protein and fibrinogen [16,17]. Brought about by particulate matter increments, inflammation is thought to exacerbate preexisting inflammatory diseases. Experimental evidence suggested a hierarchical oxidative stress model, in which a weakened antioxidant defense, as observed in disease or induced by inhaled particles, increased the particulate matter ability to cause lung inflammation, accounting for exacerbations that occur in asthmatics and in patients with chronic obstructive lung disease. In the lungs, the secretion of adhesion molecules by inflamed endothelial cells resulted in binding and activation of leukocytes and platelets, formation of platelet-leukocyte conjugates, and generation of hemostatically active, tissue factor-bearing microparticles [18]. The role of particulate matter-induced systemic inflammation leading to acute cardiovascular events such as arrhythmia, heart failure, and myocardial infarction is more speculative. As a whole, data in humans indicated that short-term inflammatory responses to particulate matter were not always detected; they were usually mild and loosely correlated with functional changes. Among these studies, the diversity of particulate matter characteristics, dose metrics, and endpoints hampered a clear discerning of inflammatory mechanism(s). Therefore, research on controlled exposure needed expanding, so that the results of time-series and panel studies would be better understood and short-term standards for human exposure might be more confidently allocated [19]. But different findings showed that in vivo daily exposure to concentrated urban $PM_{2.5}$ could decrease endothelium-dependent relaxation and eNOS expression on pulmonary arteries associated with local high TNF-alpha level but not systemic pro-inflammatory factors [20].

The pathogenic mechanisms has been demonstrated that particulate matter exposure triggers massive oxidative stress in vascular endothelial cells (ECs), resulting in the loss of endothelial cells integrity and lung vascular hyperpermeability. And the experimental results suggested a potentially protective role for hydrogen sulfide in particulate matter-induced inflammatory lung injury and vascular hyperpermeability [21]. Previously work also suggested that the particulate matter induced genotoxicity in human lung bronchial epithelial cells and definitely DNA damage in A549 cells [22,23]. Recently work also suggested that the associations noted between certain pollution types and sources and oxidative stress might reflect a mechanism by which these pollutants accelerated aging via enhanced erosion of telomeres. Not only would pollution reduction imperatives be more focused, but interventions which could reduce oxidative stress would become more important [24].

Numerous reports indicated the role of oxidative stress and inflammation in impairing the function of lung exposed to particulate matter. Probably, the ability of particulate matter to cause oxidative stress underlay underlaid the association between increased exposure to particulate matter and exacerbations of lung diseases. Mostly because of their large surface area, ultrafine particles have been shown to cause oxidative stress and proinflammatory effects in different pathways in vivo and in vitro studies. Particle components and surface area may act synergistically inducing lung inflammation. In this vein, reactive oxygen species elicited upon particulate matter exposure have been shown to activate a number of redox-responsive signaling pathways and Ca(2+) influx in lung target cells that were involved in the expression of genes that modulate relevant responses to lung inflammation and disease [25].

Plenty of studies also suggested that effects on lung, or pulmonary vascular, or endothelial barrier were associated with particulate matter exposure. The airway epithelium is the first line of defense against inhaled insults and therefore must be capable of coordinating appropriate inflammatory and immune responses. Immune responses to particulate matter exposure mediated by the airway epithelial nucleotide-binding domain and leucine-rich repeat protein 3 inflammasome might have implications in patients with asthma and other lung diseases [26].

Besides the enhanced oxidative stress and inflammation, particulate matter exposure was also linked to lung dysfunction. Particulate matter induced reactive oxygen species generation in human lung endothelium, resulting in oxidative stress-mediated endothelial cell barrier disruption via p38 MAPK- and HSP27-dependent pathways [27].

Recently works on the effects of particulate matter on lung surfactant system leads to another pathway. One of the reasons for cellular changes in the lung tissue exposed to the particulate matter, especially with adsorbed volatile organic molecules is the reduction of the clearance rate in the pulmonary region of the respiratory system. The interaction of the fractal-like particles and organic substances with a surfactant monolayer limits limited its dynamic activity. The work suggested a significant lowering of the dynamics of the surfactant monolayer. Additional measurements of surface pressure during the monotonic compression of the air-water interface containing the major lung surfactant phospholipid, dipalmitoylphosphatidylcholine, showed that the presence of benzo [a]pyrene (BaP) molecules in the system influenced its stability. The simulation results indicated the insertion of BaP molecules into the lipid layer, which explained the measured effects [28]. Even the pathways or the mechanisms of the particulate matter linked to the occurrence of pulmonary diseases were still in debate, clinical evidences showed that particulate matter was associated with the progress of the diseases. Based on the surgical lung tissues, the retained particulate matter is widely distributed in lung tissues, including the lung parenchyma, blood vessel walls, airways, lymphoid follicles, and alveolar macrophages, in the subjects with COPD and that cigarette smoke exposure and airflow obstruction are associated with retention of particulate matter in lung tissues. The downward trend in particulate matter burden in severe COPD to either less deposition and retention or selective removal of particulate matter containing tissues by emphysematous destruction was present [29].

Apart from cardiovascular and respiratory disease, particulate matter also affects the intestine. Together with evidence of increases in incidence of inflammatory bowel diseases (IBD) in the past few decades of enhanced industrialization, the recent discovery of genes linked to susceptibility to IBD explaining only a fraction of the hereditary variance suggested that environmental factors, especially particulate matter, might contribute to disease pathogenesis. Plausible mechanisms mediating the effects of particulate matter on the bowel could include direct effects on epithelial cells, systemic inflammation and immune activation, and modulation of the intestinal microbiota [30].

In the psychological studies, a novel finding presented the association of particulate matter and the risk of suicide. Thousands of subjects were observed, and a transient increase in particulate matter was associated with increased suicide risk, especially for individuals with preexisting cardiovascular disease [31].

PM_{10} is regulated as a specific type of pollutant, because the special size range is considered respirable. In other words, when inhaled, PM_{10} evades the respiratory system's natural defenses and is lodged deep in the lungs. In forensic practices, it is very common to find the anthracotic pigmentation with microscopy in the lungs of the subjects who never smoke. Health problems begin as the body reacts to these foreign particles. PM_{10} can increase the number and severity of asthma attacks, cause or aggravate bronchitis and other lung diseases, and reduce the body's ability to fight infections.

Metabolic neuropathophysiology underlying the prediabetic state may confer susceptibility to the adverse health effects of PM_{10}. Ten years of epidemiologic evidences suggested that insulin and insulin resistance exacerbate the adverse effects of PM_{10} on cardiac autonomic control and thus risk of coronary heart disease among nondiabetic, postmenopausal women with impaired fasting glucose [32].

Ultrafine particles are not only toxic, but also can be a precursor of ozone, which can coexist along with other photochemically generated oxidants. Although exposure to single pollutants e. g. particulate matter is associated with adverse health effects, scientists and policy makers have started to focus on the toxicity of different components and characteristics of the particle mixture. Studies on the synergistic interaction of multiple pollutants have mimicked a real world scenario. NO(2) exposure alone increased cholesterol and high density lipoprotein (HDL) after short-term exposure, decreased high frequency component of HRV after short-term exposure, decreased QT variability index after short-term exposure, and increased lactate dehydrogenase in bronchoalveolar lavage (BAL) fluid. The only significant change with $PM_{2.5}$ CAPs was an increase in HDL after short-term exposure, likely due to the low concentration of $PM_{2.5}$ CAPs in the exposure chamber. Exposure to both NO(2) and $PM_{2.5}$ CAPs increased BALα1- antitrypsin, mean T wave amplitude, the low frequency components of HRV and the LF/HF ratio. The study also presented that NO(2) exposure might produce and enhance acute cardiovascular effects of $PM_{2.5}$ CAPs [33]. Therefore, it is useful to consider the interactions of ambient particulate matter and gaseous co-pollutants during assessment of health effects.

How Does Particulate Matter Linking to Cigarette Smoke Cause Adverse Effects?

People are also exposed to particulate matter indoors, mostly from cigarette smoke, home heating sources (such as wood burning stoves), and cooking, but also from outdoor particulate matter sources that easily penetrate the indoor environment. Indoor exposure may be substantial because this is where most people spend the majority of their time. There are many studies about the cigarette smokers and non-smokers exposed to second hand cigarette smoke.

A recent study demonstrated that in vitro cigarette smoke extract exposure induced osteopontin expression in human endothelial cells in an oxidative stress-dependent manner.

In humans, serum osteopontin was decreased with short-term smoking cessation. It signified that endothelial-derived osteopontin might contribute to inflammation in smokers, and might also contribute to atherosclerosis and cardiovascular disease-related processes [34].

For children and youth under 18 years, second hand smoke exposure has detrimental effects on their health, particularly for those in low socioeconomic circumstances, for their environment accentuates a higher baseline risk [35].

Which Population Subgroups are Particularly Susceptible?

Epidemiological, controlled human exposure and toxicological studies have demonstrated a variety of health effects in response to particulate matter exposure with some of these studies indicating that populations with certain characteristics may be disproportionately affected.

In addition, investigators crafted a comprehensive definition of susceptibility that can be used to encompass all populations potentially at increased risk of adverse health effects as a consequence of exposure to an air pollutant.

Overall, the epidemiological studies evaluated with supporting evidence from controlled human exposure and toxicological studies, identifies characteristics of populations that may lead to increased susceptibility to particulate matter-related health effects.

It included life stage, specifically children and older adults; preexisting cardiovascular (i. e. CAD) and respiratory (i. e. asthma) diseases; genetic polymorphisms; and low socioeconomic circumstances, as measured by educational attainment and income.

Additionally, more limited evidence suggested an increase in particulate matter-related health effects in individuals with diabetes, COPD, and increased body mass index. Although not clearly established, the evidence evaluated also indicated potentially increased risk of particulate matter-related health effects by sex and race/ethnicity, but these associations were not consistent across particulate matter size fractions, health effects, and in some cases study locations [35]. Meanwhile, further studies may enable the identification of specific particulate matter size fractions, sources, or components that render a population more susceptible.

Epidemiological studies and animal experiments have shown that individuals with preexisting diseases, such as asthma, chronic obstructive pulmonary disease (COPD), and diabetes mellitus (DM) are more susceptible to particulate matter-related health problems. Particulate matter has been shown to affect macrophage functions, suggesting a hypothesis that exposure to particulate matter in the setting of DM and high glucose levels would result in enhanced macrophage activation arouse. Animal experiment demonstrated that urban particulate matter SRM 1648 caused severe oxidative stress in macrophages from DM rabbits and up-regulation of cytokine expression and MMP-9 activity [36].

Moreover, epidemiologic studies have suggested that the particulate matter may affect pregnant women and their fetuses and infants. The evidences included increases in low birth weight and more infants born prematurely, and even the increase in infant and child mortality, perhaps including sudden infant death syndrome.

What Has Been Done and is to be Done to Reduce the Particulate Matter Level?

In 1969, the U. S. Environmental Protection Agency issued the "Criteria Document", which summarized findings from previous studies on health effects related to exposure to particulate matter, total suspended particles (TSP) and sulfur dioxide (SO_2). This led to the establishment of the Clean Air Act in 1970 in the USA, followed by the first National Ambient Air Quality Standards. At the same time, the World Health Organization (WHO) set in its guideline a standard for the levels of suspended particles followed by global guideline for the levels of ambient particles. Hence, the increasing interest among scientists in particulate matter levels and health implications culminated in an increase by more than 5,000-fold in publications over the last decades. Air quality agencies in several states in U. S. have developed, or are now developing air quality plans to bring PM_{10} concentrations down to healthful levels. These plans include a variety of programs to reduce emissions, including: dust control for roads, construction, and landfills; landscaping, barriers, and fencing to reduce windblown dust; programs to reduce emissions from wood stoves and fireplaces; cleaner-burning gasoline and diesel fuel; emission control devices for motor vehicles; controls for industrial facilities. United States and Canada have completed a joint transboundary particulate matter science assessment report in support of the Canada-U. S. Air Quality Agreement.

When the National Ambient Air Quality Objective (NAAQO) for Total Suspended Particles (TSP) was established under the Clean Air Act (now subsumed into the *Canadian Environmental Protection Act, 1999 (CEPA, 1999)*) in the 1970s, the health and environmental effects related to the finer fractions of PM were not well understood. Even in the 1980s, smog was mainly considered to consist of ground-level ozone, and the role of PM as a major component of smog was not recognized. Throughout the 1990s, evidence of the serious health implications of inhaling fine particles grew with scientific studies linking fine PM to premature mortality and a range of morbidity effects such as hospital emergency room visits and asthma symptom days. The Phase 2 Federal Smog Plan released by the Government of Canada in 1997 recognized the mounting concern with fine PM but still focused primarily on ozone.

In 1998, the Canadian Council of Ministers of the Environment (CCME) selected PM as one of the first round of substances for which a Canada-Wide Standard (CWS) would be developed under the newly adopted Accord on Environmental Harmonization and its Environmental Standards Sub-Agreement. A CWS for the finer fraction of PM (PM less than 2. 5 microns in diameter ($PM_{2.5}$)) was developed and endorsed by the CCME in 2000. In 2001, the federal government declared PM less than 10 microns in diameter (PM10) to be toxic and included in CEPA 1999, with an emphasis on the finer fraction $PM_{2.5}$. In 2003, the primary precursor pollutants to the secondary formation of $PM_{2.5}$ (sulphur dioxide (SO2), nitrogen oxides (NOx), volatile organic compounds (VOCs) and ammonia (NH3)) were also declared to be toxic and added to Schedule 1 of CEPA, the List of Toxic Substances, on the basis of their contribution to PM formation.

In 2002, "Air Quality Strategy for England, Scotland, Wales and Northern Ireland" was published to describe the plans drawn up by the Government and Devolved Administrations to protect and improve air quality in the U. K. Then, the Air Quality Strategy for England, Scotland, Wales and Northern Ireland (AQEG) was set up, aiming at help the UK Government tackle air pollution by examining where pollutants came from and what their concentrations were in the UK [1].

All these guidelines are intended to inform policy-makers and to provide appropriate targets for a broad range of policy options for air quality management in different parts of the world. For the general population, to get a healthy living environment, a lot of work needs to be done in the future.

References

[1] AQEG, (2005). Particulate Matter in the UK: Summary. Defra, London. 1-28.

[2] Masiol, M., Rampazzo, G., Ceccato, D., Squizzato, S., Pavoni, B., (2010). Characterization of PM10 sources in a coastal area near Venice (Italy): an application of factor-cluster analysis. *Chemosphere.* 80, 771-8.

[3] Lee, P. K., Brook, J. R., Dabet-Zlotorzynska, E., Mabury, S. A., (2003). Identification of the major sources contributing to PM2. 5 observed in Toronto. *Environ. Sci. Technol.* 37, 4831-40.

[4] Slayback, J., Berry, K. , Hawks, R., Downs, D., Mesing, G., (2008). Final new source review (NSR) rules for $PM_{2.5}$. *Environmental Quality Management,* Inc. 1-3.

[5] HEI, (2002). Understanding the Health Effects of Components of the Particulate Matter Mix: Progress and Next Steps. 1-20.

[6] World Health Organization, (2006). WHO air quality guidelines for particulate matter, ozone, nitrogen dioxide and sultur dioxide. WHO Press, Switzerland. 1-22.

[7] Ying, Z., Yue, P., Xu, X., Zhong, M., Sun, Q., Mikolaj, M., Wang, A., Brook, R. D., Chen, L. C., Rajagopalan, S., (2009). Air pollution and cardiac remoding. a role for RhoA/Rho-kinase. *Am. J. Physiol. Heart. Circ. Physiol.* 296, H1540-50.

[8] Nelin, T. D., Joseph, A. M., Gorr, M. W., Wold, L. E., (2012). Direct and indirect effects of particulate matter on the cardiovascular system. *Toxicology Letters.* 208, 293-9.

[9] Wang, T., Lang, G. D., Moreno-Vinasco, L., Huang, Y., Goonewardena, S. N., Peng, Y. J., Svensson, E. C., Natarajan, V., Lang, R. M., Linares, J. D., Breysse, P. N., Geyh, A. S., Samet, J. M., Lussier, Y. A., Dadley, S., Prabhakar, N. R., Garcia, J. G., (2012). Particulate Matter Induces Cardiac Arrhythmias via Dysregulation of Carotid Body Sensitivity and Cardiac Sodium Channels. *Am. J. Respir. Cell. Mol. Biol.* 46, 524-31.

[10] Knaapen, A. M., den Hartog, G. J., Bast, A., Borm, P. J., (2001). Ambient particulate matter induces relaxation of rat aortic rings in vitro. *Hum. Exp. Toxicol.* 20, 259-65.

[11] Tsai, D. H., Riediker, M., Wuerzner, G., Maillard, M., Marques-Vidal, P., Paccaud, F., Vollenweider, P., Burnier, M., Bochud, M., (2012). Short-term increase in particulate matter blunts nocturnal blood pressure dipping and daytime urinary sodium excretion. *Hypertension.* 60, 1061-9.

[12] Martinelli, N., Girelli, D., Cigolini, D., Sandri, M., Ricci, G., ROcca, G., Olivieri, O., (2012). Access rate to the emergency department for venous thromboembolism in relationship with coarse and fine particulate matter air pollution. *Plos One*. 7, e34831.

[13] Stone, P. H., Godleski, J. J, (1999). First steps toward understanding the pathophysiologic link between air pollution and cardiac mortality. *Am. Heart J.* 138, 804-7.

[14] Gurgueira, S. A., Lawrence, J., Coull, B., Murthy, G. G. K., Gonzalez-Flecha, B., (2002). Rapid increase in the steady state concentration of reactive oxygen species in the lungs and heart after particulate air pollution inhalation. *Environ. Health. Perspect.* 110, 749-755.

[15] Tsai, D. H., Amyai, N., Marques-Vidal, P., Wang, J. L., Riediker, M., Mooser, V., Paccaud, F., Waeber, G., Vollenweider, P., Bochud, M., (2012). Effects of particulate matter on inflammatory markers in the general adult population. *Part. Fibre. Toxicol.* 9, 24.

[16] Su, T. C., Wu, C. F., Chan, C. C., Chen, M. F., (2011). C-reaction protein and particulate matter predict plasma fibrinogen levels. *Int. J. Cardiol.* 153, 100-1.

[17] Gardner, S. Y., Lehmann, J. R., Costa, D. L., (2000). Oil fly ashinduced elevation of plasma fibrinogen levels in rats. *Toxicol. Sci.* 56, 175-180.

[18] Vermylen, J., Hoylaerts, M. F., (2007). The procoagulant effects of air pollution. *J. Thromb . Haemost.* 5, 250-1.

[19] Scapellato, M. L., Lotti, M., (2007). Short-term effects of particulate matter: An inflammatory mechanism?. *Crit. Rev. Toxicol.* 37, 461-87.

[20] Davel, A. P., Lemos, M. P., Luciana, M., Pedro, S. C., de André, P. A., Hebeda, C., Farsky, S. H., Saldiva, P. H., Rossoni, L. V., (2012). Endothelial dysfunction in the pulmonary artery induced by concentrated fine particulate matter exposure is associated with local but not systemic inflammation. *Toxicology*. 295, 39-46.

[21] Wang, T., Wang, L., Zaidi, S. R., Sammani, S., Siegler, J., Moreno-Vinasco, L., Mathew, B., Natarajan, V., Garcia, J. G., (2012). Hydrogen Sulfide Attenuates Particulate Matter-Induced Human Lung Endothelial Barrier Disruption via Combined Reactive Oxygen Species Scavenging and Akt Activation. *Am. J. Respir. Cell. Mol. Biol.* 47, 491-6.

[22] Hemmingsen, J. G., Moller, P., Nojgaard, J. K., Roursgaard, M., Loft, S., (2011). Oxidative stress, genotoxicity, and vascular cell adhesion molecule expression in cells exposed to particulate matter from combustion of conventional diesel and methyl ester biodiesel blends. *Environ. Sci. Technol.* 45, 8545-51.

[23] Oh, S. M. , Kim, H. R. , Park, Y. J. , Lee, S. Y. , Chung, K. H. , (2011). Organic extracts of urban air pollution particulate matter (PM2. 5)-induced genotoxicity and oxidative stress in human lung bronchial epithelial cells (BEAS-2B cells). *Mutat. Res.* 723, 142-51.

[24] Grahame, T. J., Schlesinger, R. B., (2012). Oxidative stress-induced telomeric erosion as a mechanism underlying airborne particulate matter-related cardiovascular disease. *Part. Fibre. Toxicol.* 19, 21.

[25] Mazzoli-Rocha, F., Fernandes, S., Einicker-Lamas, M., Zin, W. A., (2010). Roles of oxidative stress in signaling and inflammation induced by particulate matter. *Cell. Biol. Toxicol.* 26, 481-98.

[26] Hirota, J. A., Hirota, S. A., Warner, S. M., Stefanowica, D., Shaheen, F., Beck, P. L., Macdonald, J. A., Hackett, T. L., Sin, D. D., Van Eeden, S., Knight, D. A., (2012). The airway epithelium nucleotide-binding domain and leucine-rich repeat protein 3 inflammasome is activated by urban particulate matter. *J. Allergy. Clin. Immunol.* 129, 1116-25.

[27] Wang, T., Chiang, E. T., Moreno-Vinasco, L., Lang, G. D., Pendyala, S., Samet, J. M., Geyh, A. S., Breysse, P. N., Chillrud, S. N., Natarajan, V., Garcia, J. G., (2010). Particulate Matter Disrupts Human Lung Endothelial Barrier Integrity via ROS- and p38 MAPK-Dependent Pathways. *Am. J. Resp. Cell. Mol.* 42, 442-9.

[28] Sosnowski, T. R., Kolinski, M., Gradon, L., (2011). Interactions of benzo [a]pyrene and diesel exhaust particulate matter with the lung surfactant system. *Ann. Occup. Hyg.* 55, 329-38.

[29] Ling, S. H., McDonough, J. E., Gosselink, J. V., Elliott, W. M., Hayashi, S., Hogg, J. C., van Eeden, S. F., (2011). Patterns of retention of particulate matter in lung tissue of patients with COPD potential role in disease progression. *Chest.* 140,1540-9.

[30] Beamish, L. A., Osornio-Vargas, A. R., Wine, E., (2011). Air pollution: An environmental factor contributing to intestinal disease. *J. Crohns. Colitis.* 5, 279-86.

[31] Kim, C., Jung, S. H., Kang, D. R., Kim, H. C., Moon, K. T., Hur, N. W., Shin, D. C., Suh, I. , (2010). Ambient particulate matter as a risk factor for suicide. *Am. J. Psychiat.* 167, 1100-7.

[32] Whitsel, E. A., Quibrera, P. M., Christ, S. L., Liao, D., Prineas, R. J., Anderson, G. L., Heiss, G., (2009). Heart Rate Variability, Ambient Particulate Matter Air Pollution, and Glucose Homeostasis: The Environmental Epidemiology of Arrhythmogenesis in the Women's Health Initiative. *Am. J. Epidemiol.* 169, 693-703.

[33] Huang, Y. C., Rappold, A. G., Graff, D. W., Ghio, A. J., Devlin, R. B., (2012). Synergistic effects of exposure to concentrated ambient fine pollution particles and nitrogen dioxide in humans. *Inhal. Toxicol.* 24, 790-7.

[34] Bishop, E., Theophilus, E. H., Fearon, I. M., (2012). In vitro and clinical studies examining the expression of osteopontin in cigarette smoke-exposed endothelial cells and cigarette smokers. *BMC. Cardiovasc. Disord.* 12, 75.

[35] Sacks, J. D., Stanek, L. W., Luben, T. J., Johns, D. O., Buckley, B. J., Brown, J. S., Ross, M., (2011). Particulate matter-induced health effects: who is susceptible?. *Environ. Health. Perspect.* 119, 446-54.

[36] Mo, Y., Wan, R., Wang, J., Chien, S., Tollerud, D. J., Zhang, Q., (2009). Diabetes is associated with increased sensitivity of alveolar macrophages to urban particulate matter exposure. *Toxicology.* 262, 130-7.

In: Sudden Death
Editors: Jiashin Wu and Jessica Wu
ISBN: 978-1-62618-825-9

Chapter XII

Biochemical, Cytological and Histopathological Examination of Sudden Unexpected Death in Infancy

Iwao Emura[*]
Department of Surgical Pathology, Japanese Red Cross Nagaoka Hospital, Niigata Prefecture, Japan

Abstract

We reported that scavenger receptor A (SRA) positive cells and neutrophils in peripheral blood (PB) might play an important role in the development of multiple organ injury. SRA^+ cells also increased in PB of autopsy cases with sudden unexpected death in infancy (SUDI) and sudden deaths (SD) in those over 1 year of age. To evaluate the pathophysiologic mechanisms underlying sudden infant death syndrome (SIDS), 4 SUDI and 3 SD cases were examined.

Cases were classified into Group A and B. Numerous platelet emboli were extensively distributed in both ventricular walls in group A, but small in number in group B. Contraction band necrosis were very small in number in group A, but were large in group B. Many neutrophils were accumulated in capillaries, and capillary endothelial cells were injured extensively in both groups. There were minute foci of alveolar epithelial cell injury (MFAECI) where alveolar epithelial cells had disappeared from the surface of the alveoli with intra-alveolar edema fluid and cell debris. These foci were juxtaposed next to normal lung tissue without an intervening transitional zone, and scattered in all lobes.

[*] Address for corresponding author: Iwao Emura MD, Department of Surgical Pathology, Japanese Red Cross Nagaoka Hospital, 2-297-1 Sensyuu Nagaoka city, Niigata Prefecture, 940-2085, Japan; emura@nagaoka.jrc.or.jp.

Neutrophils were accumulated mainly in capillaries, and various sized emboli of platelet aggregates were observed in group A. Gram positive cocci were detected in pulmonary tissue of all cases.

Large numbers of platelet aggregates were presented in PB of group A. Increase of SRA^+ cell and presence of TNF-α^+ cell in PB were confirmed in all cases.

All cases had M-CSF, IL-6, IL-8, TNF-α, and IL-1β levels above the normal threshold.

We considered the mechanisms underlying the death of our cases as follows. 1) SRA^-monocytes differentiated into SRA^+ cells by the stimulation of microbes translocated into PB via MFAECI. 2) Abnormalities of cytokines induced by SAR^+ cells in PB played an important role on the development of organ injury. 3) Platelet emboli or contraction band necrosis were the leading causes of death.

All our present SUDI cases seemed not to satisfy the diagnostic criteria of SIDS since pathological findings of the heart were thought to be leading causes of death. However, Patients similar to our SUDI cases were considered to be included in SIDS.

Introduction

Sudden unexpected death in infancy (SUDI) is defined as the sudden death of an apparently healthy infant aged <1 year (usually 7-365 days). In some, the autopsy determines a cause of death (explained SUDI), whereas in most, a definite cause of death cannot be found (unexplained SUDI); following current autopsy protocols, almost two-thirds of SUDI remain unexplained[1], most being synonymous with sudden infant death syndrome (SIDS)[2]. Recently, new hypotheses that inflammatory responses (such as overwhelming pro-inflammatory response) [3-5] are underlying mechanism in SIDS have been proposed.

We previously reported that scavenger receptor A positive (SRA^+) cells in peripheral blood (PB) might play an important role in the development of multiple organ injury [6]. As a result of examining autopsy cases of SUDI and of sudden deaths (SD) in those over 1 year of age, we noticed that SRA^+ cells increased in PB. To the best of our knowledge, there are no published data on the significance of SRA^+ cells in PB of SUDI. We thus decided to explore the significance of SRA^+ cells in PB to understand the pathophysiological mechanisms of SIDS.

Study Subjects

Four SUDI patients (cases 1 to 4) and 4 SD patients were drawn from 419 autopsy cases from 1999 to 2009 (Table 1). All subjects showed normal growth and development after birth, and they had no similar deaths in their siblings or relatives. A history of a mild common cold preceded death in 4 cases.

Bloody oronasal secretions were observed in 2 cases at autopsy. All infants appeared normal and healthy when they were put to bed, but they died quietly in their sleep. The clinical diagnoses of cases 1 to 5 were SIDS, and those of cases 6, 7 and 8 were SD. The central nervous systems of cases 4, 7 and 8 were not examined.

Table 1. Clinical findings in patients with sudden unexplained death in infancy and sudden deaths

case	Sex	Age	C.D.	Fatal episode	G.A.(W)	Growth	Com. cold	Secretion
1	Male	4M	SIDS	During sleep	34	Normal	(-)	(-)
2	Female	4M	SIDS	During sleep	37	Normal	(-)	(+)
3	Male	5M	SIDS	During sleep	39	Normal	(+)	(-)
4	Female	9M	SIDS	During sleep	40	Normal	(+)	(-)
5	Female	1Y	SIDS	During sleep	38	Normal	(-)	(+)
6	Female	2Y	SD	During sleep	40	Normal	(+)	(-)
7	Male	3Y	SD	During sleep	40	Normal	(+)	(-)
8	Male	3Y	SD	During sleep	40	Normal	(-)	(-)

Footnotes: M; month, Y; year, C.D.; clinical diagnosis, SIDS; sudden infant death syndrome, SD; sudden death, G.A.(W); Gestational age (week), Com.cold; Common cold.

Tissue Processing and Histopathological Procedure

Autopsy was performed 2 or 3 hours after death. Organs were fixed in 10 % neutral formalin, embedded in paraffin, and examined using hematoxylin and eosin (HE), the reticulin silver impregnation method, elastica van Gieson, and phosphotungstic acid hematoxylin (PTAH) sections.

Cytological Methods

PBs obtained from the right atrium at autopsy were examined. Cord blood from 24 placentas (gestational age of ≧37 weeks) were examined as a control of cytological and immunocytochemical examination of SRA^+ cells in PB, since we could not obtained PB from the age-matched healthy babies. All PB were collected into tubes containing EDTA (Vacutainer plastic, EDTA 2K; Becton Dickinson, Franklin Lakes NJ, USA). I believe that the method of cytological examination of peripheral blood is my original method [7]. Briefly, red blood cells were lysed with lysing reagent (826 mg of NH_4CL + 3.7 mg of EDTA-4Na + 100 mg of $KHCO_3$ in 100 ml H_2O), then nucleated cells were suspended in isotonic sodium chloride solution, and the suspensions containing about $5x10^6$ nucleated cells were smeared on glass slides using Auto smear CF-12 (Sakura Seiki, Tokyo, Japan). Cells that did not adhere to the glass slides were gently washed away with 95% ethanol solution. Smear preparations were fixed in 95% ethanol solution and stained with the Papanicolaou method. Smear preparation of PB is shown in Figure 6a. About one million and two hundred thousand nucleated cells were smeared in one slide. Nucleated cells are smeared evenly and precise nuclear structures are excellently preserved. About one thousand nucleated cells were observed in one high power field (×400).

Immunohistochemical and -cytochemical Examination

Papanicolaou-stained smears and paraffin sections were used for the examination, which was performed with the simple stain MAX-PO method (Nichirei Co., Tokyo, Japan) and with diaminobenzidine as the chromogen using mouse monoclonal anti-human glycoprotein 1b (CD42b, a platelet marker, 1:100; Novo Castra, Newcastle upon Tyne, UK), mouse monoclonal anti-human 3-Fucosyl-N-acetyllacetosamine (CD15, a neutrophil marker, 1:100; Novo Castra), mouse monoclonal anti-human keratin (AE1/AE3, an epithelial cell marker1:150, DAKO USA, Carpinteria, CA, USA), mouse monoclonal anti-human transmembrane glycoprotein (CD34, an endothelial cell marker, Immunotech, Marseille, France), mouse monoclonal anti-human tumor necrosis factor (TNF)-α (1:100; Abcam, Cambridge, UK), mouse monoclonal anti-human surfactant apoprotein A (1:100 DAKO Japan, Kyoto, Japan) and mouse monoclonal anti-human SRA (CD204, a macrophage SRA marker, 1:200; Trans Genic Inc., Kumamoto, Japan) antibodies. An antigen retrieval method using citrate buffer and microwave heating was employed for all antibodies. As a negative control, the primary antibody was substituted by phosphate-buffered saline, and a positive stain was not observed in these controls.

Cytokine Test of PB

PB obtained from the right atrium was collected into Venoject II tubes (TERUMO, Tokyo, Japan), and centrifuged as soon as possible. Plasma components were stored at – 80°C until analysis. We used the following parameters, reference values, and measurement methods: serum interleukin (IL)-1β, <0.928 pg/ml, (human IL-1β enzyme- linked immunosorbent assay: ELISA kit), macrophage colony stimulating factor (M-CSF), 362−515 pg/ml, (human M-CSF ELISA kit), tumor necrosis factor (TNF)-α, <1.79 pg/ml, (human TNF-α chemiluminescent ELISA kit) and IL-6, <2.41 pg/ml (human IL-6 chemiluminescent ELISA, kit), all from R&D Systems (Minneapolis MN, USA), and IL-8, <8.0pg/ml, (enzyme amplified sensitivity immunoassay: EASIA, human EASIA kit, BioSourcs Europe S.A. Nivelles, Belgium).

Definitions

SRA^+ cells in PB that were over twice as large as monocytes were defined as large SRA^+ cells. SRA^+ cells in PB that were smaller than large SRA^+ cells were defined as small SRA^+ cells. The SRA index was defined as the number of small SRA^+ cells in 10 high power fields (×400). The number of large SRA^+ cells was defined as the number of large SRA^+ cells on one slide. Based on the SRA index of apparently healthy people in their 20s, we temporarily set the normal upper limit of the SRA index at 30[8]. We examined the number of necrotic cardiac myocytes in 1 cm^2 of a PTAH section. When necrotic cardiac myocytes were observed as a small group and the exact number could not be counted, we described this as "many".

The following criteria were used to define injured capillary, platelet thrombus and platelet aggregate: injured capillaries, if the tube-like structure of the capillary was destroyed; platelet thrombi or emboli, aggregate of platelets that plugged capillary or small vessels; aggregate of platelets in PB, aggregation of platelets that was over twice as large as that of neutrophils. We examined the number of injured capillaries and platelet thrombi or emboli in 10 high power fields (×400), and that of platelet aggregates in PB on one slide. When capillaries were severely injured and the exact number could not be counted, we described this as "many."

Histopathological Findings

All subjects had a normal nutritional status with no underlying dysmorphism or injuries. The results of histopathological examinations are shown in Table 2. Cases were classified into 2 groups according to the pathological findings of the heart (Group A: case 1, 2, 3, and Group B: case 4, 5, 7, 8). Renal tubular necrosis and necrosis of hepatocytes were observed in 1 and 3 cases. Severe respiratory syncytial virus infection was confirmed as the leading cause of death in case 6.

Table 2. Pathological and cytological findings

Case	Lung		Heart			PB		
	Mic.Organism	Patho.	Inj. Capi.	E. Pl.	CBN	SRA index	L SRA$^+$ C	Pl. Agg.
1	G+ cocci	MFAECI+LSDAD	many	187	< 1	35	171	283
2	G+ cocci	MFAECI+LSDAD	many	231	< 1	67	495	138
3	G+ cocci	MFAECI+LSDAD	many	204	< 1	318	1178	264
4	G+ cocci	MFAECI	many	7	52	795	483	2
5	G+ cocci	MFAECI	many	12	many	54	483	5
6	RSV	RVS	many	46	< 1	675	0	69
7	G+ cocci	MFAECI+LSDAD	many	20	many	318	92	1
8	G+ cocci	MFAECI	many	37	many	ND	ND	ND
Control	ND	ND	ND	ND	ND	1-19	0	0-10

Footnote: PB: Perioheral blood, Mic.organism; Micro organism, Patho.; Pathology, Inj. Capi; Injured capillary, E.PL; Emboli of platelet aggregates, CBN; Contraction band necrosis, SRA; Scavenger receptor A, L SRA$^+$ C; Large scavenger receptor A$^+$ cell, Pl. Agg.; Platelet aggregate, G+ cocci: Gram positive cocci, RSV; Respiratory syncytial virus, MFAECI; Minute focus of alveolar epithelial injury, LSDAD; Less severe diffuse alveolar damage, ND; No data.

Heart

Macroscopically, no abnormalities were found.

Group A: No conspicuous pathological findings were found under low magnifications except for congestion and edema (Figure 1a). However, careful examination revealed numerous platelet emboli or thrombi in capillaries of both ventricular walls (Figure 1b, 1c). Contraction band necrosis was very small in number (Figure 1d).

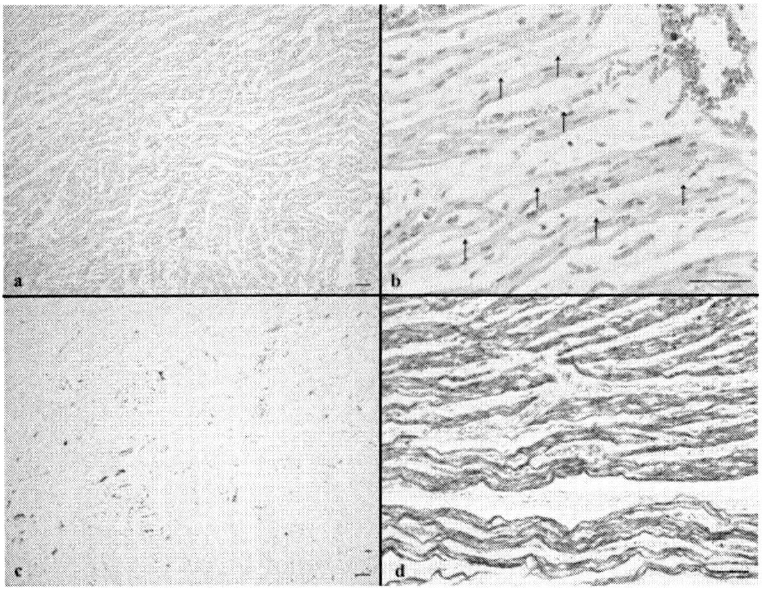

Figure 1. Histopathological findings of heart of group A patients. a) No conspicuous pathological findings are found under low magnifications except for congestion and edema. B) Numerous platelet emboli are extensively distributed in capillaries of both ventricular walls (arrows). C) Numerous platelet thrombi or emboli (brown). d: Contraction band necrosis are very small in number. Hematoxylin and eosin stain (a, b), phosphotungstic acid hematoxylin (d), Immunohistochemistry for CD42b (c). Bar, 50 μm (a~d).

Group B: Similarly, no conspicuous pathological findings were found under low magnifications (Figure 2a). However, numerous small groups of contraction band necrosis were observed with high magnification, and were extensively distributed in both ventricular walls (Figure 2b, 2d). Platelet emboli or thrombus were very small in number (Figure 2c).

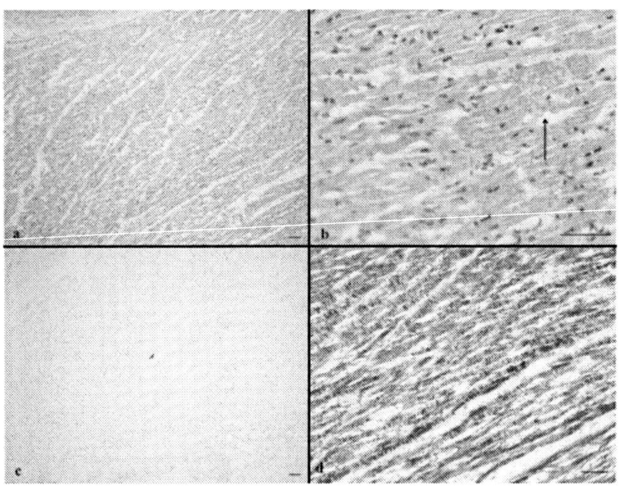

Figure 2. Histopathological findings of heart of group B patients. A) No conspicuous pathological findings are found under low magnifications. B) Small group of contraction band necrosis (arrow). C) Platelet emboli or thrombus are very small in number . d: Numerous small groups of contraction band necrosis. Hematoxylin and eosin stain (a, b), phosphotungstic acid hematoxylin (d), Immunohistochemistry for CD42b (c). Bar, 50 μm (a~d).

Many neutrophils were accumulated in capillaries among cardiac myocytes (Figure 3a), and capillaries were injured extensively in both groups (Figure 3b).

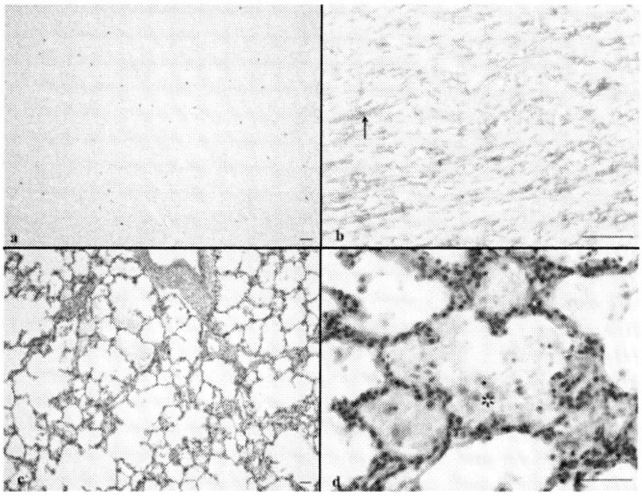

Figure 3. Histopathological findings of heart and lung. A) Many neutrophils are accumulated in capillaries among cardiac myocytes (Brown). B) Capillaries are injured extensively and only one nearly normal capillary is observed (arrow). C) Pulmonary congestion and edema are observed in all cases. d: A minute foci of alveolar epithelial cell injury (⁎). Hematoxylin and eosin stain (c, d), Immunohistochemistry for CD15 (a), CD34 (b). Bar, 50 μm (a~d).

Lung

Pulmonary congestion and edema were observed in all cases (Figure 3c).

There were minute foci of alveolar epithelial cell injury (MFAECI) where alveolar epithelial cells had disappeared from the surface of the alveoli with intra-alveolar edema fluid, and cytokeratin positive cell debris in case 1-5, 7, and 8 (Figure 3d, 4b). These foci were juxtaposed next to normal lung tissue without an intervening transitional zone, and scattered in all lobes (Figure 4a).

Besides of MFAECI, alveolar epithelial cells are fragmented, and congestion, slight extravasation, interstitial and intra alveolar edema are observed in cases 1, 2, 3, 7 (Figure 4c, 4d). Hyaline membranes, the histologic hallmark of the acute stage of diffuse alveolar damage (DAD), were not observed. These lesions were widely spread in lung. Similar pulmonary findings were detected in MODS cases and classified as less severe form of DAD induced by cytokine abnormality [6]. Because of the hisopathological similarities, the present pulmonary lesion was considered to be same lesion as less severe form of DAD observed in MODS patients.

Neutrophils were accumulated mainly in capillaries of all cases (Figure 5a), and various sized emboli of platelet aggregates or platelet thrombi were extensively observed in case 1, 2, and 3 (Figure 5b). Very mild aspiration (Figure 5c) and Gram positive cocci (Figure 5d) were detected in pulmonary tissue of cases 1-5 and 7, 8, but inflammatory cell reaction was hardly observed.

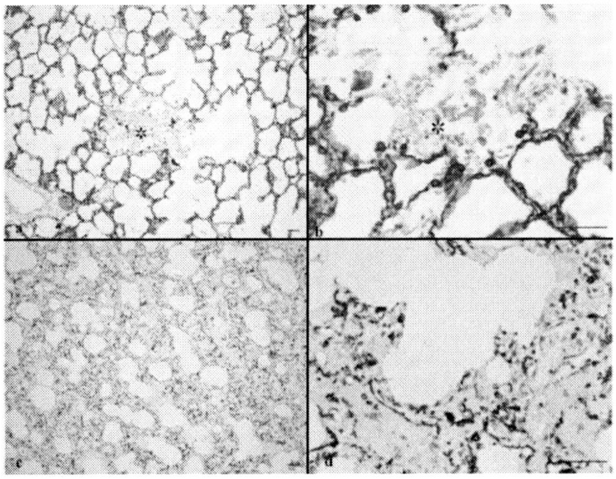

Figure 4. Histopathological findings of lungs. a, b) Minute foci of alveolar epithelial cell injury (*) in nearly normal lung tissue. These foci are juxtaposed next to normal lung tissue without an intervening transitional zone (a), and alveolar epithelial cells have disappeared from the surface of the alveoli with intra-alveolar edema fluid, and cytokeratin positive cell debris (b). c, d: Less severe form of diffuse alveolar damage. These lesions are widely spread in lung (c),and alveolar epithelial cells are fragmented, and congestion, slight extravasation, interstitial and intraalveolar edema are observed (d). Immunohistochemistry for AE1/AE3. 5 (a~d). Bar, 50 μm (a~d).

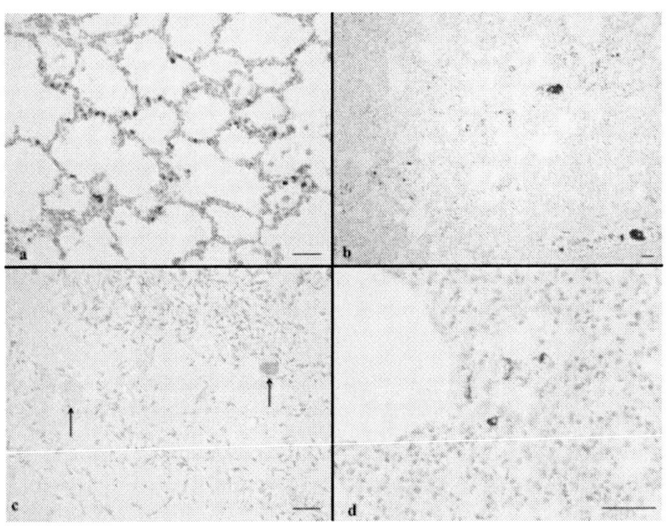

Figure 5. Histopathological findings of lungs. A) Neutrophils are accumulated mainly in capillaries of all cases. B) various sized emboli of platelet aggregates or platelet thrombi are extensively observed. c: Very mild aspiration (arrow). D: Gram positive cocci. Immunohistochemistry for and CD15 (a), CD42b (b). Hematoxylin and eosin stain (c) and Gram stain (d). Bar, 50 μm (a~d).

Cytological Findings of PB

About 1.2×10^6 nucleated cells are evenly smeared in a $1.4 \times 1.4\ cm^2$ area (Figure 6a). The SRA index and the number of aggregates of platelets of 24 control cases ranged from 1 to

19 (mean±SD= 4.9±5.6) and 0 to 10 (mean±SD=2.5±2.6) respectively. Large SRA^+ cells and TNF-α^+ cells were not observed in control cases (Table 2). The SRA index exceeded 30 in all examined cases and large SRA^+ cells were detected in cases 1 to 5 and 7 (Figure 6b). TNF-α-positive cells were detected in all examined cases (Figure 6c). Large numbers of platelet aggregates were presented in cases 1, 2 and 3 (Figure 6d).

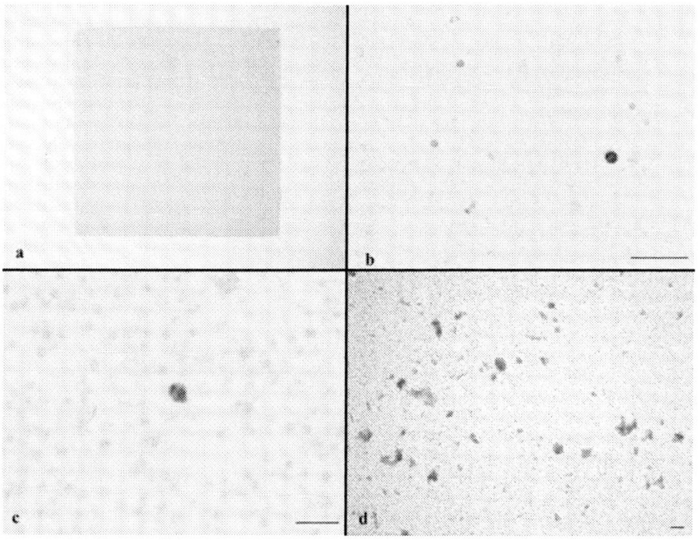

Figure 6. Cytological findings of peripheral blood. A) About 1.2×10^6 nucleated cells are evenly smeared in 1.4×1.4 cm^2. b: Small and large scavenger receptor A positive cells (Brown). c: A tumor necrosis factor-α positive cell (Brown) d: aggregates of platelets in peripheral blood. Papanicolaou stain (a, d), Immunohistochemistry for scavenger receptor A (b), and tumor necrosis factor-α (c). Bar, 50 μm (b, d) and 30 μm (c).

Cytokine Levels

All examined cases had M-CSF, IL-6, IL-8, TNF-α, and IL-1β levels above the normal threshold (Table 3).

Differentiation of SRA^+ Cells in PB

In spite of above mentioned abnormalities of SRA^+ cells and cytokines, all SUDI subjects had no underlying foci of infection or large focus of injury such as trauma. SRA^+ macrophages are known to arise from SRA^- monocytes. SRA^- monocytes became positive for SRA after 5 days in culture with M-CSF[9], and had differentiated into large macrophages by 10 days [10]. Recent retrospective studies typically pathogenic bacteria in normally sterile sites of infants succumbing to SUDI [11, 12], and a proportion of SUDI might be triggered by bacteraemia [13]. We did not examine pathogenic bacteria in PB at autopsy. However Gram-positive cocci were detected in the lungs of 7 cases.

Table 3. Cytokine levels

	IL1-β	IL-6	IL-8	TNF-α	M-CSF
1	ND	ND	ND	ND	ND
2	21.1	90.4	57.5	2.14	31800
3	3.5	855	36.3	2.67	13400
4	ND	ND	ND	ND	ND
5	3.2	6900	2690	5.58	6590
6	ND	ND	ND	ND	ND
7	17.2	319	688	9.36	7730
8	2.9	330	23.8	2.61	4740

Footnote: IL: Interleukin, TNF: Tumor necrosis factor, M-CSF: macrophage colony stimulating factor, ND; No data.

SRA index more than 30, and presence of large SRA^+ cells and TNF-α^+ cells were observed in all examined cases with MFAECI. All examined cases had M-CSF levels above the normal threshold. Some of the particles or solutes from particles may reach the lymphatics or the blood stream and invoke systemic responses [14]. Increase of MFAECI is increase of injured alveolar epithelial cells, and is a severe insult. Systemic inflammatory response is induced by insult [15]. From these data, we considered the mechanisms underlying SRA^+ cell differentiation and cytokine production as follows. 1) Translocation of microbes or solutes from microbes in PB or injury of alveolar epithelial cells induced production of M-CSF. 2) SRA^-monocytes were stimulated by M-CSF and differentiated into small and large SRA^+ cells. 3) A large number of cytokines were abruptly released into the systemic circulation from these SRA^+ cells.

Pathogenesis of SIDS

Although the pathological findings and degree of organ injury in MODS[6] were somewhat different from those in the present SUDI cases, accumulation of neutrophils mainly in capillaries, increase of SRA^+ cells and appearance of TNF-α^+ cells in PB, and abnormally high levels of IL-1β, IL-6, IL-8, TNF-α and M-CSF were observed both in the MODS[6] cases and present SUDI cases. Platelet emboli or thrombi were observed in lungs and heart of all cases, and many contraction band necrosis and less severe form of DAD were observed in 4 of 8 and 4 of 8 examined cases respectively, and renal tubular necrosis and necrosis of hepatocytes were observed in 1 and 3 cases. Therefore, pathology of our present cases was considered to be multiple organ injury. Multiple organ injury is caused by an imbalance of pro-inflammatory (such as IL-1β, IL-6, IL-8 and THF-α etc.) and anti-inflammatory mediators [16, 17]. From these findings, pathophysiological substrate of the present SUDI was considered to be common in the MODS[6], and abnormalities of cytokines induced by SRA^+ cells in PB were considered to play an important role on the development of multiple organ injury in the present SUDI cases.

Pulmonary congestion and intra-alveolar edema were observed in all of our cases. Congestion and edema were commonly present in SIDS cases, and these changes were considered to represent agonal events [18]. However, MFAECI were scattered in all lobes, and less severe form of DAD was observed in 4 of 8 cases. Numerous platelet emboli or thrombi were diffusely observed. We therefore considered that congestion and intra-alveolar edema represented alveolar epithelial cell injury, inflammatory lung injury and/or circulation disturbance. MFAECI and less severe form of DAD were microscopically similar to each other, but were different in distribution pattern. We therefore could not determine whether the MFAECI of the present SUDI were a result of systemic cytokine abnormalities or not.

Leading Cause of Death

Numerous emboli of platelet aggregates were detected in 3 of 4 SUDI cases (Case 1-4). Many platelet aggregates were observed in PB of these 3 cases, so most of these platelet aggregates in capillaries were thought to be emboli. These aggregates were considered to be formed as a result of systemic inflammation, since systemic inflammation results in activation of coagulation due to tissue factor-mediated thrombin generation [19].

To the best of our knowledge, there has been only one paper on the contraction band necrosis in SIDS [20]. However, numerous contraction band necrosis were observed in 1 SUDI and 3 of 4 SD cases. Numerous contraction band necrosis were observed in MODS patients. Distribution pattern and microscopical findings of contraction band necrosis of our present cases were quite similar to those of MODS cases. Therefore we surmised these contraction band necrosis were developed as a result of capillary injury and platelet emboli or thrombi induced by cytokine abnormality.

The number of platelet emboli or contraction band necrosis was so large in number that cardiac failure induced by these emboli or contraction band necrosis was considered to be the leading cause of death of our SUDI and SD cases. Severe respiratory syncytial virus infection was considered to be the principal cause of death of case 6. Emboli of platelet aggregates were observed mainly in cases under 1 year of age, and contraction band necrosis in cases over 1 year. Further studies are necessary to clarify whether this trend is repeated in most SUDI and SD cases.

SIDS and Our Present Cases

All our present SUDI cases seemed not to satisfy the diagnostic criteria of SIDS since pathological findings of the heart were thought to be leading causes of death. However, the biochemical, cytological, immunocytochemical and immunohistochemical studies in our present examination were not performed in the previous papers[21, 22, 23]. Therefore, we believe that 1. Cases 1 to 4 may be classified as SIDS if sufficient examination is not performed, 2. Patients with similar histopathological findings may be included in SIDS, and 3. Cytokine abnormality may be one of the underlying mechanisms in SIDS.

References

[1] Weber MA, Ashworth MT, Risdon RA et al. The role of post-mortem investigations in determining the cause of sudden unexpected death in infancy (SUDI). Arch Dis Child 2008;93:1048-53.

[2] Krous HF, Beckwith JB, Byard RW, et al. Sudden infant death syndrome and unclassified sudden infant death: a definition and diagnostic approach. Pediatrics 2004; 114: 234-8.

[3] Vege A, Rognum TO. Sudden infant death syndrome, infection and inflammatory response. *FEMS Immunol Med Microbiol* 2004;42:3-10.

[4] Goldwater PN. SIDS pathogenesis: pathological findings indicate infection and inflammatory responses are involved. *FEMS Immunol Med Microbiol* 2004;42:11-20.

[5] Blood-Siegfried J, Rambaud C, Nyska A, Germolec D. Evidence for infection, inflammation and shock in sudden infant death: parallels between a neonatal rat model of sudden death and infants who died of sudden infant death syndrome. *Innate Immun* 2008;14:145-52.)

[6] Emura I, Usuda H. Histological and cytological examination of autopsy cases with multiple organ dysfunction syndromes. *Pathology International* 2010;60:443-451.

[7] Emura I. High incidence of apoptosis in peripheral blood of myelodysplastic

[8] syndrome patients determined by Papanicolaou-stained preparations. *Laboratory Hematology* 2003;9:42-6.

[9] Emura I, Usuda H, Fujita T, et al. Increase of scavenger receptor A-positive monocytes in patients with coronary syndromes. *Pathology International* 2007;57:502-8.

[10] Naito M, Kodama T, Matsumoto A, Doi T, Takahashi K. Tissue distribution, intracellular localization, and in Vitro expression of Bovine macrophage scavenger receptor. *Am J Pathol* 1991;139:1411-23.

[11] Young DA, Lowe LD, Clark SC. Comparison of the effects of IL-3, granulocyte-macrophage colony- stimulating factor, and macrophage colony-stimulating factor in supporting monocytes differentiation in culture. *J Immunol* 1990;145:607-15.

[12] Weber MA, Klein NJ, Hartley JC, Lock PE, Malone M, Sebire NJ. Infection and sudden unexpected death in infancy : a systematic retrospective case review. *Lancet* 2008;371:1848-53.

[13] Goldwater P. Sterile site infection at autopsy in sudden unexpected deaths in infancy. *Arch Dis Child* 2009;94:303-7.

[14] Highet AR, Berry AM, Goldwater PN. Novel hypothesis for unexplained sudden unexpected death in infancy (SUDI). *Arch Dis Child* 2009;94:841-3.

[15] Borm PJ. Particle toxicology: from coal mining to nanotechnology. *Inhal Toxicol* 2002;14:311-24.

[16] American College of Chest physicians/Society of Critical Care Medicine Consensus Conference: Definitions for sepsis and organ failure and guidelines for the use of innovative therapies in sepsis. Crit Care Med 1992;20:864-874.

[17] Bone RC, Grodzin CJ, Balk RA. Sepsis: A new hypothesis for pathogenesis of the disease process. *Chest* 1997;112:235-43.

[18] Ware LB. Pathophysiology of acute lung injury and the acute respiratory distress syndrome. *Semin Respir Crit Care Med* 2006;27:337-49.

[19] Thompson MW, Hunt CE. Control of breathing: development, apnea of prematurity, apparent life-threatening events, SIDS. In: MacDonald MG, Mullett MD, Seshia MMK, editors. *Avery's neonatology: pathophysiology and management of the newborn.* 6th ed. Philadelphia: Lippincott Williams & Wilkins; 2005. p535-52.

[20] Levi M, Keller TT, van Gorp E, and ten Cate H. Infection and inflammation and coagulation system. *Cardiovascular Research* 2003;60:26-39.

[21] Kariks J. Cardiac lesions in sudden infant death syndrome. *Forensic Sci Int* 1988; 39:211-225.

[22] Berry PJ. Pathological findings in SIDS. *J Clin Pathol* 1992;45(Suppl 11):11-16.

[23] Krous HF. Sudden infant death syndrome: Pathology and pathophysiology. *Pathol Annu* 1984;19Pt 1:1-14.

[24] Valdes-Dapena M. The sudden infant death syndrome: pathologic findings. *Clin Perinatol* 1992;19:701-716.

In: Sudden Death
Editors: Jiashin Wu and Jessica Wu
ISBN: 978-1-62618-825-9

Chapter XIII

Diagnostic Efficacy of Biochemical Markers in Sudden Cardiac Death

Esperanza Navarro Escayola*
Forensic Doctor, Head of Toxicology Department,
Institute of Legal Medicine, Alicante, Spain

Abstract

Sudden unexpected death is one of the main topics in forensic pathology, largely due to its rapid development and the effects of cellular autolysis. Several studies have investigated the use of biochemical assays for serum cardiac markers as a complement to the histological study of the heart, including the investigation of different fluids preserved from hemolitical processes, such as pericardial fluid, cerebrospinal fluid, vitreous humor, and so on.The aim of this paper is to review published studies of postmortem cardiac markers in different fluids and their application to the study of sudden cardiac death.

Introduction

Sudden cardiac death is one of the first causes of natural death in industrialized countries. It mainly stems from coronary pathology and, specifically, from coronary atheromatosis disease, whose frequency increases with the age of the deceased.

At times, the speed of the onset of the symptomatology can affect the development of the necrosis and tissue repair phenomena that characterize myocardial infarction. This process interferes with the postmortem diagnosis, making it one of the most difficult problems to resolve in legal medical autopsies.

* Correspondence with Author: Esperanza Navarro Escayola C/ Radiofonista Raúl Álvarez Antón nº2 escalera 5 2º Dcha. (03005) Alicante, España. Telephone: 965126616; 606749415; Fax: 965935827; E-mail: enavarro@infomed.es.

Establishing a conclusive diagnosis is not always easy, above all in cases of cardiac diseases that cause sudden death but occur without coronary artery disease [17].

To complement the diagnosis of sudden cardiac death, in forensic medicine the use of biochemical markers of myocardial necrosis has been proposed, along with the histopathological study of the heart.

The search for a specific and early molecular marker of myocardial ischemic damage is an objective that has been pursued by forensic pathology research, as in cadaveric specimens the results are generally limited by the autolytic phenomena produced after death. These phenomena influence the sensitivity and specificity of the markers commonly used in clinical practice, reducing their diagnostic efficacy when compared to their clinical performance.

The biochemical markers of myocardial necrosis applied in clinical practice, such as myoglobin, creatine kinase (CK-MB) and troponin, have also been used in forensic samples. New markers have also been tried out, such as the natriuretic peptides, which are used in the clinic to study heart failure.

This chapter will provide a review of different studies published on the use of postmortem markers of heart damage in different fluids, and their usefulness in the study of sudden cardiac death.

Biochemical Markers of Cardiac Damage

Biochemical markers play a principal role in the diagnosis and treatment of patients with Acute Coronary Syndrome, as has been demonstrated by the incorporation of cardiac troponins in the new protocols for the treatment of patients with Acute Coronary Syndrome and in the redefinition of myocardial infarction. (AMI) [4,51].

In the case of cell injury necrosis, there is a loss of the integrity of the cell membrane, causing a release of its constituents. Particles dissolved in the cytoplasm and of a reduced size are the ones that more easily access the circulation; they are, therefore, the earliest markers of cell damage. If this damage continues, from the injured cell there will be a release of cytoplasmatic macromolecules of greater cardio-specificity, such as myglobin or creatine kinase. Finally, structural molecules such as troponin will spread first to the interstitium and then through lymphatic vessels and capillaries to the peripheral circulation, where they can be detected.

The World Health Organization (WHO) has defined AMI based on the presence of two of three diagnostic criteria, which are:

- An appropriate clinical presentation,
- Typical changes in the electrocardiogram, and
- An increase in the levels of cardiac enzymes

However, since the year 2000, the joint *European Society of Cardiology (ESC)* and *American College of Cardiology (ACC) Committee* has published their consensual recommendations for the new Universal definition of Myocardial infarction [4,51]. According to this document, the diagnosis of AMI requires an increase and decrease in the indicators for myocardial necrosis markers (troponin), with at least a value above the 99th percentile as the upper limit of reference, along with at least one of the following criteria:

- Symptoms of ischemia,
- Development of pathological Q waves on the electrocardiogram
- Ischemic changes in the electrocardiogram
- Evidence by imaging of new loss of viable myocardia or the presence of a new abnormality in the regional contraction.

Although the WHO's definition makes it possible to diagnose a myocardial infarction in the absence of elevated biochemical markers, in the consensus document the ESC/ACC stipulates as a mandatory criterion that the biomarkers must be elevated and then show a decline in the appropriate clinical context.

The new consensus on the definition of Myocardial Infarction has placed the diagnosis in biochemical territory, a choice that was adopted after the appearance of the new markers of myocardial necrosis. Among them, the Troponins stand out, as they have been shown to have diagnostic specificity in cardiac injury. [20, 21].

This development is important because a significant proportion of patients with AMI present with atypical clinical symptomatology. On the other hand, although the usefulness of the electrocardiogram in the diagnosis of Acute Coronary Syndrome is indisputable, there are cases where patients have shown symptoms of ischemia without elevation of the ST segment of the electrocardiogram, but with positive results for cardiac troponins. These results have some clear therapeutic consequences, and they are of legal medical interest in the evaluation of sudden death situations with a normal electrocardiogram [7, 8].

From a clinical point of view, the ideal marker would fulfill the following characteristics [24]: High sensitivity or abundance in cardiac tissue; high specificity or absence in non myocardial tissue; rapid release, which would allow an early diagnosis, and a long half-life for a late diagnosis; moreover, it should also be a rapid, precise and low-cost technique.

Troponin

The troponin complex is a large globular protein located in the fine filament of the tropomyosin complex of the contractile cells. It is formed by three subunits (troponin T (TnT), troponin I (TnI) and troponin C (TnC), which are involved in the actomyosin interaction for muscle contraction.

The TnT is a 37.000 D molecule that fixes the tropomyosin. The TnI is a 23.000D molecule that inhibits the contraction of the myofibril at rest, by inhibiting the interaction of the actin with the myosin. The TnC is an 18.000D molecule that binds calcium, and it initiates the contraction after uniting with the calcium.

There are specific isoforms of TnT and TnI for the heart muscle (cTnT and cTnI), with an amino acid sequence that differs from that of non cardiac striated muscle. This permits the development of specific immunoassays.

In contrast to the myoglobin and the CK-MB [39], which are dissolved in the cellular cytoplasm, most of the troponin is attached structurally to the tropomyosin complex, although a small portion (6-8% of cTnT and 3-8% of cTnI) is also dissolved in the cellular cytoplasm. The molecular weight of the cardiac troponin is similar to that of the CK-MB. These factors suggest that, in spite of being a predominantly structural molecule, the cytoplasmatic fraction of troponin should be released as early as the CK-MB.

In a process of myocardial necrosis, the cardiac troponin is detected in the plasma from 4-6 hours after the onset of the symptoms, probably reflecting the early release of its cytoplasmatic component. The kinetics of the release of cTnT and cTnI are different. The cTnT reaches an initial maximum 12 hours after the symptoms, followed by a plateau and a gradual decline lasting up to 10 days. The cTnI presents a similar dynamic, but with a shorter return to normality time than that of the cTnT, although, as in the case of the cTnT, it depends on the extent of the AMI.

In addition to being more specific [23,52], both troponins have equal sensitivity and specificity, having been consolidated as high sensitivity markers in clinical practice for myocardial infarction and ischemic damage, being the biomarker of choice in these cases. One possible disadvantage of the troponin is its long half-life (10-14 days), which does not allow it to differentiate between a new infarction and an old one in this time frame. Due to its great specificity for myocardial tissue and its high sensitivity, the increase in its numbers may even reflect the presence of microscopic areas of myocardial necrosis [4, 8].

However, when applying troponin determination in the diagnosis of AMI, it is important to take into account that this marker reflects the presence of myocardial necrosis, but it does not provide information about its mechanism. Thus, a high value in the absence of obvious signs of ischemia makes it necessary to rule out other causes of cardiac injury. Many non ischemic, pathophysiological entities can cause myocardial necrosis and, consequently, elevations in the concentrations of serum cardiac Troponins [40].

The troponin elevation that occurs in cases of heart trauma, including cardiac contusion, is of great importance in forensic medicine, as has been demonstrated in several articles on this topic [1, 33, 42, 47]. Troponin elevation has also been shown in pathologies that lead to a terminal situation [3, 57] and in cases of generalized sepsis [48], which are all situations of interest in forensic investigation.

Creatine-Kinase (CK)

Creatine-kinase is an enzyme that plays an important role in transporting energy to the tissues by catalyzing a reaction of energy transference, the phosphorylation of creatine into creatine phosphate.

It is formed by two subunits (B and M) and its isoforms (BB, MM and MB). The mean concentrations of each of these isoforms vary greatly from some types of tissues to others, but the maximum concentration of CK-MB is found in the myocardium [23,24,26,39,52]. The appearance of CK-MB in serum, in the absence of muscle trauma, is indicative of cardiac damage and, more specifically, myocardial infarction. After an acute myocardial infarction, the CK-MB blood levels rise in the first 2-6 hours and peak at 24 hours. The CK-MB levels normalize two to three days after the episode [8,10,34-37,41].

Low levels of CK-MB are found in healthy people, limiting its specificity to myocardial necrosis, as it can also be elevated in cases of severe damage to skeletal muscles (myopathies, some neoplastic processes).

Until the introduction of troponins, it was the most widely-used marker in Acute Coronary Syndrome. However, due to its incomplete cardio-specificity, the new AMI definition requires that in the clinical context of coronary ischemia, at least one value of CK-MB should duplicate the upper reference limit, or two values should be above it [4].

Myoglobin

Myoglobin is the principal protein responsible for supplying oxygen to the striated muscle. It is a protein of low molecular weight (18kDa), located in the cytoplasm and found in both skeletal and heart muscle. Due to its low molecular weight and its abundance in muscle tissue, it is released quickly (even in the first hour) into the blood when there is myocardial damage. Therefore, myoglobin is the earliest among all the known markers, and its sensitivity is considered greater than that of the Troponins in the first hours after a myocardial infarction. However, its diagnostic value in acute myocardial infarction is limited by the short duration of its elevation, since it disappears from circulation in 12-24 hours due to its rapid renal clearance. Another factor worth mentioning is its lack of cardio-specificity, as there are no structural differences between the myoglobin released in the heart muscle and that of skeletal muscle.

Elevated myoglobin is also found in patients with renal failure, due to the decrease in its renal clearance.

The main use of myoglobin is based on its high sensitivity and negative predictive value in the first hours of the AMI[44].Consequently, by measuring the myoglobin, it is possible to rule out myocardial necrosis within the first 6 hours of the patient's admittance. However, its low cardio-specificity and rapid renal clearance make its positive predictive value quite low. [45] The characteristics of some of the most significant markers are shown in Table 1.

Table 1.

	Time of initial detection in plasma	Peak	Duration of the elevation
MYOGLOBIN	2-3 hours	6-12 hours	24-48 hours
CK-MB	2-6 hours	12-24 hours	2-3 days
TROPONIN T (cTnT)	4-6 hours	12-24 hours	7-10 days
TROPONIN I (cTnI)	4-6 hours	12-24 hours	6-8 days

Cardiac Natriuretic Peptides

New markers have been proposed for the diagnosis of impaired heart function in clinical practice, and they are a novelty compared to the traditional markers of myocardial ischemic injury: the natriuretic peptides [40].

Cardiac natriuretic peptides belong to the family of hormonal polypeptides that are synthesized, stored and secreted by the myocardial cells, presenting similarities in their peptide chains and their degradation pathways.

They include the arterial natriuretic peptide (ANP) and the type B natriuretic peptide (BNP) [14].

Both the ANP and BNP are derived from precursors, the pre-pro-hormones that contain a peptide signal sequence in the N-terminal extreme. These pro-hormones are subsequently split into an inactive N-terminal fragment and the biologically active hormonal peptide (NT-pro BNP and BNP) [11].

Whereas ANP is mainly secreted in the cardio-myocytes of the atrium, BNP is produced and secreted primarily in the left ventricle, although this might be a simplification, since the right cavities also synthesize and secrete BNP in pathological situations. The precise mechanisms that control the production and secretion of natriuretic peptides are still unclear, although ventricle distention and wall overload are likely to play important roles. [14].

It has been generally accepted that the plasma concentrations of these peptides increase in diseases characterized by volume expansion, such as renal failure, primary hyperaldosteronism and congestive heart failure. They also increase because of the stimulation of the production due to ventricle hypertrophy or dilatation, thyroid disease, excess circulating glucocorticoids, or hypoxia [12].

Plasma concentrations of BNP are affected by age, sex, renal failure and certain drugs, such as diuretics and beta blockers.

The determination of cardiac natriuretic peptides (especially BNP and Nt-ProBNP) has been proposed in the following situations [14]:

- Evaluation of patients with suspected heart failure.
- Prognostic classification of patients with Congestive Heart Failure
- Detection of left ventricle dysfunction, both systolic and diastolic.
- Differential diagnosis of dyspnea (differentiating the dyspnea of cardiac origin).

The concentration of NT-proBNP has also been seen to rise, even in greater quantities than the BNP, in cases of cardiac failure. This increase, coupled with its greater stability in circulating blood, is an advantage of the determination of NT-proBNP compared to BNP.

The elevation of the plasmatic concentrations of natriuretic peptides has been related to the risk of a myocardial infarction and death in apparently asymptomatic people [55]. Some authors have concluded that BNP is an independent predictor of death in patients with heart failure [50].

Hence, the *European Society of Cardiology* has proposed the incorporation of the natriuretic peptide determination in the first step of the evaluation of symptomatic patients in whom the presence of congestive heart failure is suspected [43].

The levels of BNP and Nt-ProBNP appear to have a prognostic value for long-term mortality when measured after an acute coronary accident, both in patients with ST segment elevation and in those without it, with elevation of the Troponin levels or with no modification in them, and with symptomatic or asymptomatic cardiac failure [54].

Therefore, in clinical practice the BNP peptide is a diagnostic tool that is being used more and more often as a marker for the presence of ventricular dysfunction in symptomatic and asymptomatic patients, and its concentration appears to be related to the severity of this alteration.

For this reason, many authors recommend its routine determination in heart failure patients, as a means of diagnostic confirmation in borderline cases, and as a way to assess the severity of the condition, the prognosis and the efficacy of the treatment.

Postmortem Study of Biochemical Markers of Cardiac Damage

The determination of myofibrillar proteins from the cardiac muscle in cadaveric tissues is not problem-free. The majority of authors warn about the problems arising from their use in postmortem diagnosis.

The blood from a cadaver is different from blood collected before death, due to the effects produced by the cessation of normal metabolism and excretion, autolysis, microbial degradation, etc. Hemolysis can occur hours after death, and hemoglobin can interfere in the analysis of biomarkers such as troponin, affecting the results [59]. For all of these reasons, some authors warn that these determinations should not be used to make diagnostic deductions about the cause of death when cadaveric blood is used [16], restricting their use to confirming the diagnosis of death due to cardiac causes only in certain cases.

The use of different biomarkers that can be useful in the diagnosis of sudden cardiac death has been tested in postmortem studies.

Likewise, different fluids have been tested, such as cerebrospinal fluid, pericardial fluid, and vitreous humor, in order to try to minimize the effects of autolysis in the determination of markers of myocardial damage in cadavers.

The ideal fluid must be one that is preserved for post mortal processes, without the presence of cellular elements in suspension, and with easy accessibility. Recently, Immunohistochemical techniques have been used for the diagnosis of acute myocardial damage in cadavers. For this purpose, different antigenic markers have been used (troponin, Myoglobin, CK), and results showed that the reduction in these cardiac markers can be detected in cardiac tissues before they are deposited in serum. Most of them can be visible even minutes after the onset of the symptoms. Although there is no single ideal marker for the diagnosis of acute myocardial ischemia, the combination of several of them has been used to detect the presence of ischemic areas when there is no macroscopic or microscopic evidence. However, it must be kept in mind that some factors, such as the phenomena surrounding the death or cardiopulmonary resuscitation, may affect the expression of each marker [9, 19, 27, 38].

Troponin

Although troponin is currently considered the most specific biomarker for the diagnosis of heart damage in clinical practice, the usefulness of the determination of Troponin in the diagnosis of cardiac death is disputed. Some authors have proposed its use as a test-type *Point-of-care* to be used even in cases of external examination of the body without a visceral study [10]. Other studies invoke its high specificity to defend its effective diagnostic role, although in no case can it replace performing a complete postmortem examination[18,41].

Although both troponins have equal sensitivity and specificity, some authors [23,52] have found that the determination of cTnI is the most suitable marker in patients with chronic renal failure or myopathies when myocardial damage is suspected.

Blood

Batalis et al. [6], using blood from different locations (blood from the left ventricle and right ventricle, aorta and femoral) from a sample of deaths due to myocardial infarction and a control group, found that results obtained for cTnI in femoral venous blood, although with significantly higher values, is the one that more closely approaches antemortem physiological levels, while blood from central locations, such as the aorta and both ventricles, obtains much higher values [60,61].

Survival time has a significant influence on the venous blood results for cTnT and cTnI, producing an increase in the values obtained when survival time increases. This increase is related to the severity of the morphological cardiac damage [42, 62].

In the laboratory of the Institute of Legal Medicine in Alicante, we performed a study on the utility of the use of various biomarkers of sudden cardiac death (troponin, myoglobin, and CK-MB) in peripheral blood samples (femoral) from 97 autopsies. In our study, as in the case of other authors [22], the average levels of cTnI were significantly higher in the groups with cardiac-produced death, thereby demonstrating its diagnostic utility in this type of deaths.

The sensitivity of the cTnI obtained for the cut-off value proposed for cases of death due to cardiac causes (0.74 ng/ml) was 73%, and the specificity was 70%, lower values than those obtained in clinical practice [32].

Our results show that, unlike what happens with CK-MB, whose values are influenced by the postmortem interval, the mean concentration of cTnI is not affected by the postmortem interval or by other parameters such as age or sex. These results coincide with those obtained by other authors in previous studies using this marker in blood from cadavers [2,28,29,35,37,41], but it differs from those obtained by Zhu et al. [60.61], who found higher values of cTnT when the postmortem interval increased. These authors found that this correlation was greater in the results obtained in blood from the right ventricle and pericardial fluid, while it was lower in peripheral blood. Zhu et al. [62] found that the cTnI/CK-MB ratio, in both cardiac blood and pericardial fluid, was not affected by the postmortem interval, and it had higher values in Myocardial Infarction, among others. Therefore, these authors say that this ratio can be used as an index for the existence of heart damage in these fluids, regardless of how much time has elapsed after death.

In our study, there were no significant variations in the presence of cardio-pulmonary resuscitation maneuvers, agreeing with findings published by Cina et al. [10.41].

The existence of a number of diseases that produce an elevation in the Troponin figures obliges the pathologist to determine whether the myocardial damage occurs in situations of acute myocardial ischemia and, therefore, leads to the diagnosis of AMI, or whether it has another cause instead [58].

Zhu et al. [60,61,62] observed elevated values of cTnT in hypothermia, electrocution[22] carbon monoxide poisoning, and methamphetamine intoxication, in the blood as well as in the pericardial fluid. This increase can be explained by the production of a diffuse cardiomyolysis. This damage to the membrane of the heart cells could be due to the systemic hypoxia that occurs during the period of agony.

Due to its importance in forensic medicine, it is worth highlighting the elevation that occurs in cases of heart trauma, including cardiac contusion, as has been pointed out in several articles on this topic [1,33,42,47].

In our experience, we found a significant elevation of cTnI in the group with severe thoracic trauma with cardiac contusion, which agrees with published works, thus limiting its diagnostic usefulness in these cases. Therefore, it would be advisable to use cTnI along with other markers that are not affected by this circumstance.

Different alternatives to blood fluids have been used to try to avoid factors such as hemolysis, which may affect the result obtained.

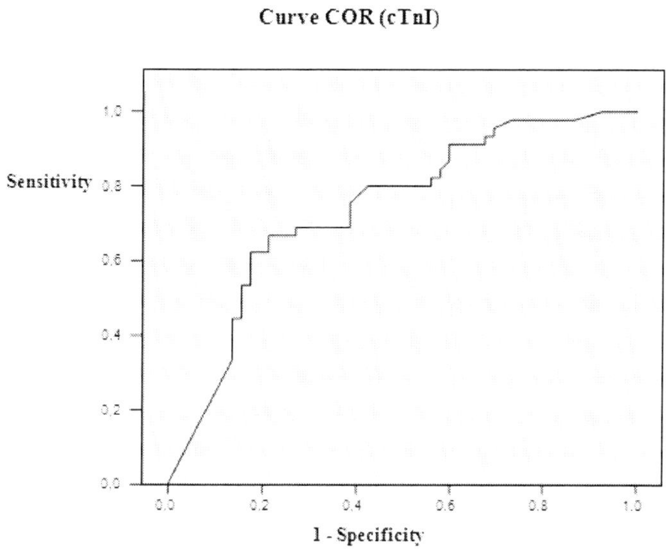

Figure 1.

Pericardial Fluid

Pericardial fluid has been used in numerous investigations. Represents a different matrix than blood and is a filtrate produced via the serous layer of the pericardium. Being so, chemicals and other markers should become elevated in pericardial fluid after becoming elevated in peripheral blood. However, as the fluid also bathes the myocardium, enzymes and proteins may also be released directly into the pericardial fluid from the cardiac muscle and some studies have shown elevated concentrations of (PMC) in pericardial fluid when compared to peripheral blood [6,60,61].

As in the case of blood, in pericardial fluid, the levels of cTnI and cTnT are higher in cases of death due to acute myocardial infarction and recurrent myocardial infarction. This elevation increases with the severity of the cardiac damage [62] and with the increase in the postmortem interval, just as occurs in the case of CK-MB [60.61].

The determination of cTnI in pericardial fluid is especially useful to exclude possible myocardial damage, and it has a high negative predictive value (96.4%). [27].

Cerebrospinal Fluid

Wang et al. [56] found in cerebrospinal fluid that levels for cTnI and myoglobin are higher when there is an increase in the postmortem interval. Nevertheless, this does not occur with the determination of the CK-MB in this substratum.

Vitreous Humor

The study of vitreous humor presents a series of advantages and disadvantages: Some advantage are that it is a readily available fluid with no hematic content and, therefore, not affected by hemolysis, it has a good diffusion to the extracellular space, and it directly reflects alterations in the concentrations of metabolites in a stable way. The disadvantages are that it presents the effect of dehydration that occurs as time elapses after death, and that diffusion through the membrane is limited to a certain molecular size. Thus, certain biochemical markers made up of proteins or enzymes with high molecular weight do not penetrate into the intraocular space and are undetectable in this fluid, even in the case of high serum concentrations.

In vitreous humor, the troponin T was undetectable. This absence can be explained by the large size of the molecule, and it renders the evaluation of this marker useless in cadaverous vitreous humor, given the impossibility of obtaining a useful concentration [5].

Despite the proven usefulness of cardiac troponin in clinical studies, there is still a need to develop earlier and more specific markers capable of detecting cases of ischemia or myocardial injury without objective myocyte injury [13].

Two other markers of wide clinical use, myoglobin and the MB fraction of the CK enzyme, have been proposed for the postmortem diagnosis of heart disease.

Creatine-Kinase (CK-MB)

Blood

The CK-MB determined in cadaveric serum is not very specific to myocardial damage, since high levels can be found in cases of striated muscle necrosis, as well as in traumas, rhabdomyolysis, convulsions, acute and chronic muscular dystrophies and renal failure in dialysis. Our data coincide with those of other authors [1,23,29,42], who found that the specificity of CK-MB is questionable, as high values of this isozyme appear in cases in which there is skeletal muscular damage without detectable heart damage [32]. We have also found significant differences in the amounts of CK-MB as the postmortem interval increases ($p<0.01$), with these values being greater when the time elapsed after death is greater. These results would indicate that this marker is altered by the effect of the autolysis, showing less reliability in blood samples from corpses.

Therefore, in the case of CK-MB, its low specificity and molecular characteristics make it particularly sensitive to the influence of the postmortem interval, which reduces its usefulness in the forensic field, with poor results from the point of view of its diagnostic value in cardiac impairment.

Pericardial Fluid

The determination of CK-MB in pericardial fluid, whose proximity to the infarction makes it particularly sensitive, offers better prospects in postmortem diagnosis than its determination in serum [34,35]. Batalis et al. [6] found a correlation between the findings obtained for CK-MB in pericardial fluid in deaths of cardiac origin when compared to control groups. However, Zhu et al. [62] found that the correlation between levels of CK-MB and severe cardiac damage was lower, both in blood and in pericardial fluid, than the cTnI levels obtained. This finding justifies the preference for other markers (such as troponin) in the study of sudden cardiac death. However, in cases in which death occurs quickly, some authors recommend the additional determination of CK-MB, both in serum and in pericardial fluid, given its early release [27].

Vitreous Humor

The determination of CKMB in vitreous humor, as occurs in other substrates, presents a poor correlation with causes of death [5].

Myoglobin

Blood

Myoglobin shows low specificity as a marker of cardiac necrosis in clinical practice, so that its use requires the association of Troponin measurements to confirm the myocardial injury and exclude false positives.

In forensic samples, the lack of specificity due to the molecular characteristics of this marker, together with the modifications that the autolysis phenomena produce in the results, discourages its study in cadaveric serum [30, 32].

Vitreous Humor

Its study in vitreous humor was not useful either, as minimal and invariable quantities were obtained that seem to lie between the lower limit of detection and the upper limit of normalcy. This circumstance makes it devoid of discriminatory value [5].

Cardiac Natriuretic Peptides

Type B natriuretic peptides (BNP and NT-proBNP) present some molecular characteristics that justify the investigation of its behavior in cadaveric serum from forensic samples: It is released in response to the increase in wall tension and to cardiac pressure overload, and its levels increase consistently in cases of congestive heart failure.

BNP y NT-proBNP differ in their biochemical and physiological characteristics. BNP is hormonally active, with a half-life of approximately 22 min, whereas NT-proBNP, the inactive precursor of BNP, lacks a clearance receptor and, therefore, has a longer half-life (about 120 min). The circulating concentration for NT-proBNP is believed is taken. In addition, NT-proBNP appears to be more discerning marker of early cardiac dysfunction than BNP [31]

Some authors have observed that the use of NT- proBNP, both in femoral serum and pericardial fluid, is a good biomarker of cardiac function [31], even though it is not very useful in detecting acute myocardial ischemia. These data are consistent with the results from a study carried out in our laboratory to determine serum BNP levels in a total of 133 samples from forensic autopsies. In our study, there were statistically significant differences ($p < 0,05$) in the BNP values between the deaths of cardiac origin and the rest of the groups studied.[1]

The atrial natriuretic peptide (ANF) showed little efficacy in the diagnosis of myocardial infarction and sudden cardiac death in forensic samples, mainly due to its short half-life [25].

Table 2. Description of the sample by causes

Characteristics of the sample	Number
Causes of death	132
Group 1. Causes of death of cardiac origin	n=58
Aortic Disorders:	n=4
Congestive heart failure:	n=11
Dilated cardiopathy:	n=3
Hypertrophic cardiopathy:	n=3
Ischemic Cardiopathy:	n=37
Group 2. Causes of death of traumatic origin	n=17
Polytrauma:	n=12
Craneal trauma :	n=5
Group 3. Causes of death from Asphyxiation	n=19
Strangulation:	n=8
CO poisoning:	n=2
Intrinsic airway occlusion:	n=2
Submersion:	n=5
Electrocution:	n=1
Thoracic compression:	n=1
Group 4. Natural non-cardiac deaths and Intoxications,	n=38
Digestive causes:	n=3
Non-traumatic intracranial hemorrhages:	n=6
Respiratory Causes:	n=12
Infectious causes:	n=8
Multi-organ failure	n=2
Intoxications:	n=7

[1] Communication presented in the *Oporto International Congress* 2007.

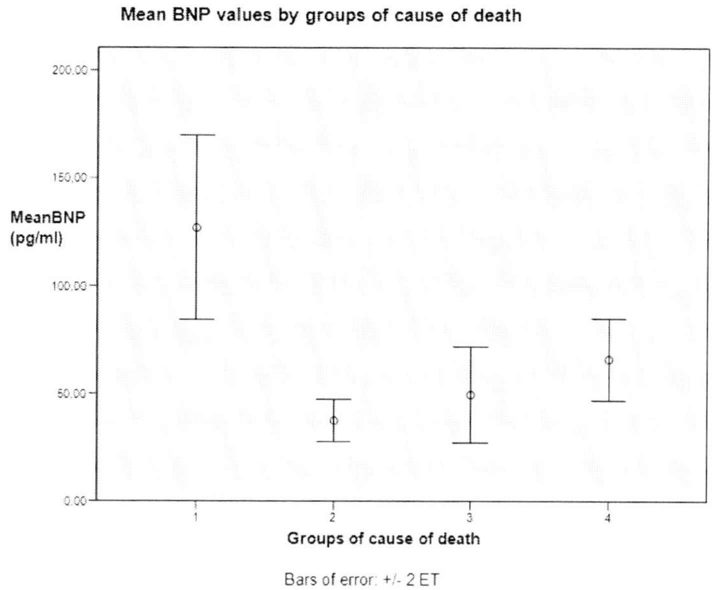

Figure 2.

Vitreous Humor

Michaud et al. [31] showed that the NT-proBNP values obtained in vitreous humor did not correlate well with those obtained in other body fluids. In our experience in a study carried out with 40 cases from forensic autopsies, we obtained a mean concentration of NT-proBNP in vitreous humor that was higher in individuals who died from cardiac causes (133.4 4 8.8 compared to 87.3 34.7 pg/ml; p=0.002) [5].

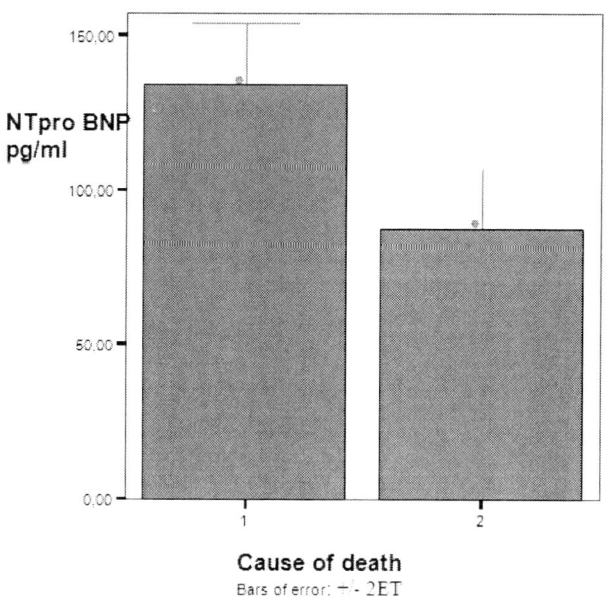

Figure 3. Mean of NT-proBNP cause of death (1:Cardiac; 2: Non cardiac).

Discussion

Sudden cardiac death is one of the principal causes of natural death in industrialized countries. Finding a biochemical marker for myocardial necrosis that would be useful in postmortem studies and in clinical practice has been the objective of numerous research studies.

However, the clinical criteria for the determination of these markers in peripheral blood may not be applicable to postmortem research, mainly due to the specific myocardial damage that occurs during the agony period. The markers that produced the best results in both postmortem studies and clinical practice were the troponins, mainly cTnI.

CK-MB and, above all, Myoglobin were less specific to myocardial damage. Some authors recommend the additional determination of CK-MB when the death occurred rapidly.

A new biomarker, the type B natriuretic peptide (BNP and NT-proBNP), has been found to be a good marker of cardiac function, even though it is not useful in acute myocardial ischemia.

Different fluids have been used, such as blood from different locations, pericardial fluid, cerebrospinal fluid and vitreous humor, to try to minimize the autolysis phenomena and find a more suitable matrix.

The best results were obtained with peripheral blood and pericardial fluid for troponin and CK-MB, although with levels higher than those obtained ante mortem, resulting in an increase in the values directly related to the postmortem interval. Some authors have found that the cTnI/CK-MB ratio, both in cardiac blood and in pericardial fluid, is not modified by the postmortem interval, so that it can be used in these fluids as an index for the existence of heart damage, regardless of the time elapsed after death.

The study of the cTnI in pericardial fluid has a high negative predictive value, serving to exclude cardiac pathology as a cause of sudden death. In recent years immunohistochemical techniques have been employed for the diagnosis of myocardial damage using different markers such as troponins, since it has been demonstrated that the majority of them can be visible, even serologically, minutes after the onset of the symptoms. Although there is no single ideal marker for the diagnosis of acute myocardial ischemia, the combined use of several of them has been utilized to detect the presence of ischemic areas when there is no macroscopic or microscopic evidence.

The determination of myocardial damage markers can be useful in the postmortem diagnosis of ischemic cardiac death only when other causes of myocardial damage (hyperthermia, methamphetamine and carbon monoxide poisoning, intense thoracic injuries) have been ruled out.

The findings from the biochemical study alone should not be used to establish a diagnosis of sudden cardiac death. These results should be integrated with the clinical history, autopsy findings, histological studies, and toxicological studies to help determine heart disease as the cause of death.

However, there is a need for a greater number of studies to obtain definitive evidence on the use of these markers.

Conclusion

- The marker that has produced the best results in postmortem studies is cardiac troponin I (cTnI) in peripheral blood and pericardial fluid.
- The additional determination of CK-MB is recommended when the death occurred suddenly.
- The study of the BNP and NT-proBNP can be useful for the diagnosis of heart failure, but it is not very useful in acute myocardial ischemia.
- The study of these markers in different body fluids is recommended, basically peripheral blood and pericardial fluid.
- The immunohistochemical study of the markers of heart damage can help detect early myocardial damage.
- There is a need for further studies in order to draw definitive conclusions about the use of these markers.

References

[1] J.E. Adams, V. Davila-Roman and P. Bessey, Improved detection of cardiac contusion with troponin I, *Am. Heart. J.* (1996); 131: 308-12

[2] Adams, J.E. III, Schechtman, K.B. Landt, Y. Ladenson J.H., Jaffe. A.: "Comparable detection of acute myocardial infarction by creatine kinase MB isoenzyme and cardiac troponin I. *Clin Chem* (1994); 40:1291-5

[3] Arlati S, Brenna S, Prencipe L et al. Myocardial necrosis in ICU patients with acute non-cardiac disease: a prospective study. *Intensive Care Med* (2000); 26:31-7.

[4] Alpert J, Thygesen K for the Joint European Society of Cardiology/ American College of Cardiology Committee. Myocardial infarction redefined – a consensus document of the Joint European Society of Cardiology/American College of Cardiology Committee for the Redefinition of Myocardial Infarction. *Eur Heart J* (2000);21:1502–13.

[5] Bañón R, Navarro E, Noguera JA, Benali L, Osuna E. Utilidad de la determinación de Troponina T, CK-MB, NT pro-BNP y mioglobina en humor vítreo en autopsias forenses. *Rev Esp Med legal.* (2008); 34:18-24.

[6] Batalis NK, Bradley JM, Papadea CN, Collins KA. The role of postmortem cardiac markers in the diagnosis of acute myocardial infarction. *J Forensic Sc.* (2010); 55(4):1088-91.

[7] Braunwald, E. et al.:ACC/AHA 2002 guideline update for the management of patients with unstable angina and non-ST-segment elevation myocardial infarction. A report of the American College of Cardiology/American Heart Association Task Force on Practice Guidelines *J. Am Coll Cardiol* (2002) 2;40(7):1366-74.

[8] Bertrand, M.E, et al.: Management of acute coronary syndromes in patients presenting without persistent ST-segment elevation. The Task Force on the Management of Acute Coronary Syndromes of the European Society of Cardiology. *Eur. Heart J* (2002); 23:1809-40.

[9] Campobasso CP, Dell Erba AS, Addante A, Zotti F, Marzullo A, Colonna MF. Sudden cardiac death and myocardial ischemia indicators: a comparative study of four immunohistochemical markers. *Am J Forensic Med Pathol.(*2008);29(2):154-61

[10] Cina, S.J., Brown, D.K., Smialek, J.E. Collins. K.A.: A rapid postmortem cardiac troponin T assay: laboratory evidence of sudden cardiac death. *Am J Forensic Med Pathol.*(2001) ;Jun22(2):173-6

[11] Clerico A. Pathophysiological and clinical relevance of circulating levels of cardiac natriuretic hormones: are they merely markers of cardiac disease? *Clin Chem Lab Med* (2002);40:752-60.

[12] Clerico A, Iervasi G, Mariani G. Pathophysiologic relevance of measuring the plasma levels of cardiac natriuretic peptide hormones in humans. *Horm Metab Res* (1999);31:487-98.

[13] Collinson PO. Early diagnosis of myocardial infarction: why measure cardiac enzymes? *J Clin Pathol* 1998;51:2-4.

[14] Cowie MR, Mendez GF. BNP and congestive heart failure. *Progr Cardiovasc Dis* (2002);44:293-321.

[15] Cowie MR, Jourdain P, Maisel A et al. Clinical applications of B-type natriuretic peptide (BNP) testing. *Eur Heart J* (2003);24:1710– 8.

[16] Davies SJ, Gaze DC, Collinson PO.: Investigation of cardiac troponins in postmortem subjects: comparing antemortem and postmortem levels. *Am J Forensic Med Pathol.* (2005);26(3):213-5.

[17] Davies MJ. The investigation of sudden cardiac death. *Histopathology*. 1999;34: 93-8.

[18] Ellingsen et al. Serum concentrations of cardiac troponin T in sudden death. *Am J Forensic Med Pathol.*(2004);25:213-5.

[19] Fishbein MC, Wang T, Matijasevic M, Hong L, Apple FS. Myocardial tissue troponis T and I. An immunohistochemical study in experimental models of myocardial ischemia. *Cardiovascular Pathology*.(2003); 12:65-71

[20] Hamm CW. Acute coronary syndromes. The diagnostic role of troponins. *Thromb Res* (2001);103:S63-9.

[21] Jaffe AS, Ravkilde J, Roberts R et al. It's time for a change to a troponin standard. *Circulation* (2000);102:1216–20.

[22] Khalifa AB, Najjar M, Addad F, Turki E, Mghirbi T. Cardiac troponin T (cTnT) and the postmortem diagnosis of sudden death. *Am.J Forensic Med Pathol.* (2006); 27(2):175-7.

[23] Katus, H.A Haller, C. Müller-Bardoff, M. Scheffold, T. Remppis A.: Cardiac troponin T in end-stage renal disease patients undergoing chronic maintenance hemodialysis. *Clin.Chem* (1995).41:1201-2.

[24] M. Kemp, J. Donovan, H. Higham and S. Hooper.: Biochemical markers of myocardial injury.*Br J Anaesth.* (2004); 93(1): 63-73

[25] Lorente JA, Villanueva E, Hernandez-Cueto C, Luna JD.: Plasmatic levels of atrial natriuretic peptide (ANP) in drowning. A pilot study. *Forensic Sci Int.*(1990);44(1):69-75.

[26] Lott, J.A.: Serum Enzyme Determinations in the Diagnosis of Acute Myocardial Infarction: An Update. *Hum Pathol* (1984);15:706-16

[27] Luna A. Is post-mortem biochemistry really useful? Why is it not widely used in forensic pathology?. *Leg med* (2009);11 Suppl1:S27-30

[28] Mair. J.: Clinical significance of cardiac contractile proteins for the diagnosis of myocardial injury. *Adv Clin Chem* (1994); 31:63-98

[29] Mair, J., Morandell, D., Genser, N., Lechleitner, P., Dienstl, F., Puschendorf. B.: Equivalent early sensitivities of myoglobin, creatine kinase MB mass, creatine kinase isoforms rations, and cardiac troponins I and T for acute myocardial infarction. *Clin Chem* (1995); 41:1266-72

[30] McCord J, Nowak RM, Hudson MP et al. The prognostic significance of serial myoglobin, troponin I, and creatine kinase-MB measurements in patients evaluated in the emergency department for acute coronary syndrome. *Ann Emerg Med* (2003);42:343–50.

[31] Michaud K, Augsburger M, Donzé N, et al. Evaluation of postmortem measurement of NT-proBNP as a marker for cardiac function. *Int J Legal Med.*(2008); 122(5):415-20

[32] Navarro E, Bañon RM, Giner S, Cardona B, Devesa MA. Utilidad de la determinación de la fracción I de la Troponina cardíaca en el diagnóstico de la muerte súbita de origen cardiaco en autopsias forenses. *Cuad. Med. Forense.* (2007);13:131-42

[33] Obnibene, F. Mori and R. Santoni, Cardiac troponin I in myocardial contusion, *Clin. Chem*. 44 (1998); 44: 889–90.

[34] Osuna E, Pérez-Cárceles MD, Vieira DN, Luna A.: Distribution of biochemical markers in biologic fluids: application to the postmortem diagnosis of myocardial infarction. *Am J Forensic Med Pathol.* (1998); 19(2):123-8.

[35] Osuna, E. Pérez-Cárceles, M.D., Alvarez, M.V., Noguera, J. Luna A.: Cardiac troponin I (cTnI) and the postmortem diagnosis of myocardial infarction. *Int J Legal Med* (1998):173-6

[36] Osuna, E., Pérez Cárceles, M.D., Jakobsson, S.W., Luna. A.: Biochemical and morphological markers in the post mortem diagnosis of ischemic heart distress. *Acta Med Leg Soc* (Liege) (1990); 40:275-83

[37] Ooi, D.S., Isotalo, P.A, Veinot J.P.: Correlation of antemortem serum creatine kinase, creatine kinase-MB, troponin I and troponin T with cardiac pathology. *Clin.Chem.* (2000); 46: 338-344

[38] Ortmann C, Pfeiffer H, Brinkmann B. A comparative study on the immunohistochemical detection of early myocardial damage. *Int J Legal Med* (2000); 113:215-20.

[39] Owen, A.: Cardiac troponins: improved diagnosis and cost benefits. *Clin Lab* (2001);25 (8):14-15.

[40] Panteghini, M.: Role and importance of biochemical markers in clinical cardiology. *European Heart Journal* (2004) 25, 1187-96

[41] Pérez-Cárceles MD, Noguera J, Jiménez JL, Martínez P, Luna A, Osuna E.: Diagnostic efficacy of biochemical markers in diagnosis post-mortem of ischaemic heart disease. *Forensic Sci Int.* (2004) ;28,142(1):1-7.

[42] Peter, J., Kirchner, A., Kuhlisch, E., Menschikowski, M., Neef, B., Dreßler. J.: The relevance of the detection of troponins to the forensic diagnosis of cardiac contusion. *Forensic Sc.i Int.*(2006) ;160(2-3):127-33

[43] Remme WJ, Swedberg K. Guidelines for the diagnosis and treatment of chronic heart failure. *Eur Heart J* (2001);22:1527-60

[44] Roxin LE, Culled I, Groth T, Hallgren T, VengeP. The value of serum myoglobin determinations in the early diagnosis of acute myocardial infarction. *Acta Med Scand.* (1984);215:417-25

[45] Santaló Bel M, Gindo Soldevila J, Ordoñez Llanos J. Marcadores biológicos de necrosis miocárdica.*Rev.Esp Cardiol* (2003);56(7):703-20.

[46] Simons ML, Fox KA et al. Management of acute coronary syndromes in patients presenting without persistent STsegment elevation. *Eur Heart J*(2002);23:1809-40.

[47] Sybrandy KC, Cramer MJM, Burgersdijk C. Diagnosing cardiac contusion: old wisdom and new insights. *Heart* (2003);89:458–89.

[48] Spies C, Haude V, Fitzner R et al. Serum cardiac troponin T as a prognostic marker in early sepsis. Chest (1998);113:1055–63.

[49] Struthers AD. Introducing a new role for BNP: as a general indicator of cardiac structural disease rather than a specific indicator of systolic dysfunction only. *Heart* (2002);87:97–8.

[50] Tsutamoto T, Wada A, Maeda K,Hisanaga T, Maeda Y, Fukai D, et al.Attenuation of compensation of endogenous cardiac natriuretic peptide system in chronic heart failure: prognostic role of plasma brain natriuretic peptide concentration in patients with chronic symptomatic left ventricular dysfunction. *Circulation* (1997);96:509-16

[51] Thygesen K, Alpert J, White HD Universal Definition of Myocardial Infarction. On behalf of the Joint ESC/ACCF/ AHA/WHF Task Force for the Redefinition of Myocardial Infarction. *Circulation* (2007);116:2634-53

[52] Thome-Kromer, B. Michel. G.: Human cardiac troponin I: detectability after myocardial infarction and severe skeletal muscle damage. *Clin.Chem.* (1993) 39:1248

[53] Van der Veen, K.J., Willebrands, A.F.: Isoenzymes of Creatine Phosphokinase in Tissue Extracts and in Normal and Pathological Sera. *Clin Chim Acta* (1966);13: 312-6

[54] White HD, French JK. Use of brain natriuretic peptide levels for risk assessment in non-ST-elevation acute coronary syndromes. *J Am Coll Cardiol* (2003);42: 1917–20.

[55] Wang TJ, Larson MG, Levy D et al. Plasma natriuretic peptide levels and the risk of cardiovascular events and death. *N Engl J Med* (2004);350: 655–63.

[56] Wang Q, Michiue T, Ishikawa T, Zhu BL, Maeda H. Combined analyses of creatine kinase MB, cardiac troponin I and myoglobin in pericardial and cerebrospinal fluids to investigate myocardial and skeletal muscle injury in medicolegal autopsy cases. *Leg Med* (Tokyo). (2011); 13(5) 226-32.

[57] Wright RS, Williams BA, Cramner H et al. Elevations of cardiac troponin I are associated with increased short-term mortality in noncardiac critically ill emergency department patients. *Am J Cardiol* (2002);90: 634-6.

[58] Wu AH, Ford L. Release of cardiac troponin in acute coronary syndromes: ischemia or necrosis? *Clin Chim Acta.*(1999);284:161-74.

[59] Yucel, Dalva. Effects of in vitro hemolysis on 25 common biochemical tests. *Clin Chem.* (1992);38:575–77.

[60] Zhu BL, , Ishikawa T, Michiue T, et al. Postmortem cardiac troponin T levels in the blood ad pericardial fluid.Part 1. Analysis with special regard to traumatic causes of death. Leg Med (Tokyo).(2006);8(2):86-93

[61] Zhu BL, , Ishikawa T, Michiue T, et al. Postmortem cardiac troponin T levels in the blood ad pericardial fluid.Part 2:Analysis for application in the diagnosis of sudden cardiac death with regard to pathology. *Leg Med* (Tokyo). 2006:1-8.

[62] Zhu BL, Ishikawa T, Michiue T, et al. Postmortem cardiac troponin I and creatine kinase MB levels in the blood and pericardial fluid as markers of myocardial damage in medicolegal autopsy. *Legal Medicine*.(2007);9:241-50.

Index

A

B

C

D

F

G

H

I

J

K

L

M

N

O

P

Q

R

S

T

U